The
Whole Life Nutrition
C O O K B O O K

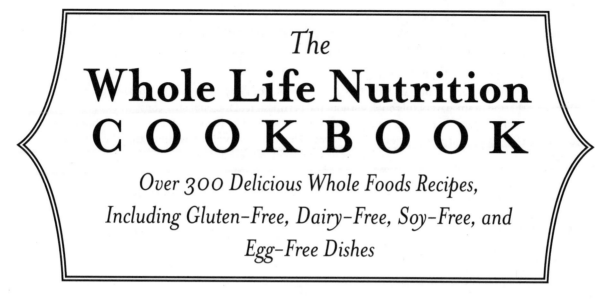

The
Whole Life Nutrition
C O O K B O O K

Over 300 Delicious Whole Foods Recipes,
Including Gluten–Free, Dairy–Free, Soy–Free, and
Egg–Free Dishes

Alissa Segersten
and
Tom Malterre, MS, CN

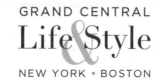

GRAND CENTRAL
Life & Style
NEW YORK • BOSTON

Grand Central Life & Style
Hachette Book Group
1290 Avenue of the Americas
New York, NY 10104

www.GrandCentralLifeandStyle.com

Printed in the United States of America

LSC-W

First Edition: April 2014
10 9 8 7 6

Grand Central Life & Style is an imprint of Grand Central Publishing.
The Grand Central Life & Style name and logo are trademarks of Hachette Book Group, Inc.

The Hachette Speakers Bureau provides a wide range of authors for speaking events. To find out more, go to www.HachetteSpeakersBureau.com or call (866) 376-6591.

The publisher is not responsible for websites (or their content) that are not owned by the publisher.

Library of Congress Cataloging-in-Publication Data

Malterre, Tom.
   The whole life nutrition cookbook : over 300 delicious whole foods recipes, including gluten-free, dairy-free, soy-free, and egg-free dishes / Alissa Segersten and Tom Malterre, MS, CN. — First edition.
      pages cm
   Reprint of: Bellingham, WA : Whole Life Press, [2008].
   Includes bibliographical references and index.
      ISBN 978-1-4555-8189-4 (paperback) — ISBN 978-1-4555-8190-0 (ebook)   1. Cooking (Natural foods)
2. Natural foods.   3. Gluten-free diet—Recipes.   4. Milk-free diet—Recipes.
5. Egg-free diet—Recipes.   I. Title.
   TX741.S44 2014
   641.3'02—dc23
                                                                                              2013045589

This book is dedicated to our five children,
Lily, Grace, Sam, Ben, and Camille
and to my mother who filled my childhood
with healthy, nourishing meals.

—Alissa

This book is dedicated to all of our clients.
May you find nourishment, healing, and hope
within these pages.
And to our children,
and the next seven generations.

—Tom

ACKNOWLEDGMENTS

First, I would like to thank my family for their encouragement to create this book; my children for being my recipe testers day in and day out; my parents for encouraging me to start this book in the first place and then for their continued support throughout this entire project; and of course, Tom, for his depth of knowledge on the subject of food and health, which continually inspires me to create new and delicious recipes for the benefit of all.

Many thanks to all of my recipe testers—especially my mom and dear friend April Brown—for testing so many of the recipes in this book and encouraging me throughout the whole process. I am so grateful for our agent, Celeste Fine, for believing in us and seeing our goals through. Much gratitude to our editor, Diana Baroni, and the whole team at Grand Central Publishing for creating a flowing, beautiful book.

A very special thanks to those of you who contributed so many hours of childcare for our children. Thank you to my two Bastyr University cooking instructors, Cynthia Lair and Mary Shaw, who have inspired me to be where I am today. And a special thanks to Mary Shaw for permitting me to use some of her delicious recipes in this book.

—Alissa

I would like to thank my clients. I have learned so much from you over the years. You have shown me that anything is possible and that food really is medicine.

To the researchers and clinicians I call teachers, mentors, and friends: your desire for helping people and the planet is what has me waking every day with excitement and anticipation. The stories you tell in your articles and books are writing a new chapter of history for my children.

To my children, I adore you. You inspire me to be a better father, nutritionist, and steward of the earth. I long for you to live in a beautiful world that leaves you in awe as it has done for me.

To Ali, you are my superhero. You never cease to amaze me with your intuitive knack for recipe creation and your amazing multitasking skills as a mother, author, and chef.

—Tom

CONTENTS

INTRODUCTION

Let food be thy medicine and medicine be thy food.
—*Hippocrates*

The diet and environment that humans have evolved with over the last tens of thousands of years have changed drastically within the last several decades. With these changes have come rising rates of obesity, skin disorders, childhood and adult cancers, heart disease, diabetes, and more. There is overwhelming evidence now that our food choices drastically affect our state of health. Humans are not meant to have high cholesterol, high blood pressure, high blood sugar, chronic pain, or other common health problems. These health conditions are often a result of dietary, environmental, and lifestyle factors.

Food is powerful medicine. It is energy and information. Every molecule that exists in our body was created from the food we eat, the water we drink, and the air we breathe; we quite literally are what we eat! Whole foods, or foods in their natural unrefined forms, offer us the vitamins, minerals, and antioxidants we need to prevent and treat most diseases while creating a state of balance and health within us. Whole grains, beans, nuts, seeds, vegetables, and fruits provide thousands of important phytochemicals that work with our bodies to maintain and build optimal health. Eating food is so much more than a way to fill our bellies. Food affects our quality of life, how we look, how we feel, how much we weigh, how much energy we have, how we age, and how healthy we are.

HARD-WIRED FOR HEALTHY EATING

As children, we both learned that food is powerful medicine. Healthy eating was hard-wired in our brains from the time we were very young.

When I was 10 years old, Dr. John McDougall, the renowned physician and nutrition expert, was my family doctor. I watched and learned as he treated his patients, including my family, using food as medicine. Seeing people reclaiming their health with each and every forkful of food shifted my life's purpose. This interaction inspired me to learn all I could about nutritional sciences. While I was attending Bastyr University for my first degree in nutrition, I met Ali. At the time, I thought health food was reserved for people that had relatively inactive taste buds. My personal meals were extremely healthy, but they never tasted very good. I clearly remember my first dinner date over at Ali's apartment where I got to assist in preparing food. She taught me how to chop vegetables properly and how to time the addition of every single ingredient to bring out the best color, texture, and flavor of the dish. I found the food (and the company) absolutely stunning! And I knew then that it would be possible for people to find bliss in eating their way to optimal health. Early in 2004, while working on my master's degree in nutritional sciences, I decided to try a raw food cleanse to see if it would help with my digestive discomforts. Within a week, 90% of my issues had either subsided or disappeared altogether. Upon the reintroduction of gluten, my symptoms started to reappear. I began to delve deeply into the science behind food sensitivities and health in order to help more people like myself. Could eliminating gluten really be the answer for millions of people dealing with so many health problems? I found that it did indeed play a very large role. My studies at Bastyr reaffirmed how powerful nutrition really is and deepened my awareness of food sensitivities and numerous other topics.

I, Alissa, feel grateful that my mother took the time to research nutrition and health before I was born. She made the decision to make all of my baby food from scratch instead of feeding me something that came in a jar. Looking at my baby book, I noticed that some of my first foods were stewed beef, homemade plain yogurt, and puréed steamed vegetables. It's no wonder I've never liked processed foods! My taste buds developed to prefer fresh, home-cooked whole foods. By the time I was 10 years old I had taken over the kitchen and was creating recipes using every ingredient imaginable. Some of those early creations actually tasted good, but I'm sure many did not. When I moved away and went to college I had to eat the required meal plan food for the first 2 years. After the first year of eating processed cafeteria meals I petitioned the school to allow me to stay off the meal plan and prepare my own food in my dorm room. That's when I first started shopping at small health food stores. I loved being in charge of what I put in my body. The more research I did,

the more I became interested in food and nutrition. I decided to pursue a degree in nutrition to deepen my understanding of everything I had learned thus far. That's when I met Tom. He had such a knack for nutritional biochemistry that I thought I better study with him! He was able to break down hard-to-understand information into something easy to digest. My studies in nutrition at Bastyr University deepened my respect for food and its role in either keeping us healthy or making us sick.

WHAT IS HEALTH?

Your health is your wealth. It's like your personal bank account. You can make deposits or withdrawals to it every day. The more deposits you make, the larger your account, and hence the greater your health. The more withdrawals you make—by eating processed foods or not getting enough sleep, for instance—the smaller your bank account gets, and hence your health slowly begins to deteriorate.

Disease doesn't happen overnight. Small withdrawals to your health happen daily, depleting your health reserves over time. A child eating a diet filled with processed foods may appear vibrant and healthy—they may even avoid seasonal colds and flus—but what's happening inside the body is a different story. That child is slowly being depleted of what she needs to thrive. Health problems might not occur right away—perhaps not until her mid-twenties—but eventually things may begin to run amuck in her body: digestive distress, food allergies, thyroid disorders, unexplained weight gain, or maybe even a cancer diagnosis. The foods that most people are accustomed to eating are slowly killing them. Our government—our taxpayer dollars—supports the production of many of these toxic "foods." These "food-like" substances that are sold in our grocery stores and that are on the menus of restaurants nationwide are not compatible with our human biology. Just walk down any grocery store aisle and pick up a package. How many ingredients are on there that you can't pronounce? You may also see some ingredients you can pronounce, like wheat flour, soybean oil, and sugar. Those don't sound so bad, right? Maybe even healthy? What if we told you that the wheat flour was sprayed with toxic herbicides—ones that damage your digestive health—causing a leaky gut. Or that the soybean oil was genetically engineered to withstand massive spraying of these herbicides? It was then processed using solvents to extract the oil, then bleached and deodorized with more toxic chemicals. And the sugar? When a label says sugar it most likely means it came from genetically engineered sugar beets, which are grown using a chemical soup of pesticides known to kill off honeybee colonies and damage human health.

Our current food system is not designed for the health and well-being of the people and the planet. Luckily, there are many healthy options you can choose to build up your personal health bank account. In this book, we'll help you do just that. We want to guide you toward a Whole Life Nutrition lifestyle—a way of eating that can change your health and life for the better. If you are running on empty, it might take some time to repair your body, but it can happen!

WHAT IS WHOLE LIFE NUTRITION?

We are all unique individuals, with different backgrounds, unique genetics (and epigenetics), particular nutrient deficiencies, and accumulated environmental toxins. It is of utmost importance to take into consideration this greater whole—the bigger picture. We can no longer simply look at diet and its impact on health. Many of the earlier studies in nutritional sciences were geared toward the elementary thinking that nutrition was about counting calories, determining optimal ratios of macronutrients like carbohydrates, proteins, and fats, along with ingesting adequate amounts of vitamins and minerals. While these tasks have their merits, we also need to consider the potential adverse effects of the more than 80,000 chemicals that have been introduced into the natural world by industries.

Whole Life Nutrition takes into account everything that is being ingested by an individual—whether it is coming from the food we eat, the air we breathe, or the water we drink. After taking into account the body's toxicity from industry and nonorganic food, we look at immune function and digestive health—many of the toxins in our environment cause digestive distress. Intestinal health plays a key role in most modern diseases, including diabetes, obesity, heart disease, mental disorders, and autoimmune disorders. When digestion and immune functions are compromised, food sensitivities can manifest. Whole Life Nutrition understands that removing food irritants like gluten, dairy, corn, eggs, and soy provides an opportunity for the intestines to begin the healing process.

There isn't a perfect diet or one perfect approach to healing. There are just too many variables. You can let an organic, whole foods diet be your starting point and then refine it to meet your needs. Each individual is unique, and some people benefit tremendously from a plant-based diet, while others benefit by using an animal-based diet for healing. This book is meant to guide you in choosing what is right for you in this moment and beyond, and provide you with many delicious, nourishing recipes to assist you on your journey.

We have developed over 300 fabulous-tasting recipes using nutritious whole foods that promote optimal health. All the recipes in this book are gluten-free. Most recipes are free of dairy, soy, and eggs as well; however, there are various options for using these ingredients in some recipes. Many of the recipes in this book are healthier versions of traditional favorites and some may be very new to you. If you feel overwhelmed and don't know where to begin, then simply start by making a few of the recipes that look familiar to you. As your cooking repertoire builds, so will your confidence, and soon you will want to try other recipes.

In this book, you will also find useful information about environmental toxicity and how to protect yourself, how food sensitivities affect your health, the basics of a whole foods diet, stocking your whole foods pantry, quick nutritious break-fasts, cooking beans and whole grains, selecting and storing fresh produce, adding more vegetables to your diet, and nutritious snack ideas!

Lasting dietary change takes time. You don't need to do it all at once. Remember that nourishing ourselves is a process and that making small changes can be enough to begin. *The Whole Life Nutrition Cookbook* was created under the premise that food can be both healing and delicious. Food is pleasure and eating is something we do throughout the day, every day, for our entire lives. Why not create a daily diet that heals our bodies and is absolutely satisfying to all of our senses? As we partake in the joy of eating nutritious organic food, we share this experience with others and together we build a healthier community, country, and planet.

Part I

WHOLE LIFE
NUTRITION

1

THE WHOLE DIET STORY

Everyone should be his own physician. We ought to assist and not force nature. Eat with moderation what agrees with your constitution. Nothing is good for the body but what we can digest. What medicine can produce digestion? Exercise. What will recruit strength? Sleep. What will alleviate incurable ills? Patience.

—Voltaire

Everyone is confused about how to eat these days. There are many different diets ranging from eating only plants to eating a diet primarily of animal foods—vegan, vegetarian, Mediterranean, Paleo, grain-free, raw food diet, and everything in between. Proponents of each diet proclaim that they know the ticket to health, justifying their points with well-documented research and case studies. For many, creating nourishing meals has become confusing and stressful rather than a joyous process.

I am sure by now most of you have heard that eating a lot of meat is going to cause heart disease, that animal fat clogs your arteries, that grains and beans are slowly killing you, and that too many raw greens are dangerous! Oh my, this is getting quite confusing! We are trying to peg all of our modern health problems on these beautiful, healing whole foods! Focusing on the minutiae of diet is only a small fragment of the bigger health picture.

One common denominator with all of the different diets is that they are centered on eating whole foods. We believe in eating by the principles of Whole Life Nutrition. That means the basis of any eating plan should be organic, whole foods. Whole foods are foods in their natural, unrefined form, such as vegetables, fruits, whole grains, beans, meat, fish, nuts, and seeds. These foods offer us the vitamins, minerals, and antioxidants we need to thrive.

We also believe in eating a balanced diet—one that includes a variety of whole foods—rather than the latest and greatest "superfood" or lifestyle trend. Have you noticed that with each new food hype, people begin consuming this new popular food in excess, thinking that if a little is good, then a lot must be better. Take soy for instance. Research showed health benefits from consuming it so everyone started eating a lot of it—soy protein powder shakes, fake soy meats, and soy milk by the gallon! If we look at traditional Asian cultures that consumed soy, we see that they ate small amounts of organic, fermented soy foods in balance with other vegetables, grains, fish, and sea vegetables. The bottom line to a nutritious diet is that each person has a unique balance point.

Everyone's body is different. Digestion and immune functions can be compromised by what we eat and how we live. Food sensitivities—to gluten, dairy, corn, and soy—are a reality for many. As a result, some people thrive on one diet while others don't. Your goal should not be to try the hot new lifestyle trend, but to find a way of eating that is best for you. A few decades ago, vegetarianism was in. Meat was "bad" and grains and beans were the way to go! Soy foods were becoming the popular health food. People started eating more plants and losing weight. Heart disease, cancer, and diabetes were being reversed on a whole foods plant-based diet. Now, the pendulum is swinging toward the other side—many experts are saying that eating a diet high in animal foods heals everything from autoimmune diseases to obesity. The reality is that both sides of the diet spectrum can offer healing and life-long health when used appropriately.

Let's review the principles of some of these popular eating philosophies in order to better understand the theories behind them, as well as some of their health benefits and risks.

VEGANISM AND VEGETARIANISM

Principles: The basics of a vegan diet include whole plant foods such as whole grains, legumes, vegetables, fruits, nuts, and seeds. No animal products are consumed (no meat, fish, eggs, or dairy products). Vegetarians will often add in eggs (ovo), and dairy (lacto), and sometimes fish (pesco).

Both choose not to consume meat for a variety of reasons—preserving the environment, choosing not to harm animals, and maintaining optimal health are high on the list for many.

The production of factory-farmed animals is resource-intensive, requiring a lot of fossil fuels, water, pesticides, and raw land (possibly rainforest). Comparisons between animal protein–based diets and plant-based diets have shown a significant decrease in environmental impacts when plants are the primary food source. Many vegans and vegetarians also feel a connection to animals on a spiritual level and would prefer not to eat them. They will often question whether or not the death and suffering of an animal is justified so they can have a meal.

Many people who have followed whole foods vegan diets have helped to reverse the progression of heart disease, diabetes, and various forms of cancer. Dean Ornish has 30 years of research showing that his vegan and vegetarian diet programs, which also include fitness, stress management, and lifestyle changes, can do all these things and more.

Theory: Animal fat and protein is going to cause heart disease, obesity, and cancer, and increase your risk for type 2 diabetes. You can get all of the nutrients you need from a plant-based diet.

Considerations: Fresh, organic, plant-rich vegan diets are indeed beneficial as they provide a wide array of miraculous compounds that are protective against numerous diseases. However, our bodies are not biologically designed to eat solely a vegan diet over a lifetime. Our bodies have specific requirements for vitamin B12, essential fatty acids, and fat-soluble vitamins, such as A, K2, and D, that are not possible to get from entirely plant-based diets.

Vitamin B12, which can only be found in animal foods, is likely to be low in long-term vegans and vegetarians. Vegans and vegetarians who don't supplement with vitamin B12 often have higher levels of homocysteine, a potential risk factor for heart disease and stroke. One study showed that 68% of vegetarians and 77% of vegans had B12 deficiencies. Contrary to popular belief, you cannot get B12 in tempeh, seaweed, or unwashed organic vegetables. Therefore, vitamin B12 supplementation is essential when planning a vegan diet.

Vegan and vegetarian diets are also often low in essential fatty acids. Essential fatty acids (EFAs) are found in wild Alaskan cold-water fish and in other animal fats in smaller amounts, and they include the hard-to-come-by EFAs, EPA, DHA, and CLA. It is extremely difficult to attain higher therapeutic amounts of these fats from plant foods unless you are taking an algae supplement rich in DHA. The conversion rate from omega-3's (ALA) in plants (like flaxseeds) to DHA is small, and 7% of woman have genes that do not allow them to convert much at all. Infants and children with low DHA are showing memory and brain abnormalities. Although new research is showing that the fats from chia seeds can be converted into EPA at a decent rate in the body (up to 60%), the conversion rate to DHA is nominal. The brain of a developing fetus and young child needs these fats, especially DHA, for proper development. At least during pregnancy and early childhood, dietary sources of DHA from animals (like wild salmon, purified fish oil, and krill oil) or algae may be helpful.

In summary, diets high in plants, as in true vegan and vegetarian diets, can reverse diabetes and heart disease, and stop or slow the progression of certain cancers; however, a vegan diet may not be adequate during pregnancy, lactation, and early childhood. Our bodies are biologically designed to be consuming a small amount of animal foods, or at the very least, supplementing with the nutrients found in them.

A plant-rich vegan or vegetarian diet is beneficial for:

✓ Reversing diabetes
✓ Lowering cholesterol
✓ Reversing heart disease
✓ Slowing the aging process
✓ Slowing the progression of prostate cancer

RAW VEGAN

Principles: A raw food vegan is one who abstains from all animal foods and chooses to eat plant foods in the raw, uncooked form. Although these diets may be high in carbohydrates, Dr. Gabriel Cousens has demonstrated a reversal of diabetes with a raw vegan diet. This is attributed to the multitude of positive effects plant chemicals have on the human body. People have cured incurable diseases by consuming a diet of raw vegetable and fruit juices for an extended period, giving the digestive system a break and allowing the body's healing mechanisms to take over.

Theory: Cooked food is less nutritious. Raw food has all the necessary enzymes to digest your meals, and by eating raw, all of the nutrients found in plants are preserved by preparing food at or below 115°F.

Considerations: If there is one thing every nutrition expert will agree on it is the fact that human health improves with the consumption of fresh organic vegetables and fruits. New research comes out every month talking about the miraculous healing compounds found in plants, reassuring us that humans are meant to be consuming large amounts of plants for optimal health.

While certain beneficial compounds like sulforaphane from broccoli are most potent in raw or lightly steamed foods, other compounds such as carotenoids (beta-carotene and lycopene) show improved absorption from consuming cooked foods. Plants also contain defensive compounds (antinutrients) that they use to repel animals that try to eat them. Some of these may be mildly toxic when eaten raw, such as lectins found in dry beans, but are often neutralized by the cooking process. Thankfully, many raw food lovers are conscious of this and take care in preparing foods in ways that neutralize or reduce these compounds.

Additionally, some people with digestive disorders may have a difficult time digesting large amounts of raw food, which can lead to excessive gas, bloating, digestive upset, and nutrient deficiencies.

In summary, a raw foods diet can be quite healing for some people, especially when used therapeutically, like in juice fasting. However, it may not be ideal for growing children and pregnant women, unless one is taking a variety of nutritional supplements. Eating a diet high in raw foods can't be underestimated—for some this may be the ticket to vibrant, disease-free living.

A raw vegan diet is beneficial for:

✓ Cancer prevention
✓ Healing diabetes
✓ Regulating blood sugar
✓ Weight loss
✓ Reducing inflammation

MEDITERRANEAN DIET

Principles: The Mediterranean diet is a lifestyle and way of eating similar to those living in regions around the Mediterranean Sea—the coastal areas in Greece, Turkey, and Italy. Some of the cultures from this region have the healthiest and longest-living people on the planet today. The Mediterranean diet is heavy in fresh vegetables, fruits, whole grains, nuts, and high-quality extra-virgin olive oil. Typically, fish is consumed about twice a week, and meat and sweets are consumed only about once per month. Emphasis is placed on maintaining a low-stress lifestyle, connecting and sharing meals with others, and weaving plenty of exercise into daily activities. A study on Europeans demonstrated that elderly patients who ate a Mediterranean diet and took walks regularly could reduce their risk of dying from ALL diseases by 50%!

Theory: If we replicate a diet similar to those living around the Mediterranean region, we can lower the prevalence of metabolic syndrome and heart disease, and increase our life span. The healthy fats from olive oil, fish, and nuts, as well as the potent antioxidants from the wine, olive oil, and tomatoes, are particularly protective against disease.

Considerations: Many people are trying to mimic the benefits of a Mediterranean diet by adopting key features talked about in the news. Lycopene found in tomatoes has been touted as a heart-protective antioxidant, olive oil as the perfect oil, and wine as a longevity elixir. As a result, people will purchase these Mediterranean diet ingredients and readily add them to their current diets. The quality and quantity of these ingredients must be considered for optimal outcomes. For example, pouring more ketchup on your foods will not improve your weight. Ketchup is often laden with high fructose corn syrup, which is theorized to be one of the primary causes of weight gain and the increased incidence of diabetes in the United States. High-quality, organic extra-virgin olive oil coming from a reputable source will contain potent anti-inflammatory antioxidants that are proven to be protective to your heart; a lesser-quality oil will often contain much lower levels of these antioxidants. While the Mediterranean diet does include wine, it recommends only 1 to 2 glasses per day. An excess of alcohol consumption may negate any positive benefits from drinking wine.

In summary, a Mediterranean diet is ideal for those wanting to eat healthier, lower their risk of most diseases, and live a long, healthy life. It is important to remember that the benefits of this diet happen when it is adopted fully—eating a completely unprocessed, whole foods diet full of a variety of fresh vegetables, fruits, whole grains, nuts, and a high-quality extra-virgin olive oil, as well as getting plenty of exercise and maintaining a low-stress lifestyle.

A Mediterranean diet is beneficial for:

- ✓ Lowering the incidence of metabolic syndrome
- ✓ Decreasing the risk for diabetes
- ✓ Decreasing the risk for heart disease
- ✓ Increasing life span

TRADITIONAL FOODS: WESTON A. PRICE FOUNDATION

Principles: In the early 1930s a dentist named Weston A. Price started to investigate healthy populations around the globe untouched by Western civilization and modern diets of white flour, sugar, refined vegetable oils, and processed foods. For over a decade he traveled to unique regions of the world trying to understand what factors contributed to healthy teeth that were free of cavities and deformed dental arches. What he found were villages of people in all areas of the globe that had beautiful, healthy, straight teeth, robust physical structures, and resistance to disease. When these native diets were analyzed, Dr. Price found them to have ten times the amount of fat-soluble vitamins compared to the diet of most Americans at the time, all coming from animal foods such as butter, organ meats, eggs, fish, and animal fats. Fat-soluble vitamins, such as A, D, and K, are needed to absorb minerals which form strong teeth and bones, and keep the immune system strong.

Eating a traditional diet would include organic whole foods, soaked whole grains and legumes, fermented foods, raw dairy products, seafood, organ meats, and animal fats from grass-fed animals. Emphasis is placed on consumption of the fat-soluble vitamins A, D, and K coming from the animal foods during the preconception time for both parents, as well as during pregnancy, breastfeeding, and early childhood. Recommendations include a diet with higher amounts of butter, full-fat milk and cheese, cod liver oil, and animal organs.

Theory: Processed foods and industrial agriculture have led to the downfall of human health. Diets high in whole-grain products that have not been soaked or fermented can lead to mineral deficiencies. The consumption of a high-fat, preindustrial whole foods diet will restore health and vitality to humans.

Considerations: Eating a whole foods diet free of processed foods and harmful agricultural chemicals is extremely important for both personal and planetary health. The Weston A. Price Foundation has done an amazing job of raising awareness of centralized animal feeding operations, the hazards of pasteurized dairy, and numerous other atrocities of our modern diets.

Unfortunately, our earth is increasingly bombarded with toxins that bioaccumulate in animal fats. Butter, farmed salmon, and other animal fats have been shown to contain levels of environmental persistent organic pollutants (POPs) like PCBs, dioxins, furans, and brominated flame retardants that are much higher than their lower-fat counterparts. Animal fats concentrate these POP chemicals that have been shown to disrupt our hormones in our endocrine system. People with higher levels of these endocrine disrupting chemicals (EDCs) in their bodies have shown a significant increase in type 2 diabetes and obesity. Because of their ability to make both humans and animals fat, EDCs are often called "obesogens." Unfortunately, negative effects from EDCs are usually not seen for quite some time. Studies on animals have found that it may take up to one-sixth of the animal's lifetime before significant adverse effects of these chemicals are seen. If the average life expectancy in the United States is around 79 years old, it could take up to 13 years before the harmful effects from our EDC exposure becomes apparent. The exception is fetal exposure. Science is now finding that minute amounts of these EDCs can alter fetal development, changing immune system function and causing subsequent disease risk over the life of the child. It is unfortunate to think that foods once considered to be the most nourishing are now becoming potentially dangerous.

In summary, a traditional foods diet is ideal for those wanting to gain the most nutrition from their food, for those wanting to replenish their bodies with nutrient-dense foods in preparation for conception and pregnancy, and for those with chronic mood disorders like depression or anxiety. It is of utmost importance to consider the amount and source of animal fats being consumed, as environmental toxins bioaccumulate in animal fat. The toxins found in certain fish are especially dangerous when consumed during the preconception time, pregnancy, and early childhood. As always, it is important to also eat a lot of vegetables when you are consuming animal products.

A traditional foods diet is beneficial for:

✓ Healing nutrient deficiencies that are often passed down generationally
✓ Helping to build strong teeth and bones
✓ Helping to heal and reverse dental caries

✓ Healing infertility
✓ Stabilizing moods

PALEO

Principles: Proponents of the Paleo diet follow a nutritional plan based on the eating habits of our ancestors in the Paleolithic period, between 2.5 million and 10,000 years ago. They believe that our genetics has not evolved to consume foods of modern society and therefore we should not eat them.

Theory: Grains, legumes, and dairy products were not part of our Paleolithic ancestry and therefore should be avoided. Fossil records show that when humans switched from the hunter-gatherer lifestyle to agrarian societies 10,000 years ago, there was more prevalence of disease, shorter statures, and a decline in dental health and jaw size. Grains and legumes contain antinutrients that degrade the digestive system and cause a leaky gut. The carbohydrates in grains and beans increase blood sugar too much and too fast, and are responsible for the rise in diabetes and obesity. Lectins—specific proteins that bind to carbohydrates—are also found in grains and beans. These compounds can cause something called leptin resistance, or a consistent increase in appetite, and weight gain. Phytic acid in grains and beans can decrease the amount of minerals we can absorb. Our bodies are biologically designed to be eating vegetables, meat and organs, fruits, nuts, and seeds.

Considerations: By thinking like a Paleo woman or man, we naturally avoid all processed and refined foods, and eat a diet rich in healthy, whole foods. In fact, a true Paleo diet would revolve around fresh vegetables and wild game. We would also get plenty of fresh air, exercise, and sunshine. By nature, Paleo diets would be entirely and totally gluten-free and dairy-free. Interestingly, the original grains of agrarian societies were primarily gluten-containing grains. Gluten is extremely hard to get out of the diet as cross contamination is everywhere when a person is eating processed grain products. We now know that many people cannot properly digest gluten. True Paleo diets eliminate gluten and dairy, which will completely cease a person's exposure to two of the most reactive foods. By eliminating processed foods and all grain products, you will ensure a complete elimination of gluten.

But are organic, gluten-free whole grains really that bad? Is the consumption of these foods behind the pandemic-type increase in chronic diseases we are seeing? Cultures around the world have been consuming plant-based diets rich in whole grains for thousands of years—rice and millet in Asia, teff in Africa, quinoa in South America, and corn in North America—without the diseases we see today. Decades of research have proven that diabetes and obesity can be reversed on a plant-based diet rich in whole grains and beans.

Do the lectins found in grains and beans really cause a leaky gut and weight and appetite issues (leptin resistance)? Lectins are mostly broken down by soaking, sprouting, and cooking, and by the beneficial bacteria in your digestive system. Those with imbalanced gut microflora are likely to have a harder time breaking down lectins. Is phytic acid responsible for significant reductions in nutrition that would warrant complete elimination of beans and grains from our food supply? Similar to lectins, phytic acid is readily broken down by soaking and cooking, and by the beneficial bacteria in our guts. Interestingly, phytic acid also has shown to be beneficial in treating cancer. Problems can arise when grains are eaten in excess for a person with intestinal imbalances.

Conventionally grown grains and beans often have elevated levels of herbicides and other agricultural chemicals. Farmers will use glyphosate (the active ingredient in Roundup and other herbicides) to kill weeds, and as a preharvest desiccant on their bean and grain crops. This can lead to high residues on these specific crops. So much so that the EPA recently raised acceptable levels of these chemical residues in order to sell crops often saturated with them. Glyphosate was patented as a potent biocidal shown to knock out beneficial species of bacterium, leaving pathogens to flourish. By avoiding conventionally grown beans and grains, and by purchasing organic options, a person can drastically lower his or her exposure to glyphosate and protect the microbial balance in the gut.

When people have severe intestinal imbalances (ulcerative colitis, Crohn's disease, celiac disease), they may not be able to digest complex carbohydrates effectively at all. Your intestinal cells secrete enzymes that digest carbohydrates; if the intestinal surface is damaged by food sensitivities, pathogenic microbes, or chemical exposure, these enzymes may not function well at all. As a result, complex carbohydrates are not broken down properly and used by the body. Instead they are used by nonbeneficial bacteria and yeasts. These same organisms can cause damage to intestinal cells. This continued damage inhibits more carbohydrate-digesting enzymes from being secreted, and thus more yeast and bacterial overgrowth, contributing to a vicious cycle. Along with using digestive enzymes and antimicrobial plant compounds, like berberine and oregano oil, some people benefit from eliminating specific complex carbohydrates in order to break this cycle. *The Specific Carbohydrate Diet* (SCD Diet) and *Gut and Psychology Syndrome* (GAPS Diet) are two amazing books for addressing these issues.

In summary, a Paleo diet is ideal for those wanting to eat healthier and remove all processed foods from their diets. Eating a plant-rich Paleo diet—one that revolves around fresh vegetables and fruits—assures optimal nutrition. Consider avoiding grains and beans if your gut is damaged and you have severe microbial imbalances. Remember to also consider how much animal fat you are consuming—as the levels of certain toxins build up in our world, they will concentrate in animal fat. These toxins can cause an increased risk for diabetes, obesity, and a leaky gut.

A Paleo diet is beneficial for:

- ✓ Those who have celiac disease or a gluten sensitivity
- ✓ Healing food and environmental allergies
- ✓ Healing autoimmune disorders
- ✓ Nourishing a weak, depleted child or adult
- ✓ Providing key nutrients for the brain development of a fetus and growing child
- ✓ Weight loss
- ✓ Reducing inflammation
- ✓ Treating acne and other skin conditions

GETTING STARTED WITH WHOLE LIFE NUTRITION

Consider completing an Elimination Diet at www.WholeLifeNutrition.net to determine the foods that you may be sensitive to. We have found that an organic whole foods, gluten-free diet that is completely free of foods you are sensitive to can do wonders for your health. However, everyone is unique. Some people thrive on vegan diets, while others do best on a Paleo diet. There are recipes in this book that will appeal to all audiences. We recommend you listen to your body as you try different dietary choices, as it will tell you what is working best and what is not. You may want to give a new diet some time as your body adjusts to the changes. If your symptoms of discomfort persist, we suggest you consult a Functional Medicine–trained doctor. You can find a practitioner by going to www.Functional Medicine.org and clicking on the "Find a Practitioner" button.

If you're still feeling confused as to what to eat, consider this: When researchers look at "blue zones," or areas around the planet where people live the longest and with the greatest health, they notice a dietary pattern. People living in these blue zones are consuming a plant-rich diet, full of unrefined whole grains, legumes, vegetables, and fresh fruit, along with a small amount of animal foods. The recipes in this book follow these guidelines. So living a healthy lifestyle has never been easier! Just choose from the 300 recipes in this book and you'll be living healthier and feeling better in no time!

2

THE WHOLE FOOD SENSITIVITY STORY

A journey of a thousand miles must begin with a single step.
—*Lao Tzu*

Current research suggests that food allergies and sensitivities are far more common than we might have imagined. The number of people having immune reactions to foods is increasing. This is due to the many changes our immune systems are experiencing. Changing levels of beneficial bacteria, drastic increases in chemical exposure, and poor nutrition are making our immune cells more reactive to their environment.

Gluten, dairy, and eggs are some of the most common foods that people can be sensitive to. The majority of clients that we see are sensitive to at least one of these food groups. Upon providing them with options that are gluten-, dairy-, and egg-free, their lives change.

The following conditions can be associated with a food sensitivity:

✓ Acid reflux
✓ Constipation
✓ Chronic fatigue
✓ Diarrhea
✓ Chronic headaches
✓ Migraines
✓ Sinus problems
✓ Arthritis
✓ Eczema
✓ Asthma
✓ ADD/ADHD
✓ Irritable bowel disease
✓ Type 1 diabetes
✓ Osteoporosis
✓ Multiple sclerosis
✓ Dementia
✓ Hypothyroidism

People often don't realize just how much of their health concerns are associated with the foods they eat. Moods, intestinal health, body weight, and other issues can be directly correlated with food sensitivity reactions. I see it time and time again in my practice—someone has a host of symptoms and, in the end, it's actually a food sensitivity that's wreaking havoc on his or her body. For instance, in December of 2006, Sally came into my office with a laundry list of symptoms. She had been diagnosed with asthma, acid reflux and other digestive imbalances, chronic fatigue, and a host of psychiatric disorders, including atypical bipolar disorder, anxiety, and depression. Due to Sally's chronic fatigue, she could only function for about 5 to 6 hours per day. After bouncing around from specialist to specialist for 10 years, Sally was referred to my office by one of her neurologists. It appeared obvious from her symptoms list that she was reacting to gluten and potentially a few other food proteins. After three sessions, Sally (and her husband) reluctantly agreed to try an Elimination Diet to identify possible foods that could be making her symptoms worse. On day 12 of the diet, Sally's chronic fatigue all but disappeared. The asthma vanished and her mood stabilized. After 9 months of dietary changes, Sally is healthier than ever and experiences 15 hours of abundant energy per day as long as she avoids gluten, dairy, eggs, yeast, and soy. In addition to cooking many of the recipes from this book as daily staples, Sally also added a number of cultured and fermented foods to her diet, including kombucha, cultured vegetables, and homemade, gluten-free sourdough bread. The only complaint she has now is that she needs to spend money on new clothes as she continues to lose weight.

WHAT IS A FOOD SENSITIVITY?

A food sensitivity can occur when the immune system considers a food a potential threat to the body. As a response, the immune cells secrete chemicals called inflammatory cytokines. These chemicals are signaling molecules that alert other cells of the body of the perceived foreign invader—the food you just ate. This starts a cascade of events, which can lead to inflammation and disease in the body. The term "food sensitivity" literally means that your body is sensitive to eating a particular food. We are all biochemically unique. It seems logical that we would all respond differently to the biological chemicals in food. As world-renowned nutritional biochemist Dr. Jeffrey Bland often says, "The food of one can be the poison of another."

10 Common Food Sensitivities:

- ✓ Gluten
- ✓ Dairy
- ✓ Soy
- ✓ Eggs
- ✓ Corn
- ✓ Yeast
- ✓ Nightshade vegetables
- ✓ Citrus
- ✓ Nuts
- ✓ Chocolate

Let's look a little more closely at three of the most common food sensitivities: gluten, dairy, and eggs. If everyone in my clinical practice were to remove just these three foods from their diets for 28 days or more, I can confidently say that many of their health concerns would improve. These foods all contain higher levels of proteins that are not always easily broken down. If there are imbalances in a person's digestive capacities (their ability to break food down from large pieces to small pieces) partnered with a leaky gut (openings in the intestinal wall), these proteins can sneak into their bodies and wreak havoc on the entire system.

GLUTEN

Gluten is a protein complex that is found in wheat, spelt, kamut, barley, and rye. The immune system in people who are either celiac positive, gluten sensitive, or allergic to wheat perceives gluten as a foreign invader. This leads to an activation of the immune cells in the intestines when exposed to gluten. These immune cells release chemicals that lead to a host of symptoms (see list on page 14). One particular problem caused by gluten intolerance is destruction or disruption of the surface, or *villi*, of the intestines.

When the intestinal villi are not functioning, there is a decreased ability to absorb nutrients from food. This can lead to malnutrition conditions including anemia and osteoporosis. One can also be sensitive to gluten and not have any damage to the intestines with reactions ranging from foggy thinking and joint pain to skin disorders.

There are three primary gluten-related disorders that are commonly researched. According to scientific studies, wheat allergy accounts of .4% of gluten-related reactions, celiac disease is around 1%, and non-celiac wheat sensitivity accounts for around 6%. If there were no crossovers in these groups, that would imply that over 7% of the general population would have a negative reaction every time they ate gluten-associated foods. From what we are seeing in our clinical practice, this number seems rather low as the majority of our clients feel improvements in health when going on a gluten-free diet. Certain populations of people may be more likely to have sensitivity reactions to gluten. For example, it was shown in one study that 30% of clients presenting with irritable bowel disease were actually suffering from a sensitivity to gluten. We have witnessed that many cases of chronic diarrhea, arthritis, chronic fatigue, migraines, and irritable bowel disease are associated with a gluten sensitivity. When our clients transition to eating foods free of gluten and other irritating substances, many of these conditions either disappear entirely or improve considerably.

TRIGGERS OF CELIAC DISEASE

Celiac disease is a genetic condition, but it can be triggered by stressful events in life including pregnancy, childbirth, viral infections, death of a loved one, or even a surgery.

Common symptoms associated with a gluten sensitivity and celiac disease:

- ✓ Obesity/weight gain
- ✓ Weight loss
- ✓ Diarrhea
- ✓ Constipation
- ✓ Gas and bloating
- ✓ Nausea
- ✓ Headaches
- ✓ Fatigue
- ✓ Skin problems
- ✓ Joint pain
- ✓ Acid reflux
- ✓ Anemia
- ✓ Osteoporosis
- ✓ Numbness and tingling
- ✓ Behavior and mood changes
- ✓ Dental problems (loss of enamel)

Gluten is found *everywhere* in our food supply. Baking powder can contain gluten. So can cottage cheese, soy sauce, beer, and lentils. Many gluten-free foods may also be cross-contaminated with gluten because they are grown, stored, transported, or processed in the vicinity of gluten-containing grains. In addition, nonfood sources of gluten include lip balm, playdough, toothpaste, and baby powder.

Adhering to a gluten-free diet can be challenging. We would estimate that over 90% of our clients who attempt a gluten-free diet still consume a small source of gluten without ever knowing it. It often requires a thorough diet diary evaluation to find all the potential pitfall foods. Once these foods are replaced in a gluten-sensitive individual, changes in health are often seen immediately. See our website, www.WholeLifeNutrition.net, for more information.

We invite you to explore this topic further with your local health-care practitioner and Gluten Intolerance Group, www.Gluten.net. You can find a Certified Gluten Practitioner at www.TheDr.com. Celiac disease is now being accurately diagnosed via four blood markers (IgA anti-dpgli, IgG anti-dpgli, IgA anti-tissue transglutaminase, and IgA anti-endomysium). This negates the need for an invasive biopsy. Saliva tests, blood tests, and even biopsies are not able to diagnose a gluten sensitivity. The only diagnostic tool available for gluten sensitivity remains an Elimination Diet—eliminating gluten from the diet for a minimum of four weeks and then challenging it back in to determine if you have a reaction.

Marian, a 58-year-old busy school teacher from California, called our clinic complaining of constant arthritis pain. She had been experiencing this pain for over 8 years and had heard that dietary changes may be able to help. Her other conditions included carpal tunnel syndrome, trigger finger, frequent loose stools, and fatigue. Marian needed to have energy to keep up with her students. After our initial phone consultation I suspected that her symptoms indicated a potential sensitivity to gluten-containing foods. I recommended Marian try a gluten Elimination Diet for 2 weeks. After her initial 2-week dietary change, her symptoms and pain diminished substantially, bowel movements normalized, and she experienced increased energy. I gave Marian many of our gluten-free recipes, supplements to help heal her intestines, and continued with our phone consultations. She is now following a gluten-free diet, is living pain-free, and says she feels 20 years younger.

DAIRY

For many years, cow's milk has been advertised as the elixir of health. Whether it was for strong bones or big muscles, most of us were told to drink up. In formula, and in bottles, some of us started drinking it at birth. Because cow's milk was designed for an entirely different species of animal, a large portion of the population has an adverse reaction when consuming it. Beyond the majority of the world's population that are lactose (milk sugar) intolerant, many people also have various reactions to the proteins in cow's milk. There are at least 30 antigenic primary proteins in milk. Casein is the most commonly used milk protein in the food industry; lactalbumin, lactoglobulin, bovine albumin, and gamma globulin are other protein groups within milk. Milk proteins are listed on food labels with a variety of names such as milk solids, skim milk powder, casein, caseinates, whey, and albumin.

The feeding of cow's milk formula has been well documented as contributing to cases of eczema, colic, diarrhea, and sinus conditions in infants. When breast-feeding mothers consume dairy products, their exclusively breast-fed children may test positive to having a cow's milk protein immune reaction as well. Later in life, a cow's milk sensitivity can contribute to sinus conditions, asthma, eczema, headaches, arthritis, acid reflux, constipation, and other bowel problems.

Common symptoms associated with a dairy sensitivity include:

- ✓ Gas
- ✓ Abdominal bloating and pain
- ✓ Diarrhea
- ✓ Constipation
- ✓ Gastrointestinal bleeding
- ✓ Anemia
- ✓ Nausea and vomiting
- ✓ Acid reflux
- ✓ Chronic headaches/migraines
- ✓ Joint pain/arthritis
- ✓ Rhinitis
- ✓ Ear infections
- ✓ Hay fever

Katie, a 2-year-old girl, and her mother, Joan, came in to see me regarding Katie's asthma. Her doctor's skin prick test had identified Katie as having multiple airborne allergies, including dust, mold, and pollen. Katie also displayed behavioral problems, dark circles under her eyes, and reoccurring sinus infections. After a few visits to the emergency room, Katie's family did everything they could to eliminate the airborne allergens in their home including removing all of their carpeting and replacing it with hardwood flooring, repainting the walls, and covering all mattresses and pillows with hypoallergenic covers. After doing all of this, Katie's symptoms did not change. Katie's mother then decided to see me. I mentioned to Joan that Katie's symptoms might be associated with a dairy sensitivity. Joan was apprehensive to take cheese out of Katie's diet, considering it was her favorite food. After a few more consultations and a health food store tour, Joan felt confident that she had enough dairy-free food options for her daughter. After the second week of eating dairy-free, Katie's sinuses began to drain, and, more importantly to Joan, Katie's mood was better than it had been in the last 6 months. Joan now controls Katie's asthma attacks through dietary changes alone, and is grateful to have a happy, healthy daughter.

- ✓ Asthma
- ✓ Eczema
- ✓ Depression and mood swings
- ✓ ADHD
- ✓ Bed-wetting in children

In our own practice, we have seen that by eliminating or reducing dairy products, many health conditions resolve on their own, without the use of medications. When milk antigens get through the gut mucosa intact, they may be responsible for a host of delayed immune responses that do not depend on the standard antibodies that people associate with allergies called IgE antibodies. These delayed immune responses depend on antibodies, like IgA, IgG, IgD, and IgM antibodies, that do not show up on standard allergy skin prick tests designed to pick up IgE related reactions. To determine if you react to dairy, we recommend following a 30-day dairy Elimination Diet. See our website, www.WholeLifeNutrition.net, for more information.

EGGS

Eggs have long been known to be one of the most common allergens in children. This may be due to early exposure to egg albumin that is in vaccines. We have noticed that people with conditions such as eczema and migraines often improve on an egg-free diet. Four proteins in eggs that cause much of the problems are ovomucoid, ovalbumin, ovotransfferin, and lysozyme. Eggs can be an ingredient in many processed foods including glazes on pastries, ice cream, some margarines, noodles, processed meats, sauces, candy, a wide variety of ready-made foods, custards, and breads. Egg proteins can also hide in lotions, shampoos, vaccines, and in some medications. Always read labels to determine if a product contains eggs. Eggs listed on the label may appear as albumin, globulin, livetin, lysozyme, or lecithin. In addition, many people who react to hen's eggs will also react to eggs of another species, including duck and turkey.

Common symptoms associated with an egg sensitivity include:

- ✓ Abdominal bloating and pain
- ✓ Diarrhea
- ✓ Constipation
- ✓ Nausea and vomiting
- ✓ Chronic headaches
- ✓ Migraines
- ✓ Rhinitis
- ✓ Asthma
- ✓ Dermatitis
- ✓ Eczema
- ✓ Hives
- ✓ Itching of the mouth and tongue
- ✓ Wheezing

Christy, a 48-year-old business woman, came in to my office with chronic migraines and chronic back pain. I suspected a food sensitivity and advised her to see her doctor to get an updated ELISA (enzyme-linked immunosorbent assay) blood allergy test. The test results showed positive IgG and IgE antibodies for eggs and dairy. Ali then provided cooking classes, recipes, and meal planning. After 3 weeks of eliminating all dairy and egg products, Christy's chronic migraines disappeared. Christy then had laboratory tests done for both vitamin D deficiency and gluten sensitivity, which both showed imbalances. She then went on a gluten-free diet and supplemented with vitamin D, and is now free of her back pain as well.

THE ELIMINATION DIET

We have found the process of removing potentially irritating foods from our clients' diets to be incredibly effective in improving a host of diseases and disorders. In order to find out what foods are contributing to your health disorders, it is necessary to take out the 10 most common suspect foods (see list on page 13) for at least 28 days. If your body was getting inflamed when you consumed these foods, you will likely notice a huge change when the irritating foods are removed. Many of the common symptoms of stomach upset, bowel problems, skin rashes, headaches, and mood will calm down or go away all together. At that time, you can add back in the suspect foods one at a time to see which ones are responsible for your reactions. This process of eliminating foods and then adding them back in is called an Elimination Diet. After recommending these diets to thousands of people, we have come up with some valuable resources and tasty recipes to help you get the best possible results from your dietary experiment. You can find this detailed information on the Elimination Diet at www .WholeLifeNutrition.net.

3

DIGESTIVE HEALTH

When health is absent, wisdom cannot reveal itself, art cannot manifest, strength cannot fight, wealth becomes useless, and intelligence cannot be applied.

—Herophilus, 300 BC

Your digestive tract is an important interface between your body and the outside world. It is a highly tuned mechanism designed to discern friend from foe—healthy food from things that might harm you. At the same time, it is responsible for directing the digestion and absorption of food and all the vital nutrients that come along with it.

When things go wrong with your digestive tract it has far-reaching impacts on your overall health. Scientists are discovering that there is a connection between digestive imbalances and obesity, diabetes, mental and behavioral disorders, heart disease, and autoimmune disorders. Maintaining a healthy gut is a strong support for your overall health and well-being.

In this chapter we'll explore some important, simple ways you can nourish your digestive system, which can affect your overall health and well-being.

DO YOU HAVE A HEALTHY DIGESTIVE SYSTEM?

If you have one or more of the following symptoms, your digestive system could be impaired:

✓ Eczema, acne, and other skin conditions
✓ Food and environmental allergies
✓ Frequent bowel movements (3 or more per day)
✓ Consistently loose stools
✓ Consistent constipation
✓ Stools that float, are lighter in color, or are urgent
✓ GI upset after eating fatty or greasy foods
✓ Frequent bloating, distention, gas, or belching within 15 to 45 minutes after eating
✓ Undigested food in the stools
✓ Intestinal cramping

WHAT IS DIGESTION?

The word *digestion* literally means to break from large to small. Food must be broken into smaller pieces before we can access and absorb the nutrients it contains. This process usually begins with chewing and the secretion of enzymes from our saliva.

Gastric Acid

Within seconds of swallowing, our food ends up in our stomachs where we hopefully have gastric juices with a pH similar to battery acid. Stomach acid is amazing at breaking apart food proteins and hard-to-digest items. At the same time, acid protects us from parasites, bacterium, or viruses that may be traveling on or in our food. Stomach acid also plays a prime role in preparing minerals and vitamins for absorption, and activating enzymes that will further help us break apart our food. Another interesting effect of stomach acid is the breakdown of foods into small enough fragments that our immune systems can recognize them. If we do not break down our food, and it somehow sneaks through our intestinal wall, our immune cells may not recognize these larger food fragments and instead mistake them for foreign substances. As a result, they may launch an immune attack that leads to inflammation and possibly intestinal damage.

To get an idea of how important stomach acid is, we can look at what happens when we take it out. Acid-blocking medications such as Prilosec, Nexium, and Prevacid have been shown to shift the acid levels in the stomach from a pH similar to battery acid (1.2–1.6) to a pH of 5.0, which is the same as table vinegar! You can imagine that vinegar would be far less effective than battery acid in breaking apart foods to access nutrients and protect us from foreign invaders. Use of these medications over the long term has been associated with

> ## SYMPTOMS OF LOW GASTRIC ACID
>
> The most common immediate symptoms experienced by people with low gastric acid are gas and bloating, specifically in the stomach and upper GI tract. Some people experience nausea and cramping as well.

nutrient deficiencies such as vitamin B12, zinc, and magnesium, as well as an increased risk for hip fractures, pneumonia, and bacterial overgrowth. Research indicates that people taking acid-blocking medications have a significant increase in both food (10.5 times increase) and airborne allergies months after taking these medications.

CCK and Pancreatic Enzymes

Once food passes out of the stomach, the cells in the upper small intestine, or duodenum, "read" the food to determine what needs to happen next. Fatty acids (fats) and peptides (protein fragments) will signal the secretion of hormones that will

> ## SYMPTOMS OF A LACK OF PANCREATIC ENZYMES
>
> If you are lacking in digestive enzymes, you could likely experience gas, cramping, nausea, looser stools, frequent stools, orange-colored stools, floating stools, or see undigested food in your stools. One study looking at the ingestion of pancreatic enzymes showed that people were able to reduce from 4 bowel movements per day to 1 with enzyme supplementation.

help digest them further. One of the primary hormones used is called *cholecystokinin* or CCK. This literally means the bile (chole) sack (cyst) moving (kinin) hormone. As the name implies, CCK tells the gallbladder to secrete bile. Bile is like detergent. It splits apart, or emulsifies, fat globules into smaller groups of fatty acids.

Imagine for a second, a greasy dish in a sink of hot water. All the fat floats to the top of the sink. Squirt some liquid dish soap into the sink and... *whoooosh!* All of the fat breaks apart. Bile acts like detergent in breaking apart fats so they are ready to be absorbed into your body.

CCK also stimulates the pancreas to secrete digestive enzymes. Enzymes facilitate the breaking down of proteins, carbohydrates, and fats into smaller pieces.

Bacteria in the Role of Digestion

If you cannot break down food properly, intestinal organisms will likely do it for you. But this can come at a price as many of the beneficial organisms thrive on properly broken down foods, while pathogenic or potentially harmful organisms thrive on undigested foods. As a result, people with CCK and pancreatic enzyme insufficiencies are susceptible to a potentially uncomfortable condition called small intestinal bacterial overgrowth or SIBO.

Bacteria and other organisms in the intestinal tract play a vital role in digestive health. Studies have demonstrated that intestinal organisms can "communicate" with intestinal cells, allowing for either a calm immune system environment or a relatively volatile one. There are actual receptors, called Toll-like receptors, that stick out of the intestinal cells waiting to interact with the surrounding environment. When proteins from bacteria bind to these receptors, chemicals are released that allow for normal intestinal surface function. Inflammation is calmed down, and if an injury

does occur, there is a robust repair response. On the contrary, if certain bacteria species are not present in the intestinal tract and these receptors are not bound to bacterial proteins, then the intestinal cells are more sensitive to injury and cannot repair themselves as well. Beyond this, beneficial bacteria also protect us from toxins; help to manufacture nutrients such as vitamin K, amino acids, short-chained fatty acids, and biotin; crowd out pathogenic organisms; break down antinutrients such as lectins, phytates, oxalates, and saponins; and help in the overall digestion process. As humans, our lives and our health depend upon having a healthy inner ecosystem of bacteria.

QUICK FACTS ABOUT BENEFICIAL BACTERIA

✓ Assist with digestion, absorption, and assimilation of food nutrients
✓ Keep your immune system calm
✓ Transform toxic substances so they are less toxic
✓ Degrade antinutrients from food such as phytates, lectins, saponins, and oxalates
✓ Produce vitamins such as K and biotin
✓ Produce amino acids such as phenylalanine, tryptophan, and tyrosine (precursors to happy hormones)

Protection from a Leaky Gut

Bacteria lower inflammation in the body by keeping your gut from being leaky. When beneficial bacteria are missing, disease-causing or pathogenic bacteria can flourish. Harmful bacteria secrete chemicals that break down our intestinal barriers, causing a leaky gut. This is where gaps

SYMPTOMS OF ALTERED GUT MICROBIOTA

Gut microbiota is a complex of microorganism species living in your digestive tract. In fact, the human body carries about 100 trillion microorganisms in its intestines! Microbe imbalances can contribute to reflux, belching, gas, nausea, cramping, loose stools, periodontal disease, and a host of other issues. Having an imbalanced inner ecosystem of bacteria leads the immune system to be in a constant state of alert and alarm. This creates a ripe environment for diseases such as irritable bowel, diabetes, cancer, arthritis, food and airborne allergies, autism, celiac disease, eczema, and autoimmune disorders.

BLOOD SUGAR REGULATION AND YOUR DIGESTIVE SYSTEM

Bacteria and yeasts need foods to survive and thrive. Processed diets containing refined carbohydrates readily feed pathogenic yeasts and bacteria. Pathogenic organisms cause the immune system to be hyper-reactive to stimuli and contribute to a leaky gut. An inflamed and leaky gut allows chemicals that alter sugar and fat metabolism to circulate in your blood. When insulin docks onto cells, it normally signals transporters to take sugar out of the blood. Inflammatory chemicals will block the signaling from insulin. This allows sugar levels to increase in the blood, stick to proteins, and get converted to fat. At the same time, these inflammatory chemicals can sneak into your fat cells and signal them to grow.

The scientific story of "all carbs turn to sugar in your blood" is more complex than that. It may be that the microbe story actually has more importance than the blood sugar story. In fact, when microbes from a thin person are transferred to an obese person, the obese person will begin "thinning out" within a few days when they are on a high-carb, low-fat diet.

are formed between intestinal cells, allowing contents from the intestines to leak into our bodies. The primary content of our intestines is bacteria. So when our guts leak, bacteria, including the dangerous varieties, as well as food particles end up in our bloodstreams. When this happens, our protective immune cells launch an attack against these foreign invaders and secrete a barrage of harmful chemicals. Once these "alert and alarm" chemicals are in the bloodstream, they can affect the entire body. They can cause damage to surrounding tissue and change cellular behavior throughout your body. This includes altering your appetite, shuttling fat in your fat cells, and decreasing your cells'

ability to utilize blood sugar. These very same inflammatory chemicals lead to obesity, diabetes, cardiovascular disease, arthritis, and other inflammatory diseases. Isn't it amazing how much we depend on bacteria for all aspects of our health?

WHAT'S INVOLVED IN DAMAGING YOUR DIGESTIVE HEALTH?

1. Food Sensitivities

Food sensitivity reactions, such as to gluten or dairy, cause irritation and inflammation in the upper intestines. This often leads to damage of intestinal tissue, a leaky gut, and a subsequent breakdown of the digestive and absorptive processes. Without proper intestinal cell function, signals for hormones like CCK to be released never occur, causing a lack of bile and pancreatic enzymes. This leads to undigested food, bacterial imbalances, and food particles too large to be absorbed. In the presence of a leaky gut, this can cause further inflammation and exposure to food particles that can cause even more food sensitivities.

2. Cesarean Births and Formula Feeding

During a vaginal birth, bacteria from the mother immediately begins to colonize an infant's digestive tract, taking up to a month to become fully established. When an infant is born through a cesarean section, bacteria from sources in the operating room, such as the air, nurses, and doctors, colonize the infant's digestive tract. As a result, cesarean-born babies are more likely to have immune imbalance disorders like asthma, eczema, and allergies. Since some women do not have a choice on how their baby decides to come into the world, we highly recommend giving c-section newborns a special infant probiotic powder right after birth.

3. Common Toxins

Many toxins like mercury, PCBs, Roundup, triclosan (from hand sanitizers), and pesticides can kill beneficial bacteria that would normally keep the intestines calm. These chemicals can harm surrounding tissues in the intestines leading to more leaky gut symptoms and inflammation.

4. Medications

There are many medications that can cause an imbalance in your intestines that will lead to digestive upset. Three of the most common associated with intestinal disorders include acid-blocking medication, nonsteroid anti-inflammatories, and antibiotics.

Acid-Blocking Medications. Acid-blocking medications such as Prilosec, Nexium, and Zantac decrease your gastric acid significantly. Without adequate acid to burn incoming invaders, people on these medications are more susceptible to viral infections and bacterial imbalances. Acid is normally responsible for breaking down hard-to-digest food items and assists with making vitamins and minerals more absorbable. Lower acid in the stomach for long periods leads to nutrient deficiencies and undigested foods. Undigested foods can feed unfriendly bacteria leading once again to bacterial imbalances.

Nonsteroidal Anti-Inflammatories (NSAIDs). NSAIDs such as aspirin, ibuprofen (such as Advil and Motrin), and naproxen (such as Aleve) directly irritate the intestinal cells, while also lowering protective chemicals (prostaglandins) in the GI tract. As a result, the devastating effects these medications can have to the digestive tract are well-known and well documented. According to a study published in the *Journal of Therapeutics and Clinical Risk Management* in 2009, "Major adverse gastrointestinal events attributed to NSAIDs are responsible for over 100,000 hospitalizations, $2 billion in healthcare costs, and 17,000 deaths in the U.S. each year."

Antibiotics. A single course of antibiotics has been proven to cause lifelong changes in a person's bacterial colonies. A common side effect of antibiotic use indicating an immediate imbalance in the intestines is "antibiotic-associated diarrhea" (AAD). Knocking out the beneficial bacteria in the intestines can cause problems with nutrient metabolism and absorption such as with carbohydrates and short-chain fatty acids, as bacteria play a key role in these processes. When protective beneficial bacteria are killed off by antibiotics, disease-causing organisms like *Clostridium difficile* are more likely to flourish. Both of these problems cause flushing of the intestinal contents, leading to diarrhea.

SIX STEPS TO NOURISH YOUR DIGESTIVE SYSTEM

1. Test for Food Sensitivities

Look at food first! There are over 22 tons of food matter that you will consume in your lifetime. You could be taking in food substances that are irritating your intestines, are hard for your digestive system to break down, or are causing bacterial imbalances. An Elimination Diet (www.WholeLifeNutrition.net) will help you determine which foods your body is considering to be friends, and which it is considering to be foes.

2. Filter Your Water

Water that is treated with chlorine-based chemicals and that contains harmful antibiotic residues can wreak havoc on your gut. Consider a reverse osmosis filter and possibly an additional carbon block filter to remove these contaminants.

3. Remove Mercury Fillings

Mercury exposure from mercury amalgams can alter your intestinal flora and general health. A trained International Academy of Oral Medicine and Toxicology (IAOMT) dentist can consult you on the extremely important steps that are needed to replace your mercury fillings.

4. Eat Organic Foods!

Numerous agricultural chemicals cause damage to the intestines. The only way to lower your exposure today, and 10 years from today, is to purchase organic products that have never come in contact with herbicides made with glyphosate (such as Roundup).

5. Avoid Processed Foods

Processed foods often contain artificial sweeteners, flavors, and colors, along with fillers, preservatives, binders, and excipients that can irritate your intestines. Whole plant-based foods contain natural fibers that can only be broken down by bacteria in your gut. These prelife or prebiotic substances are needed before the life of bacterium can flourish in your intestines. Whole foods will also be full of protective plant chemicals (phytochemicals) that can lower inflammation and heal wounded intestinal tissues.

6. Avoid Triclosan

Choose soaps, hand sanitizers, cleaning products, toothpastes, and personal care products that are free of triclosan. As an antimicrobial, triclosan is efficient at knocking out beneficial microbes both in your intestines and in the environment. There are numerous nontoxic ingredients on the market that can replace triclosan as an antimicrobial. Once good example is the thyme oil used in the Clean Well All-Natural Hand Sanitizer.

THE WHOLE TOXICITY STORY

Your people are driven by a terrible sense of deficiency. When the last tree is cut, the last fish is caught, and the last river is polluted; when to breathe the air is sickening, you will realize, too late, that wealth is not in bank accounts and that you can't eat money.
—*Alanis Obomsawin*

Chemical companies have been producing or mining chemicals to use for fuel, pharmaceuticals, food (additives, preservatives, colorants, sweeteners), and pesticides (fungicides, insecticides, herbicides) for the last 100 years. Not including these just mentioned, there are an additional 74 billion pounds of chemicals produced or imported in the United States every single day! You will find them in products like shower curtains, foam cushions for couches, paints and varnishes, and the list goes on. That means that there are well over 250 pounds of chemicals produced per person per day in the United States.

We are finding more and more of them in the bodies of humans as well as animals. Scientists are finding that most people are walking around with a soup of industrial chemicals in their bodies. There have been studies that have demonstrated that even the cord blood of unborn infants contains hundreds of chemicals including heavy metals like lead and mercury, flame retardants like PBDEs (polybrominated diphenyl ethers), pesticides, and PCBs (polychlorinated biphenyls). Collectively, these are known to adversely affect the brains, immune systems, and reproductive systems of children, as well as contribute to cancer cell growth in both adults and children.

These chemicals circulate through our bodies at the parts per billion and parts per million levels. That doesn't seem so bad, right? Did you know that most pharmaceutical drugs work at these same levels? Ken Cook, president of the Environmental Working Group, states: "Albuterol is in the desk of every nurse because one dose of it, at 2.1 parts per billion, will stop an asthma attack. One dose of Paxil, a common antidepressant, operates at 30 parts per billion. And then there is NuvaRing, which is a commonly prescribed birth control drug. It is active at 0.035 parts per billion." Surprisingly, we all expect prescription and over-the-counter medication to work every time we take it. That means that we should expect these industrial chemicals to have an effect in the part-per-billion range as well.

These industrial compounds are building up in the air, water, and food supply. It is important to understand that many of the diseases on the rise today are likely the result of a buildup of these chemicals in the body. A Whole Life Nutrition lifestyle takes into account that our collective health goes far beyond diet. It encompasses everything we ingest, including the air we breathe, the water we drink, and the toxic chemicals we come into contact with in myriad ways. It is time to take action to not only reduce chemicals in our environment, but to find alternative ways of living that support the health of the people and the planet.

AIR

The Organization for Economic Co-operation and Development released a report in 2012 stating: "Urban air pollution is set to become the top environmental cause of mortality worldwide by 2050, ahead of dirty water and lack of sanitation. The number of premature deaths from exposure to particulate air pollutants leading to respiratory failure could double from current levels to 3.6 million every year globally, with most occurring in China and India."

Unfortunately, what starts in China and India does not stay there. Both of these nations are growing economically and plan to fuel their increased energy needs with coal. Mercury is a natural component of coal, and when burned to generate electricity, it is released through the smokestacks into the air, contributing to almost half of all mercury emissions!

The EPA and international organizations recognize that coal-fired power plants are a prime contributor to the air pollution mentioned above. Along with chlor-alkali plants, incinerators, and cement factories, coal power plants are emitting over 6,500 tons of mercury into the air every year. This "Brown Cloud" of mercury and other pollutants is tracked by NASA and other organizations and can travel across the Pacific Ocean in as little as 7 days, depositing pollution on the United States. Alaska Action states: "At least 20% of the mercury in (Alaska) is attributed to Asian coal plants and industry, and it is deposited onto coastal waters and inland where it ends up in the local food chain, threatening the health of the state's wildlife, ecosystems, and human communities."

Most of the mercury exposure we get is through consuming contaminated fish and shellfish. Microscopic organisms in the water and soil convert inorganic and elemental mercury into methylmercury, also called organic mercury, which accumulates up through the food chain in fish, animals, and people. Elemental mercury from air pollution can also be converted into methylmercury inside the body.

Quick facts about mercury contamination in our environment:

- ✓ The top 100 meters of the ocean have twice as much mercury as they did the previous century.
- ✓ Predatory fish contain 12 times the mercury now as during preindustrial times.
- ✓ When mercury samples in fish were examined in nine countries, the vast majority showed that a single serving per month would be considered toxic.
- ✓ Hair samples from Cameroon, Cook Islands, Indonesia, Japan, Mexico, Russia, Tanzania, and Thailand showed 82% of people had mercury levels higher than the U.S. EPA reference dose that would be determined safe in humans.

Mercury is a neurotoxic substance to humans and animals. Unborn babies are at the greatest risk for damage due to mercury exposure as methylmercury (usually from the mother's fish consumption) passing through the placenta. Hundreds of thousands of babies born each year in the United States are at risk for learning disabilities due to mercury exposure in utero. Common symptoms of mercury exposure include tremors, emotional instability, insomnia, memory loss, neuromuscular changes, headaches, polyneuropathy, and performance deficits in tests of cognitive and motor function.

What can you do to reduce mercury exposure?

✓ Eat more beans, greens (especially cruciferous vegetables), fruits, and brown rice, as chemicals and fibers in these foods help to lower absorption of mercury and increase the metabolism and elimination of mercury.

✓ Eat fermented foods and take a high-quality probiotic supplement. Research has shown that beneficial bacteria can reduce the absorption of mercury.

✓ Eat types of fish that are lower in mercury, such as wild salmon, anchovies, and herring. Avoid swordfish, marlin, orange roughy, shark, and ahi tuna. Parents are advised to limit their children's intake of tuna to one 3-ounce serving per month!

✓ Consider having your mercury fillings replaced by a dentist associated with the International Academy of Oral Medicine and Toxicology. The content of amalgam fillings can be up to 50% or higher in mercury, and contribute up to 50% of a person's daily mercury exposure.

✓ Consider seeking advice from an alternative medicine physician who is trained in mercury testing and oral DMSA supplementation. Research has shown this to be a safe and viable way of lowering mercury levels, even in children.

✓ If you have the option, choose Green Energy on your power bill. That way you only support the use of solar, wind, and hydroelectric power that will not contribute to more mercury release via coal power plants.

✓ Find alternatives to type 3 plastics or PVCs (polyvinyl-chlorides). These plastics are the prime use for chlorine in the United States, and often contain plasticizing agents such as phthalates that have been shown to increase breast cancer. Mercury cell chlor-alkali plants are a major contributor to mercury in our environment.

WATER

In the past, drinking water contained hydrogen, oxygen, and a host of minerals—pure water! In the present, water commonly contains pharmaceuticals, heavy metals, chlorine or chlorine metabolite-based disinfection by-products, antimicrobial soap chemicals (triclosan), pesticides and herbicides, as well as hundreds of other compounds. Chemicals released into the air will most often get pulled down to earth by rain; and the rain will collect in streams, rivers, lakes, and wells. Chemicals disposed of by industry also get washed into the very same watersheds when it rains. As a result, water is a storage area for industrial chemicals.

Studies looking at pesticide residues coming out of wastewater treatment plants have shown that the treatment process does often not reduce them. More than half of the finished drinking water samples from 19 drinking water treatment facilities contained pesticides and pharmaceuticals including a known sedative drug called *merpobamate*; an antiseizure drug called *phenytoin*, which is known to deplete folic acid and may increase suicide risk; and an herbicide called *atrazine* that alters hormone function, can increase cancer in humans, and is associated with preterm births. Although the herbicide atrazine was banned in Europe in 2004, 90% of water samples from 139 water systems in the United States in 2003 and 2004 had measurable levels of atrazine.

What can you do?

✓ Drink purified water preferably from a reverse osmosis (RO) system. Some RO systems also come with an additional carbon block to lower chemical residues. You may have to add in nutritional minerals to your diet in order to supplement losses from filtration.

✓ Consume a healthy, organic whole foods diet to decrease the global burden of chemicals used in agriculture. A diet rich in organic plant foods also supports your immune and detoxification systems to process the chemicals once you are exposed.

FOOD

Our exposure to chemicals in the food supply is increasing at an alarming rate. Eating organic is one of the best ways to reduce direct exposure to pesticides, but even if you are eating an organic diet, you may still be getting certain chemicals hidden in certain foods.

There is a class of chemicals that is extremely resistant to biological breakdown so they persist in the environment for many years. These Persistent Organic Pollutants (POPs) are all lipophilic—meaning they accumulate in fat, particularly in the fat of animals.

Dioxins, common POPs, are some of the most toxic substances known to man with clear evidence that they can alter learning in children, cause cancer, change blood sugar metabolism, suppress immune function, and alter hormonal function, such as thyroid and testosterone. According to a USDA report in 2000, a time when over a trillion pounds of dioxins had not yet been released, "dioxin is a human carcinogen and that the lifetime cancer risk associated with the average person's body burden of dioxin is between 1 in 1000 and 1 in 100. This estimate of risk is ten times higher than EPA's previous estimate, and represents a very significant public health concern."

Chlorine-based products are where dioxins come from. The production of herbicides, insecticides, fungicides, pharmaceuticals, and PVC—type

---

BLOOD SUGAR REGULATION AND CHEMICALS

Numerous chemicals are affecting our ability to metabolize sugar in the bloodstream. Phthalates and parabens are commonly found in personal care items like sunscreens, lotions, perfumes, hair gels, deodorants, and colognes that are being applied to people's skin each and every day. An increased use of one personal care product per day can increase phthalates in the urine by 33%. These chemicals have been associated with insulin resistance, diabetes, and obesity. BPA has been found to leach from even cold plastic bottles, and is now shown to be absorbed through the mouth and skin. Minute amounts of BPA in the blood affect sugar metabolism. BPA was originally used as a synthetic estrogen that was added to animal feed to fatten the animals up. We now produce over 6 billion pounds of BPA every year to use in plastics. They are in, and around, all of us.

3 plastics—contribute to the release of dioxins, as these are all made with chlorine. By living a healthy life, full of organic foods and free of pharmaceuticals and type 3 plastics, you will help to protect the planet from one of the most toxic substances known to man.

There is an increasing body of evidence showing that elevated levels of persistent organic pollutants (POPs) in humans are tightly associated with diabetes, metabolic syndrome, and obesity. In one study looking at six common POPs, those participants with the highest levels in their blood were 37.7 times more likely to have diabetes. Rat feeding studies have confirmed that diets containing higher levels of POPs, regardless of protein, carbohydrate, or fat content, will lead to an increase in insulin resistance and metabolic disorders over time. This should raise caution to the phrase "add a little protein with each meal to lower blood sugar." The source of the protein, along with the fats that come along with it, may make a significant difference in long-term health. A prime example of this is farmed salmon.

People now consume more farmed fish than wild fish. They also consume more farmed fish than beef. A common practice on salmon farms is to feed fish meal and fish fat to the farmed fish. Because POPs accumulate in fat, this causes a drastic increase of POPs in farmed fish. In fact, farmed salmon are often the primary source of POP exposure in the human diet.

What can you do to reduce exposure?

✓ Farmed salmon has over 7 times the POPs than its wild counterpart. The consumption of "Atlantic salmon" as it is commonly known has been linked to an increase in insulin resistance and diabetes. Always choose wild Alaskan salmon, as Alaskan salmon is never farmed. However, salmon just labeled "wild" can sometimes be farmed.

✓ Fish from contaminated waterways—the Great Lakes and St. Lawrence River—will be contaminated with POPs. Search online for the terms POPs + your local fishing area to determine if testing of POPs has been done.

✓ Fatty meats will naturally contain higher levels of POPs. Trimming the fat will reduce exposure to POPs.

✓ High-fat dairy products, such as butter and ice cream, have higher concentrations of POPs. Choosing coconut oil over butter will reduce exposure.

✓ Choose a fish oil supplement that is frequently tested for PCB levels.

✓ Green tea consumption has been shown to lower the absorption of fats and fat-soluble substances such as POPs.

✓ Go to www.LifeWithoutPlastic.com for options on how to reduce your consumption of PVC-based plastic products (type-3). Use of these plastics increases the global supply of dioxins.

5

ORGANICS, YOUR HEALTH, AND THE PLANET

The criteria for a sustainable agriculture can be summed up in one word—permanence, which means adopting techniques that maintain soil fertility indefinitely, that utilize, as far as possible, only renewable resources; that do not grossly pollute the environment; and that foster biological activity within the soil and throughout the cycles of all the involved food chains.

—Lady Eve Balfour

Organically grown food is an earth-friendly and health-supportive method of farming and processing foods. Weeds and pests are controlled using environmentally sound practices that sustain our personal and planetary health. A Whole Life Nutrition lifestyle is based on organic foods, which is better for you and the planet.

Organic farming methods were the only ways of farming ever used until the early 1920s, when synthetic pesticides, herbicides, fungicides, and large-scale growing techniques were developed. After the Second World War, these techniques were largely in place and the American landscape of small, earth-friendly family farms began to change.

Conventional farming methods adversely affect soil quality, water purity, biodiversity, health of farmworkers, survival of small family farms, and the taste and nutritional quality of food. Toxic chemical residues from conventional farming remain in the soil for many years and leech into the groundwater. DDT, a pesticide that is a known carcinogen, which has long been banned in the United States, is still found in our soils. Chemicals from industrial farming include not only pesticides but also heavy metals such as lead and mercury, and solvents such as benzene and toluene. Heavy metals can directly damage nerves, affecting brain function, and possibly contribute to disorders like autism and ADD, and diseases like Parkinson's, multiple sclerosis, and Alzheimer's. Solvents damage the immune system, which decreases our ability to resist infections.

For every action there is an equal or greater reaction. We are allowing millions of tons of chemicals to be sprayed on or around our food every single year. As time passes, we realize that many of the chemicals we imagined to be harmless are not harmless at all. What is worse is that we are getting bombarded by over 80,000 different chemicals throughout our lifetime. Eating organic foods dramatically lowers a child's exposure to dangerous chemicals. A study funded by the U.S. Environmental Protection Agency found that eating organic foods provides children with immediate protection from dangerous organophosphate pesticides, which can cause harmful neurological damage. In 2005, a study was published showing the presence of over 200 chemicals in the umbilical cord blood of newborn infants. From flame retardants and Teflon to pesticides, all the children tested had been exposed to potentially harmful chemicals even before they were born. An article in *The Lancet* in November 2006 warned of the potential effects these chemicals might be having on the developing brains of our children. The authors suggested that this overwhelming exposure to chemicals might be causing a "silent pandemic" of brain disorders. If our children really are our future, we might want to invest in organics.

Organic farming produces nutrient-rich, fertile soil, which nourishes the plants and keeps chemicals such as pesticides, fungicides, and fertilizers off the land to protect soil microorganisms, water quality, and wildlife. Organic farming gives us food that is safer to eat and much more likely to keep us healthy. Research shows that organic food contains substantially higher levels of vitamins, minerals, amino acids, and phytochemicals than nonorganic food. For example, you would need to eat four conventionally grown carrots today to get the same amount of magnesium that you could get from one carrot in 1940.

MORE NUTRIENTS IN THE FOOD WE EAT

Stress forces plants to make protective phytochemicals (*phyto* = plant). When plants are subjected to things like insect bites, weed competition, nutrient changes in the soil, temperature changes, parasite and bacterial infections, and radiation from sunlight, they are forced to produce protective compounds in order to survive.

Anthocyanins: The blue and purple pigments found in blueberries, black beans, and eggplant.

IN PLANTS: These compounds are used by plants to fight off infections and protect leaves from cold temperature and sunlight.

IN HUMANS: They have been shown to promote eye health and heart health, and decrease cancer risk.

Sulforaphane: The sulfur compounds found in broccoli, cauliflower, cabbage, and Brussels sprouts are natural pesticides.

IN PLANTS: Their sharp flavor repels insects.

IN HUMANS: These compounds turn on numerous detoxification and antioxidant genes that allow for protection against a multitude of diseases.

Carotenoids (like beta-carotene, lycopene, and lutein): Orange, yellow, and red pigments found in pumpkin, carrots, tomatoes, and apricots.

IN PLANTS: These compounds absorb and deflect UV radiation from the sun and act as antioxidants.

IN HUMANS: Carotenoids protect the eyes from light damage, assist in preventing cardiovascular disease and prostate cancer, and act as powerful antioxidants in the body.

Conventional agriculture, which uses herbicides, pesticides, and fertilizers, is designed to reduce the stress on crops. Do these crops then produce and pass on fewer protective compounds?

ORGANIC VS. CONVENTIONAL

The debate between organic and conventional agriculture comes down to the quality of the scientific research and the interpretation of the results.

In 2011, Kirsten Brandt and a scientific team at Newcastle University in Australia did an extensive review of scientific literature to determine if there are nutritional differences between organic and conventional produce. They found that organic produce indeed had 16% higher levels of all protective compounds tested except beta-carotene (which makes sense, as sun exposure does not change in either mode of growing). The review also cited higher essential amino acids in proteins and higher vitamin C levels—both major contributors to overall health.

Unlike the paper from Brandt, a Stanford University research article from 2012 neglected to look at nutrients that had significant differences and therefore came to the conclusion that there were none. This resulted in a huge media blitz informing the public that purchasing organics was not worth the extra money. Missing from the study were many of the nutrients that Brandt had found were significantly higher in organic produce.

What the Stanford paper did reaffirm is that 31% of conventional produce samples had significant levels of potentially harmful pesticides.

Organic food often costs slightly more, on average, than conventionally grown food. This is because the cost of production is often higher, the farming methods tend to be more labor-intensive, and yields may be less than their conventional counterparts. However, if we were to consider all of the unseen, indirect costs of conventional farm-

ing, we would find that industrial farming costs us more than organic farming. Factors such as high health-care expenses for conventional farmworkers; clean-up efforts for polluted waterways, rivers, and lakes; and the loss of quality topsoils would all need to be taken into account when comparing the cost of conventional to organically grown foods. If researchers are correct in finding that autism, Parkinson's disease, Alzheimer's disease, and many cancers are increasingly prevalent due to our exposure to environmental chemicals, then no price savings at the grocery store could justify purchasing chemically grown foods. For instance, recent studies have shown:

- *All* children eating conventional diets had elevated levels of two potent pesticides circulating through their blood.
- Children whose mothers lived within 500 meters of areas that used pesticides were 4.1 times more likely to develop autism.
- Elevated pesticide levels have been associated with reflex abnormalities in infants, lower development in 2-year-olds, ADHD-like behaviors in 5-year-olds, and lower IQ scores in 7-year-old children.

Life adapts. Species evolve. As we have poured billions of pounds of chemicals on the earth, insects have become resistant to them, requiring more and more toxins in order to be killed. Weeds have also adapted at an alarming rate. Over 50% of crops in the midwestern United States are now resistant to the most commonly used herbicide, Roundup. At the same time, microorganisms in the soil that are beneficial to both plants and humans are being killed off and replaced by potentially harmful counterparts. Combined with immune systems that are weakened by chemicals, plants are now more susceptible to infections, and we are having outbreaks of plant diseases across the United States and the globe. Instead

CERTIFIED ORGANIC IN THE UNITED STATES

As of October 21, 2002, all agricultural farms and products claiming to be organic must be guaranteed by a USDA-approved independent agency and must meet the following guidelines:

- ✓ Abstain from the application of prohibited materials (including synthetic fertilizers, pesticides, and sewage sludge) for 3 years prior to certification and then continually throughout their organic license.
- ✓ Prohibit the use of genetically modified organisms and irradiation.
- ✓ Employ positive soil building, conservation, manure management, and crop rotation practices.
- ✓ Provide outdoor access and pasture for livestock.
- ✓ Refrain from antibiotic and hormone use in animals.
- ✓ Sustain animals on 100% organic feed.
- ✓ Avoid contamination during the processing of organic products.
- ✓ Keep records of all operations.

Organic food products are grouped into these categories:

"100% Organic"	For a food product to be 100% organic and bear the USDA organic seal, it must be made with 100% organic ingredients. The food product also must have an ingredient list and list the certifying agency.
"Organic"	In order for a food product to be labeled as "organic" and bear the USDA organic seal, the product must be made from at least 95% organic ingredients and have an ingredient statement on the label where organic ingredients are listed as organic. Information on the certifying agency also needs to be listed.
"Made with Organic Ingredients"	To claim this statement, a food product must be made with at least 70% organic ingredients and have an ingredient statement on the label where organic ingredients are listed as organic. Information on the certifying agency also needs to be listed.
"Some Organic Ingredients"	Food products with less than 70% organic ingredients cannot bear the USDA seal nor have information about a certifying agency, or any reference to organic content.

of following the call from nature to resort to less harmful practices, even more chemicals are being applied to counteract the effects of the increase of disease. Our shortsightedness is having negative effects on this generation, and will affect many generations to follow.

FARMING WITHOUT PESTICIDES

Farming without pesticides or with integrated pesticide management works.

As an example, rice farmers in Vietnam in the late 1980s sprayed early and often when they saw the leaf folder (a bug that causes only superficial damage, which does not decrease rice yields). This premature and unnecessary spraying killed wasps, dragonflies, frogs, and spiders that eat another insect, the brown planthopper.

The brown planthopper does far more damage to the rice crops and arrives later in the growing season. Due to a lack of predators and chemical resistance, it eventually required 500 times higher doses of these toxic chemicals to kill the planthoppers. As you can imagine, this deluge of poison had numerous negative repercussions.

Seeing the need for a return to a natural balance in 2001, regional insect researchers challenged 950 Vietnamese rice farmers to reduce pesticides. They performed a study in which two plots of rice were grown side by side. One plot had conventional amounts of fertilizer and insecticide and the other used decreased amounts of fertilizer and no pesticide spray for 40 days after planting. The yield in the no-spray fields was as good or better, and the farmer's profits increased by 8 to 10%. Since then many farmers have adapted the low- or no-spray farming practices with equal success avoiding what *Science* magazine named a "tsunami of pesticides in Vietnam."

GENETICALLY MODIFIED FOOD

What Is a GMO?

Genetically modified organisms, or GMOs, are plants or animals that have been genetically engineered with DNA from bacteria, viruses, and/or other, normally incompatible plants and animals. The desired outcome is to create a new organism that exhibits a desired trait, such as a crop that can withstand the direct application of herbicide, or produce an insecticide to directly repel pests.

GMO Facts:

✓ Due to a lawsuit questioning the safety of GMOs in 1998, 44,000 internal memos from the FDA were made public. Dialogue between FDA scientists and their superiors tells an interesting story. One quote from the memos reads: "The processes of genetic engineering and traditional breeding are different, and according to the technical experts in the agency, they lead to different risks."

✓ To date, there have been *no* human safety trials to determine whether GMO consumption is safe for humans.

✓ Over 60 nations outside of the United States either label GMOs or outright ban them. Japan, New Zealand, and Ireland have evaluated the safety data and determined that the risks outweigh any benefits.

✓ The America Academy of Environmental Medicine recommends prescribing GMO-free diets to all patients.

✓ Numerous animal studies have shown an increase in pituitary, kidney, liver, and intestinal abnormalities, along with an increased risk for infertility and cancer.

✓ In Quebec, 93% of pregnant women and 80% of their unborn offspring had elevated levels of toxins from GMO corn in their blood.

- ✓ Extensive analysis of the most common GMO crops shows they do not offer increased yields, have caused an increased need for pesticides, and have inferior nutritional value.
- ✓ Currently over 90% of soy, sugar beets, and canola, and over 80% of corn, are genetically modified.
- ✓ GMO ingredients are present in over 70% of all processed foods with the average American consuming 193 pounds of GMO foods a year.

Vote with your dollars. By supporting organic agriculture, you cast your vote to support the production of safe, whole, and nutritious foods that are good for our planet and all of its inhabitants.

For detailed information and visuals showing a dramatic rise in numerous diseases and disorders since the introduction of genetically modified foods, visit www.WholeLifeNutrition.net. There, you can download a GMO-free shopping guide and phone app at the bottom of the "Where are GMOs found?" page.

THE TOP 12 FRUITS AND VEGETABLES TO BUY ORGANIC

Environmental Working Group, a nonprofit organization, created "The Shoppers Guide to Pesticides in Produce." The 2012 guide was based on the analysis of over 28,000 samples taken by the FDA and USDA, and evaluates ranking as either the 12 worst, or 15 best produce items. The following list contains the top 12 most pesticide-contaminated fruits and vegetables in America, or "The Dirty Dozen Plus," and the least contaminated product items, or the "The Clean Fifteen." For more information and to download the actual shoppers guide, please visit www.EWG.org.

DIRTY DOZEN PLUS	CLEAN FIFTEEN
1. Apples	1. Asparagus
2. Celery	2. Avocados
3. Cherry tomatoes	3. Cabbage
4. Cucumbers	4. Cantaloupe
5. Grapes	5. Sweet corn
6. Hot peppers	6. Eggplant
7. Nectarines	7. Grapefruit
8. Peaches	8. Kiwi
9. Potatoes	9. Mangos
10. Spinach	10. Mushrooms
11. Strawberries	11. Onions
12. Sweet bell peppers	12. Papayas
PLUS: Kale and collard greens*	13. Pineapples
PLUS: Summer squash*	14. Sweet peas, frozen
	15. Sweet potatoes

*Although they did not meet the standard "Dirty Dozen" criteria, summer squash, kale, and collard greens were added as plus items, as they were commonly contaminated with pesticides proven to be potent neurotoxins.

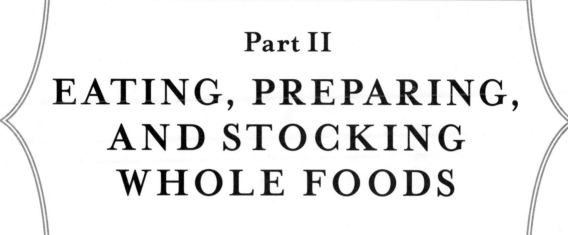

Part II

EATING, PREPARING, AND STOCKING WHOLE FOODS

6

THE BASICS OF A WHOLE FOODS DIET

The doctor of the future will give no medicine, but will instruct his patient in the care of the human frame, in diet and in the cause and prevention of disease.

—*Thomas Edison*

Eating a diet consisting largely of fresh, unrefined, whole plant foods every day is like consuming an arsenal of medicine. In an ever increasingly toxic world, our bodies can no longer afford to be exposed to processed and refined foods. They cause too much inflammation and do not provide the multitude of protective compounds found in whole organic foods. Whole foods contain all of the vitamins, minerals, antioxidants, and phytochemicals we need to prevent and reverse disease and aging.

At the same time, all people are different and some do not react well to certain foods. New research has found that a whole foods, oligoantigenic diet provides the body with all of the necessary building blocks for disease-free living and lifelong health. An oligoantigenic diet is one in which steps are taken to avoid or minimize foods that might cause a food allergy or intolerance. By eating a diet that does not irritate the immune sys-

tem at every meal, people can avoid a major contributor to disease processes. An ideal diet would consist of whole foods that are organic and locally grown.

WHAT IS A WHOLE FOOD?

Whole foods are foods that are as close to their whole or natural state as possible. If you can imagine the food growing then it is a whole food. Examples of whole foods include fresh vegetables and fruits, nuts and seeds, whole grains, dried beans, and fresh wild salmon. Whole foods have not been processed in any way that would disturb their nutrition or flavor. They are therefore free of all processing additives, such as chemical preservatives, food dyes, flavorings, solvents, and many others.

Whole foods have not had any parts removed

from them. These foods retain all of the nutrients to properly digest and metabolize themselves. For example, white rice is only part of brown rice (the nutrient-rich germ and bran parts have been removed), and cornstarch is only part of the whole corn kernel.

By choosing whole foods, you keep things out of your body that can contribute to many health problems. For example, the flavor enhancer MSG is found in many foods, including processed "health foods." It can be found in yeast extract, calcium caseinate, hydrolyzed vegetable protein, and other foods. It may be difficult to have every aspect of your diet be a whole food. Small amounts of foods that are still close to their whole form, such as extra-virgin olive oil and natural sweeteners, can be used without compromising your health.

7 Good Reasons to Eat Whole Foods

1. To Promote Intestinal Function

There are more microorganisms in the human intestinal tract than there are known stars in the universe. Certain species of bacteria help us digest our food, manufacture vitamins and amino acids, repair our intestinal cells, and even calm our immune systems. Foods such as raw cultured vegetables, raw sauerkraut, unpasteurized miso, and kombucha are sources of these beneficial bacteria. Many plant foods, such as apricots, asparagus, burdock root, Jerusalem artichokes, and onions, provide compounds that feed these bacteria, allowing them to flourish. In addition, whole plant foods, such as beans and whole grains, provide soluble fibers that regulate bowel function, bind to cholesterol and toxins, and slow the release of sugars into our bloodstream. As the prime spot for both the absorption of nutrients and elimination of wastes, taking care of your intestines is a key to optimal health.

2. To Decrease Cellular Damage

Whole foods offer potent phtyochemicals to counteract the negative effects that free radicals have on the body. Free radicals are unstable molecules that are toxic to our cells because they attack them at the molecular level, causing destruction, mutations, and cell death. Free radical damage can contribute to cancer, heart disease, arthritis, and many other diseases. Phytochemicals are naturally occurring compounds in plants. *Phyto* is the Greek word for "plant." These plant chemicals have been formed by nature and work with the body to fight disease. Phytochemicals, which give plants their color, flavor, and natural disease resistance, are very powerful in preventing and treating cancer. Diet has been found to be one of the most important lifestyle factors in the development of chronic disease and has been estimated to account for up to 80% of cancers of the large bowel, breast, and prostate. Phytochemicals work within the body to prevent cell mutation while keeping cells reproducing normally. Common phytochemicals include carotenoids, flavonoids, phytosterols, isoflavones, and phenols. Phytochemicals work synergistically with other nutrients found in foods, so supplementing with these chemicals does not produce the same effect as eating them in their whole form, in whole foods.

3. To Decrease Systemic Inflammation

Low amounts of inflammation are needed to run a healthy body. Problems arise when you take in large amounts of factory-fed animal products, refined sugar, refined vegetable oils, and refined carbohydrates. These foods promote the conversion of fats, namely arachidonic acid, into pro-inflammatory compounds. Either directly or indirectly, these foods also have the ability to trigger the gene expression of hundreds of inflammatory chemicals. This can lead to an increase in pain, swelling, and cellular damage. When you are in a state of chronic inflammation, cholesterol can collect in your arteries, causing damaging plaque to build up, fat is deposited in the abdominal region around your organs, and cancerous cells may replicate unchecked. An increase in inflammatory chemicals has been associated with most chronic diseases including arthritis, heart disease, skin disorders, diabetes, obesity, high blood pressure, osteoporosis, and various cancers. When you consume an anti-inflammatory diet, or one that comes mainly from unrefined plant foods, your body produces chemicals that cause mild, rather than excessive, inflammatory reactions, which are conducive to health.

Foods and compounds that trigger and increase inflammation:

- Refined polyunsaturated oils such as soy, canola, sunflower, safflower, and corn
- Grain-fed red meat
- Grilled and processed meats
- Refined carbohydrates and sugars
- Dairy products, especially highly processed
- Chemical additives and preservatives
- Pesticides and herbicides
- Foods to which you are allergic or sensitive

Foods that decrease inflammation:

- Ginger, turmeric, and other spices
- Green tea, nettles, and other herbs
- Omega-3 fatty acids from wild salmon, flax, walnuts, leafy greens, and purified fish oil
- Foods rich in antioxidants such as fresh fruits and vegetables, particularly the cruciferous vegetables like broccoli, cauliflower, cabbage, kale, and Brussels sprouts
- Papaya, blueberries, shiitake mushrooms, sweet potatoes, and other fresh fruits and vegetables

4. *To Support Optimum Organ Function*

Whole foods work synergistically to support the entire human body. Because whole foods have not undergone any processing, they retain all of their nutrients and fibers. These components slow the release of sugar into the bloodstream as well as optimize insulin signaling, thereby allowing for normal functioning of the pancreas. Whole foods contain all of the nutrients that are needed to support your liver. Your liver is an important organ in detoxification. Supporting your liver helps to maintain a healthy weight, keeps inflammation in check, and slows down the development of many chronic diseases. Brain function also is well supported by eating whole foods. A 2006 article from *Neurology* found that eating fresh vegetables, particularly dark leafy greens, helps to keep the brain young, improves memory, and slows the mental decline that is sometimes associated with growing old by 40%. When it comes to cardiovascular health, a diet rich in beans, whole grains, raw nuts, and plenty of fruits and vegetables has comparable benefits to many cardiovascular medications.

5. *To Assist with Hormonal Balance*

In order to produce and metabolize hormones, our bodies need the proper ingredients. Estrogen, testosterone, and even the active form of vitamin D come from cholesterol. If our liver is functioning well, we produce all the necessary cholesterol-based hormones and still have normal cholesterol levels. Did you know that our liver also breaks down and transforms hormones when we are done with them? Let's look at estrogen, for example. The liver has three choices when transforming the different forms of estrogen. It can transform estrogen into a helpful molecule, a harmful molecule, or a really harmful molecule. When we have certain foods in our diet, such as cruciferous vegetables (cabbage, broccoli, cauliflower, Brussels sprouts), flaxseeds, kudzu, green leafy vegetables, and beans, we have a tendency to transform estrogen into the beneficial form that protects our bodies. This is particularly important for women at risk with estrogen-positive cancers of the breast.

6. *To Regulate the Immune System*

Over 50% of your immune cells are located in your intestines with over 70% of the body's antibodies being produced there! By eating plants rich in fibers that feed beneficial bacteria, you ensure a calm environment for the first stage of your immune system. According to an article in the journal *Cell* in 2004, our intestines actually sense when certain bacteria are present. When an abundance of beneficial bacteria are present, we have a tendency to have mild immune reactions throughout our bodies. If the intestines are out of balance, chemicals are sent throughout the body alerting other immune cells that there is a state of alarm. These alarm chemicals can lead to collateral damage of many cells, and increase our risk for disease. Additionally, our immune cells need to be fed just like any other cell in the body. Many of us take vitamin C to boost our immunity and decrease the intensity and duration of a cold. Eating whole foods ensures a diet rich in vitamins A, C, and E, and the minerals zinc and selenium, which are all needed for optimum immune cell function.

7. *To Maintain a Healthy Weight*

Food is so much more than the calories it contains. It is a complex, life-giving substance rich in nutrients and phytochemicals that acts in our bodies to change the way our genes are expressed. Quality is the most important factor in any healthy diet and weight loss plan, not quantity. By eating a whole foods diet, you ensure that you are getting the highest-quality foods possible and all of the nutrients you need to maintain proper

functioning of vital organs and glands. Your thyroid gland, for example, can become underactive when you have a gluten sensitivity and a diet low in nutrients necessary for healthy thyroid function. Weight gain can be a sign of a dysfunctioning thyroid gland. In addition, cutting calories too severely can send your body into a state of alarm, which increases your cortisol levels, telling your body to store fat. Instead of depriving yourself to reach an ideal weight and state of health, why not nourish yourself? Depriving yourself of nutritious food and calories activates something called neuropeptide Y in your brain, which tells you to search for food. It is highest in the morning, which makes sense after a night's fast. After a nutrient-dense meal your stomach secretes a chemical called *cholecystokinin*, or *CCK*. CCK stimulates digestion, shuts down appetite, and stimulates the sensation of pleasure in part of your brain called the cerebral cortex. If you don't feel satisfied after a meal, then your body secretes neuropeptide Y to eat more food! Listen to your body's cues for hunger and honor them. Eating foods in their whole form helps to bring on that sense of satisfaction after a meal. When you eat a diet of processed and refined foods or foods that are not in their whole forms, your body, in its natural wisdom, craves the missing parts in your foods. Eating a whole foods diet full of high-quality, nutrient-dense foods will begin to reset your body's natural state of balance to gradually bring on your ideal weight and optimal state of health.

WHAT DOES A WHOLE FOODS DIET LOOK LIKE?

A whole foods diet is a balanced way of eating that promotes lifelong health. This way of eating emphasizes an abundance of fresh organic raw and cooked GREENS, fresh organic raw and cooked

VEGETABLES, fresh organic seasonal FRUIT, WHOLE GRAINS, LEGUMES, and plenty of purified WATER. Nuts and seeds, unrefined oils, natural sweeteners, and sea vegetables enhance the meals with flavor and nutrition. When animal products are included, they are sourced from humane, chemical-free organic farms.

Whatever combination of foods you choose, remember to emphasize whole, fresh, organic, local, and seasonal ingredients to the best of your ability. A whole foods diet, combined with plenty of sunshine, deep breathing, and exercise in fresh air, is your key to unlocking your unbounded health and vitality.

WHAT DO WHOLE FOODS HAVE TO OFFER?

Greens: Powerful Phytochemicals and Essential Minerals

Greens are in a category of their own because they are so vital to the daily diet. Greens provide our bodies with numerous phytochemicals, including lutein and beta-carotene, and the vitamins C, K, and E, and natural folates (as opposed to synthetic folic acid). Dark leafy greens are also a rich source of the minerals calcium and iron. The roots of green leafy plants secrete acids that dissolve rocks in the soil, freeing minerals such as calcium, magnesium, and iron. The roots then absorb these minerals into their leaf structures, which is why they are such a good source of minerals. For example, an 8-ounce serving of cooked collard greens has more calcium than an 8-ounce glass of milk.

Phytochemicals in greens support the liver in its ability to increase the production of antioxidants and excrete toxins from our bodies. This plays an important role in the prevention and treatment of heart disease, arthritis, cancers, cognitive decline, and many other ailments. Try to incorporate both raw and cooked greens into every meal.

Some common types of greens to include in your diet are kale, collard, cabbage, bok choy, Swiss chard, arugula, and many varieties of lettuce. Try adding greens to your smoothies and soups; use them as an alternative to tortillas to create healthy wraps; or use them with freshly made salad dressings to create refreshing salads.

RAW CRUCIFEROUS VEGETABLES AND THYROID HEALTH

Many nutrition "experts" are warning people not to eat raw cruciferous vegetables, such as broccoli or cabbage, because they will cause thyroid diseases. After interviewing medical experts and researching scientific articles, it looks as though many of these fears are unfounded. Thyroid issues appear to occur when a person eats over 2 pounds of raw cruciferous vegetables a day for an extended period of time *and* has an iodine insufficiency. If you eat less than a few pounds of raw cruciferous vegetables per day and have adequate iodine intake, there are no apparent causes for concern.

Vegetables: Potent Antioxidants and Vitamins

Vegetables come in so many different shapes, sizes, and colors while providing our bodies with a source for many of the essential vitamins, minerals, trace minerals, essential fatty acids, and antioxidants we need daily. Dark orange and yellow vegetables such as squash, pumpkin, yams, bell peppers, and carrots are rich in beta-carotene. Beta-carotene is fat-soluble and is converted to vitamin A in the liver. Beta-carotene is an important antioxidant that boosts the immune system, helps prevent heart disease, protects our eyes from age-related damage, and helps prevent the formation of carcinogens at the molecular level. Lycopene is another carotenoid antioxidant that gives food its reddish color; it is found in high concentrations in cooked tomato products. Lycopene plays a role in preventing prostate cancer and heart disease. In fact, much of the research available today shows that a diet high in vegetables greatly reduces the risk for many chronic diseases.

Eat a variety of raw and cooked vegetables. Balance your intake of sweet vegetables such as squash, yams, carrots, and potatoes with cleansing vegetables such as celery, cucumber, and bitter greens, with pungent vegetables such as onions and garlic. Try consuming at least 6 vegetables a day, such as 3 with lunch and 3 with dinner. Variety is key to getting your daily dose of protective phytochemicals, antioxidants, vitamins, and minerals; but for most, it will make your diet more enjoyable and sustainable over time.

Fruit: Potent Antioxidants and Vitamins

Who can resist the refreshing sweetness of peak-of-the-season organic fruit? Fresh raw fruit provides an easy and deliciously sweet way to consume a wide variety of important phytochemicals, antioxidants, and essential vitamins and minerals. Most fruits contain 80 to 95% water and adequate amounts of potassium, iron, calcium, and magnesium, and high amounts of vitamin C. Many fruits are also high in soluble fiber, which helps to lower cholesterol levels, regulate blood sugar, and improve bowel function.

Fruit is a rich source of phenols, which is a group of natural compounds that can block enzymes that cause inflammation, inhibit tumor formation, and help to prevent cell mutations, among many other things. Roughly 8,000 phenolic compounds have been identified, and many of them are flavonoids. Phenols are found in high concentrations in red grapes, apples, lemons, strawberries, blueberries, and raspberries. Fruit such as kiwi, mangos, oranges, and papayas contain the carotenoid zeaxanthin, which improves the immune response and protects the eyes against macular degeneration. All types of berries are very high in antioxidants and bioflavonoids, which work to prevent and treat many different diseases and conditions.

When shopping, choose a wide variety of organic in-season fruit. By eating fruit from all colors of the rainbow, you can be sure you're getting a wide variety of protective phytochemicals and other nutrients. Ripe, fresh fruit can be a cleansing breakfast, eaten raw as a snack, added to smoothies, or made into many fabulous desserts.

Whole Grains: Protein, Fiber, Vitamins, and Antioxidants

Whole grains have been a staple food in many cultures for thousands upon thousands of years. They are good source for fiber and a host of essential vitamins and minerals. Whole grains provide a rich source of complex carbohydrates, which are readily converted to usable energy, making them an ideal staple food.

Whole grains have not undergone processing which would remove any part of them. The bran, germ, and endosperm are all intact. Refined grains retain only the endosperm or starch—the bran and germ have been removed. The bran and germ provide fiber, which slows both the digestion of starch and release of sugar into the bloodstream. Whole grains also provide trace minerals and vitamins assisting in the digestion of the carbohydrates. Special fibers found in whole grains have the ability to bind to cholesterol, hormones, and toxins, allowing them to be excreted from our body—this is especially important in our increasingly toxic world.

Recent research from Cornell University found that whole grains contain potent disease-fighting chemicals that have equal antioxidant values to those found in fruits and vegetables. Dr. Liu, the researcher looking at these compounds in whole grains, summed it up best by saying: "Different plant foods have different phytochemicals. These substances go to different organs, tissues, and cells, where they perform different functions. What your body needs to ward off disease is this synergistic effect—this teamwork—that is produced by eating a wide variety of plant foods, including whole grains."

When whole grains are refined, say into white flour or white rice, most of the fibers, phytochemicals, vitamins, and minerals are removed in the refining process. These vital substances protect us from disease. A whole grain that has been processed is easily broken down into simple sugars and then rapidly absorbed into our bloodstream. When there is an extraordinary amount of sugar circulating in the blood, it has a tendency to stick to proteins. These altered proteins lose their normal function and may even stimulate inflammation by binding to immune cells. As stated earlier, an increase in inflammatory chemicals has been associated with many chronic diseases, including arthritis, heart disease, diabetes, high blood pressure, and osteoporosis.

Each whole grain provides a unique taste and nutrient profile, so vary the grains you cook throughout the week. Remember that some whole grains contain gluten, which is a protein that many people are sensitive to. Grains and flours containing gluten include whole wheat berries, spelt berries, rye berries, kamut, barley, and triticale. Oats may contain gluten if processed in the same facility as gluten-containing grains. Gluten-free grains include brown rice, wild rice, quinoa, amaranth, buckwheat, corn, and teff. For information on how to cook whole grains please see pages 262–264.

For increased digestibility of whole grains, soak the grains overnight in water with a little bit of apple cider vinegar, then drain and cook. When using flours, look for ones that are organic and certified gluten-free, preferably sprouted flours.

Legumes: Protein, Fiber, and Vitamins

Legumes, in addition to whole grains, have been a staple food in many cultures for thousands of years. Bean and grains help to create some of the most exciting dishes found in ethnic cuisine.

Beans are packed with an amazing amount of beneficial amino acids. They are also a good source of B vitamins, potassium, magnesium, and fibers. In fact, they are one of nature's best sources of fibers, which not only promote digestive health and relieve constipation, but also help to feed beneficial bacteria in the gut that contribute to health. These fibers also slow the absorption of glucose into the bloodstream, allowing for a slow rise in blood sugar after eating, which is why eating a diet rich in beans has been shown to help in the prevention and treatment of diabetes.

Beans work to lower blood pressure, as they are high in both magnesium and the amino acid L-arginine, which are potent regulators of smooth muscle relaxation in blood vessels. When the vessels can remain relaxed, blood pressure stays low.

A study in the *European Journal of Epidemiology* in 1999 examined food intake patterns and risk of death from coronary heart disease. Researchers followed more than 16,000 middle-aged men in the United States, Finland, the Netherlands, Italy, former Yugoslavia, Greece, and Japan for 25 years. Typical food patterns were: higher consumption of dairy products in Northern Europe; higher consumption of meat in the United States; higher consumption of vegetables, legumes, fish, and wine in Southern Europe; and higher consumption of cereals, soy products, and fish in Japan. When researchers analyzed this data, they found that beans were associated with a whopping 82% reduction in risk of death from coronary heart disease.

Choose a variety of legumes and include them in your daily diet. Beans can be made into dips, sandwich spreads, grain and bean salads, soups, stews, and more. See pages 180–183 for how to cook beans.

By consuming properly soaked and cooked beans and gluten-free grains, you increase your chances for reaching vibrant health.

Nuts and Seeds: Essential Fats, Minerals, and Protein

Nuts and seeds are the embryos from which future plants are propagated. Nuts are the edible kernels in hard shells from trees and bushes. Seeds are edible ripened plant ovules containing an embryo. Nuts and seeds are high in protein, calcium, zinc, copper, iron, selenium, folic acid, magnesium, potassium, phosphorus, vitamins E and B2, essential fatty acids, and fiber. Brazil nuts are one of the richest sources of the mineral selenium. Selenium boosts your ability to neutralize free radicals and is needed for proper thyroid function.

The essential fats in nuts and seeds are needed for proper cell function and brain development. Scientific research has shown that a daily portion of just 1 ounce of nuts rich in monounsaturated fat can reduce the risk of heart disease by up to 10%. The nuts highest in monounsaturated fat are almonds, Brazil nuts, hazelnuts, macadamia nuts, pecans, pistachios, and walnuts.

Raw nuts and seeds can be eaten as a quick snack or used to add flavor, texture, and beneficial fats to a wide variety of sweet and savory dishes. Raw nuts and seeds can be soaked, toasted, or lightly roasted with flavorings such as tamari and spices. Choose a variety of fresh raw nuts and seeds, and try to use organic whenever possible.

Sea Vegetables: Essential Minerals and Trace Minerals

The ocean contains a host of incredible plants, called sea vegetables, or seaweed. Seaweeds have been a staple in many parts of Asia for thousands of years. Sea vegetables offer us the broadest range of minerals of any food, containing all of the minerals from the ocean, which are exactly the 56 essential minerals and trace minerals that are necessary for the human body. Sea vegetables are a rich source of iodine, folic acid, and magnesium, and a good source of iron, calcium, and the B vitamins riboflavin and pantothenic acid. In addition, seaweeds contain good amounts of lignans—plant compounds with cancer-protective properties.

Use sea vegetables to add flavor, depth, and minerals to your recipes. Common sea vegetables include wakame, kombu, hijiki, arame, nori, and dulse.

Unrefined Oils: Essential Fats

In a whole foods diet, the use of certain fats and oils helps us to feel satisfied and full, thus eliminating the need to overeat and fill up on less healthful foods. Fat is needed by our cell membranes to maintain integrity and to assist in cell communication. The use of healthy fats also provides our brains with the necessary nutrients for proper cognitive function. Avoid using safflower, sunflower, soy, canola, and corn oils because they are more refined and higher in polyunsaturated fats that can feed into inflammatory pathways in the body.

The oils that we recommend using daily are organic virgin coconut oil and organic extra-virgin olive oil. Virgin coconut oil contains the medium-chain triglyceride, lauric acid. Interestingly, lauric acid is the main fat found in human milk. This fat helps to destroy unwanted pathogens in the digestive tract, while promoting the growth of friendly flora. Lauric acid is readily burned for energy rather than being stored as fat in the body. Virgin coconut oil is also a rich source of disease-preventing polyphenols. This fat remains relatively stable at higher temperatures and can be used for most of your cooking needs. Extra-virgin olive oil is high in monounsaturated fats and natural antioxidants; it can be used to make salad dressings, used for sautéing at lower temperatures, and is delicious drizzled over steamed or raw vegetables.

Natural Sweeteners: Flavor and Minerals

Natural sweeteners have undergone minimal processing. Unlike refined sweeteners, they retain much of the minerals and vitamins needed to properly metabolize the sugars they contain. Try using natural sweeteners in small amounts in your cooking to enhance the flavor of your dishes. Natural sweeteners also play an important role in creating nutritious desserts and snacks. Natural sweeteners include pure maple syrup, raw honey, dates, coconut sugar, stevia, and more.

Dairy Foods: Essential Fats, Protein, and Vitamins

Many Americans have been brought up on cow's milk. We were taught that calcium from milk helps to build strong bones. However, authors of a 2005 review article in *Pediatrics* state "we found no evidence to support the notion that milk is a preferred source of calcium." If decreasing or eliminating dairy foods from your diet leaves you concerned about not getting enough calcium, consider eating dark green leafy vegetables. After all, this is where the cows get their calcium.

Although dairy foods are not a necessary part of the human diet, they have been a part of our cultural and culinary history for many years. If you desire, dairy foods can be used in small amounts in your dishes to enhance the overall flavor. This is how dairy has traditionally been used in cultures throughout the world. Milk was used raw or cultured, and consumed in much smaller quantities than Westernized countries consume today. Modern processing of milk makes it difficult to digest and utilize. Commercial dairy products also contain high levels of residual pesticides and herbicides from the food that the animals consume. These chemicals, which are stored in their fatty tissues, are mobilized through the bloodstream and into the mammary glands when milk is produced. Fat from conventionally produced milk harbors more pesticide residues compared to nonorganic fruits and vegetables. Nonorganic, commercial milk also contains detectable levels of antibiotics used on the animal as well as many other environmental contaminants.

Many people consume a high amount of commercial dairy foods, which may be contributing to the current chronic disease problem we face in our Western culture. Furthermore, many people are sensitive or allergic to dairy foods and have symptoms ranging from joint pain to migraine headaches. If you do choose to eat dairy, choose cultured and/or raw products made from the milk of grass-fed cows, goats, or sheep raised on organic pastures and treated in an ethical fashion. Raw milk from grass-fed animals is higher in conjugated linoleic acid (CLA), essential fats, as well as the fat-soluble vitamins A, E, and K. Many health food stores and co-ops now sell organic raw and cultured dairy products. Check your local store for availability or find a local farm to buy directly from.

Meat, Poultry, Fish, and Eggs: Protein and Essential Fats

Organically raised animal products can be a very healthy part of a whole foods diet when consumed alongside a large serving of fresh vegetables. Wild game, as well as organic grass-fed meat and poultry are excellent choices when it comes to consuming meat. Wild game contains much less saturated fat than domesticated beef, and both wild game and organic grass-fed meats contain higher amounts of omega-3 fatty acids and conjugated linoleic acid (CLA). Omega-3 fatty acids and CLA assist your body in regulating weight and cholesterol. Meat and poultry are excellent sources of protein, vitamin B12, zinc, and selenium. There are many organic farms raising animals in an ethical and healthful fashion. Find a local farm that raises grass-fed beef and organic free-range chickens and buy from them. Your local co-op or health food store may also be a good place to look.

Avoid consuming grain-fed red meat because it can increase your risk for heart disease and cancer. Most meat, poultry, and fish can contain a significant amount of residual agricultural chemicals that are stored in the fatty tissues of the animal. Additionally, cured meats such as hot dogs, ham, bacon, sausages, and jerky contain sodium nitrates and/or nitrites that when eaten, react in the stomach with amino acids to form highly carcinogenic compounds called nitrosamines. These compounds pose a significant cancer risk to humans, especially children, and should be avoided at all times.

Heavy metals, such as mercury, and PCBs are among some of the chemicals that can be found in significant levels in many fish. PCBs, or poly-chlorinated biphenyls, are neurotoxic, hormone-disrupting chemicals that have been banned in the United States since 1977. Avoid farmed salmon as it is likely the most PCB-contaminated protein source in the U.S. food supply. According to a study published in *Science* in January 2004, these chemicals were found at levels seven times higher in farmed salmon than in wild ones. Also, avoid consuming tuna, swordfish, shark, king mackerel, and tilefish, as these fish also contain high levels of pollutants. For more information visit www.Got Mercury.org.

When buying fish, choose fish from a sustainable fishery in Alaska. Wild fish from Alaska are less polluted than fish from other parts of the world. Wild salmon is an ideal choice. It is an excellent source of DHA and EPA, two fatty acids that lead into anti-inflammatory pathways in the body. These healthy fats are cardio-protective as well as promote proper brain development in infants and children. A 2005 article from *Archives of Neurology* found that consuming DHA-rich fish at least once a week was associated with a 10% per year slower rate of cognitive decline in elderly people. Your local co-op or health food store is a good place to shop for fish. You can also call your local fish market and ask them where their fish comes from.

When buying eggs, choose eggs produced from a local certified organic company where the chickens have plenty of access to outdoor pasture. Chickens raised in their natural habitat and left to peck at wild grasses, mosses, and bugs will produce rich, nutritious eggs—very different from commercial factory-farmed eggs. Your local egg company may also add flaxseeds to the chickens' diet. This makes the eggs a rich source for DHA, an important fat needed for many things in the body, including proper cognitive development in developing fetuses, babies, and children.

When you eat animal foods, first and foremost

choose organic. Wild Alaskan fish, grass-fed meats and poultry, and local fresh eggs are excellent choices.

Water: Detoxification, Lubrication, and Assimilation

Drinking plenty of pure water throughout the day instead of soft drinks, juice drinks, and coffee will improve your health substantially. Every cell in your body needs water to survive. Water is used in the body to flush out waste and toxins, lubricate tissues and joints, and help assimilate the food we eat.

Pure water is increasingly difficult to find. Most of our water supply is full of potentially toxic and dangerous chemicals. Not only are chlorine and fluoride routinely added, but a wide range of toxic and organic chemicals can be found in our drinking water. These are largely agricultural and industrial wastes including PCBs, pesticide residues, nitrates, and the heavy metals lead, mercury, arsenic, and cadmium.

Our bodies need about 64 ounces of pure water each day. That's about 8 glasses. But what constitutes pure? Tap water contains chlorine, which increases free radical damage in the body, contributes to certain forms of cancer, and increases the risk for hypertension. Chlorine also contributes to magnesium deficiency while increasing urinary excretion of calcium and phosphorus, thus increasing the risk of osteoporosis. Mineral-rich, rural well water would be an ideal option if the risk for agricultural chemical contamination wasn't so high. Well water is so rich in minerals, especially magnesium and calcium, that drinking it is like taking a mineral supplement every day.

Is there a middle ground? Yes, installing an under-the-sink water filtration system would be ideal. Most systems use a solid carbon block filter, which effectively removes chlorine, bacteria, pesticides, and other organic chemicals, yet maintains dissolved minerals such as calcium and magnesium. To avoid pharmaceutical residues, many people are choosing reverse osmosis (RO) filters. The ideal would be a filter with both a carbon block and an RO system. Filling up reusable water jugs at your local co-op or health food store is a great option if you cannot invest in a home filtration system. These filters are typically the reverse osmosis type, which remove almost all contaminants and dissolved minerals.

It is important to make purified water consumption a regular daily habit. Make sure to use purified water for all of your cooking needs, including the soaking of beans and nuts, the cooking of grains, and the steaming of vegetables.

Sunshine, Fresh Air, Exercise: Bone Mineralization and Happiness

The sun is the source for all life on this planet; it connects us to our food, the earth, and life itself. Sunlight gives us vitamin D, a chemical that is actually produced in our bodies when we expose cholesterol in our skin to the sun. Upon exposure to sunlight, a substance within our skin is changed into pre-vitamin D. Our liver and kidneys convert this pre-vitamin D to its active hormone form. The hormone vitamin D binds to portions of our cells, called receptors, which allows for normal gene expression and cellular function. Research shows that vitamin D plays a role in thyroid function, prostate and breast cancer, cardiovascular disease, autoimmune diseases, arthritis, irritable bowel disease, as well as osteoporosis. In addition to maintaining normal blood calcium and phosphorus levels, active vitamin D also calms inflammation, which allows for these minerals to stay in the bones. At latitudes above the 35th parallel (Oklahoma City, OK; Raleigh, NC; and Bakersfield, CA) from about October through April, the sun's rays are at angles that are insufficient to produce significant vitamin D synthesis in our bodies. Also, in the summertime, sunscreens with a sun protection factor of 8 or greater will block UV rays that produce vitamin D. Natural food sources of vitamin D include cod liver oil, wild salmon, lard, and egg yolk, though supplementation is usually needed in the winter months.

Breathing fresh air during deep breathing or exercising relaxes our bodies and clears our minds. Breathing in deeply, we take in life—oxygen—which energizes our cells and increases our metabolism. Oxygen is needed at the cellular level to properly metabolize the energy from our food. Exercise increases your heart rate and breathing, thereby increasing your blood flow to bring needed nutrients to every cell in your body. Exercise builds muscle mass, which is needed to maintain an optimum metabolism and healthy weight. In addition, daily exercise, in combination with sun exposure or vitamin D supplementation, increases bone mineralization, thus significantly decreasing the risk for osteoporosis later in life. Daily exercise and fresh air provide a deep sense of relaxation, and in this state, you will be able to reconnect with your body more easily.

7

MAKING THE CHANGE

Peace begins with each of us taking care of our bodies and minds every day.
—Thich Nhat Hanh

Cooking real, wholesome meals for yourself and your family every day is not as difficult as it may seem. It's easy to get comfortable in our habits—buying convenience foods, stopping on the way home from work and eating out, or simply not using healthy ingredients in your own cooking. Unhealthy, disease-promoting foods leave us with a lack of energy and a sluggish feeling, so at first it can sometimes seem overwhelming to even have the energy to begin shopping for and cooking whole foods.

The food industry literally adds tons and tons of addictive food chemicals to processed foods to make sure you will keep buying their products. We understand that it can be hard to give them up. But trust us, once you start eating differently you will start feeling better and you won't want to go back to old habits. These good feelings, high energy, and clear thinking will inspire you to stick with a clean, whole foods diet.

Remember to respect yourself for where you are right now in your dietary habits. Lasting change takes time; it doesn't happen overnight. Think of eating and cooking whole foods as a daily practice—like yoga or tai chi. Every day you learn a little more and get better, and then before you know it you are doing an advanced yoga pose or cooking three wholesome meals a day! With any type of lifestyle change, but especially diet, there is this moving forward and then reverting back. Like eating a fast-food meal after you've been eating clean for a week, or eating a sandwich made with wheat bread after you've been gluten-free for a month. This push-pull type of change is perfectly normal and healthy. In fact, it can be your greatest teacher! You can take note of how you feel after these detours. Eventually there is a tipping point and there is no going back. You will only crave the foods that are good for you.

Living and eating a whole foods diet will not feel limited or strict. The needs of our bodies, our tastes, and our health are ever changing. We encourage you to listen to your body's own wisdom when choosing foods for your daily meals. Select foods that give you the most energy, the clearest thinking, the best digestion, the preferred flavors of the moment, and the most overall satisfaction. Your gut, or digestive tract, is lined with many nerves, almost as if your digestive system has its own brain! The foods you eat relay messages to your brain through your nervous system. Pay attention to the messages it sends you. Listen to the subtleties of desire for certain foods and flavors. Do you not want breakfast this morning? That's okay! Maybe you simply need to drink a quart of filtered water. Do you crave raw foods? Maybe you only want a salad for dinner. Feeling the desire for red meat? Eat a hamburger! When in balance, your body knows what it needs! If you are really craving meat, choose the cleanest forms possible and prepare it yourself, such as grass-fed and organic. If you are craving cooling, green foods, make yourself a green smoothie or large salad from organic, local produce. Realize that we don't need to eat what society tells us—we don't need meat every day, or 6 to 11 servings of whole grains a day, or a glass of milk with every meal!

Sometimes our bodies are so out of balance that we cannot remember how to eat or what foods to choose that will benefit our health. This is when following a particular diet plan, such as one of the 30-day meal plans available on our website www.WholeLifeNutrition.net, or another strict diet, can be extremely beneficial. These diet plans reset the body and act as a gateway to reawakening your own intuitive guidance in choosing what to eat and when.

Moving to a whole foods diet can take time. Remember to start small; small changes actually create more lifelong change. Start by cooking one or two recipes in this book each week, and then move up to a whole meal, then maybe a few meals a week. As you become more familiar with whole foods and how to prepare them, you will naturally want to do more.

Keeping your cooking and eating environment clean and harmonious will help you find your rhythm in preparing and eating whole meals. Your outer environment, or your living space and the people you dine with, is as much a part of your health as the food you eat. Keep your kitchen clean and work to reduce your stress. If preparing an entire meal seems stressful to you then don't do it. Begin with something very simple, maybe just a pot of cooked whole grains or a large garden salad. The more you sit down, relax, and enjoy your meals, especially if you are dining with family and friends, the more fulfilled you will feel by them. Food is pleasure; enjoy it to the fullest!

Clear your kitchen and pantry of old and unhealthy foods so it will be easy to follow the messages of your gut wisdom. Enjoy the entire process of meal preparation, including shopping, preparing, eating, and cleaning up afterward. Every meal is a celebration of life, the seasons, and rhythms of nature. Enjoy being alive and having the opportunity to eat!

Tips for making the change:

- Create a menu plan—start with 3 days on your menu, then try 5 days the following week. Include recipes and ideas for breakfast, lunch, dinner, and snacks.
- Make a grocery list every time you go to the store. It can be overwhelming to walk into a store and decide what foods to buy. After you have made a meal plan, write down all the ingredients you will need for those meals. Include in your shopping list any staple foods you might need.
- Keep your pantry, freezer, and refrigerator stocked with whole food ingredients. Having what you need in your house to create healthful meals will reduce or eliminate eating out and the consumption of unhealthy processed foods.
- Plan ahead for the following days—if you have leftovers from dinner, then pack them in a to-go container for the next day's lunch.

- Sunday morning breakfast leftovers can be used for quick breakfasts on Monday and Tuesday mornings.
- Utilize portions of the previous night's dinner for the next night's meal.
- Cook a few different pots of beans on the weekend to use throughout the week; portions of cooked beans can also easily be frozen for later use.
- Roast a whole, organic chicken so you can use it to make chicken salads, soup stock, and casseroles over the following days.
- Freeze portions of soups, stews, and casseroles into small reusable containers. Many of the recipes in this book make large batches—it is much easier to cook a larger batch of a recipe than to cook multiple recipes every day. Once you begin cooking and freezing, your freezer will soon be stocked with healthy homemade ready-to-go meals.
- Utilize the deli at your local co-op or health food store to buy wholesome prepared bean and grain dishes, vegetable dishes, or fresh soups and salads.
- Get together with others making dietary transitions or with friends who have already done so. It will be fun to share recipes and meal ideas.
- Take a guided tour of your local co-op or health food store to familiarize yourself with many of the ingredients used in this book.
- Take a cooking class at your local co-op or health food store. You can learn to prepare, cook, and ultimately taste unfamiliar foods you are curious about.
- Let your creativity flow and try developing your own tantalizing combinations of beans, whole grains, meats, and vegetables.

STOCKING YOUR WHOLE FOODS KITCHEN

Whenever you are sincerely pleased, you are nourished. The joy of the spirit indicates its strength. All healthy things are sweet-tempered.

—*Ralph Waldo Emerson*

Having a well-stocked whole foods kitchen is key to cooking daily fresh meals for you and your family. I walk into my kitchen and it's like a palette of ingredients to choose from—making cooking at home every day doable. Without a stocked pantry you might be more likely to go out to eat, which generally results in higher food bills and a lowered state of health.

It will be helpful for you to have some of the following items on hand to make the recipes in this book. Using fresh ingredients will enhance your recipes and benefit your health. You might find it beneficial to purge your house of unhealthy, processed foods. Go through your cabinets, pantry, refrigerator, and freezer and discard any old or unhealthy items you may have hiding in your kitchen, including old spices, processed oils, condiments, breakfast cereals, processed junk foods, and ready-made freezer meals. Use the following list to restock your kitchen with fresh, healthful ingredients for your meals. Begin by

adding a few items that you think you will use most often and then gradually add more as your cooking repertoire builds. Once your pantry is well stocked with whole foods it will be easier to prepare nutritious meals and snacks for yourself and your family.

UNREFINED OILS

It is important to discard any old, processed oils and replace them with a few healthful fats and oils. Fats and oils easily become rancid if stored for long periods. For example, sesame oil begins to go rancid after about 8 months, whereas extra-virgin olive oil can become rancid about 2 years after the production date. It's best to use up unrefined oils within 6 months of purchasing them. Only a few oils are needed on hand to use for all of your cooking needs. Store the following oils in a dark place, away from heat or light, which protects them from oxidative damage.

Organic Extra-Virgin Olive Oil

Extra-virgin olive oil, which is high in heart-healthy monounsaturated fats and natural antioxidants, is made from the first cold-pressing of ripe olives. When purchasing olive oil, look for unfiltered olive oil as it retains more nutrients than its filtered counterpart. Extra-virgin olive oil is good for light sautéing and works very well in salad dressings, dips, and spreads. Sometimes I prefer the flavor of olive oil to coconut oil for roasting, and therefore I use it occasionally at a higher temperature.

Organic Unrefined Virgin Coconut Oil

Lauric acid is the main fat found in coconut oil, which helps to keep our digestive systems healthy. Virgin coconut oil can be used for most of your cooking needs, from baking to sautéing, since it remains relatively stable at higher temperatures. In fact, over 90% of the fat in coconut oil is saturated—saturated fat is far more resistant to heat compared to polyunsaturated oils. Coconut oil adds a mild coconut flavor to your food, but it's not overpowering, making it very versatile.

Organic Palm Shortening

Palm shortening is derived from palm oil. Palm oil comes from the tropical palm tree, *elaeis guineensis*, which is native to tropical areas of Africa. Palm oil is a mixture of saturated and unsaturated fatty acids, with most of the unsaturated fat being monounsaturated fat. Palm shortening is palm oil that has some of its unsaturated fats removed, giving it a very firm texture and high melting point. Organic palm shortening is trans fat–free and a great replacement for butter in biscuits, shortbreads, scones, pie crusts, and other desserts. Two of our favorite brand-name products are Tropical Traditions and Spectrum.

Organic Toasted Sesame Oil

Sesame oil is very high in linoleic acid, one of the two essential fatty acids that our bodies cannot produce. Research has shown that diets high in sesame oil can lower cholesterol. Unrefined sesame oil contains an antioxidant called *sesamol*, which protects it from becoming rancid. Sesamol has been found to inhibit the damage caused by free radicals on our DNA. We like to use sesame oil in salad dressings, marinades, sauces, and as a garnish for stir-fries. If you use it for cooking, make sure it is for low temperature cooking, such as light sautéing.

Hot Pepper Sesame Oil

Hot pepper oil is delicious added to miso soup, sauces, or salad dressings, or used to garnish dark leafy green dishes.

VINEGARS

Vinegars and cooking wines are secret ingredients that will help your meals shine. Used as a garnish at the end of cooking time, they enhance the natural flavor and sweetness in foods, especially bitter greens. Store your vinegars in a dark place, away from heat or light.

Organic Raw Apple Cider Vinegar

Raw apple cider vinegar is highly regarded for its healing, cleansing, and energizing properties. It is made from the juice of fresh, crushed, organically grown apples and allowed to age in natural wooden barrels. Apple cider vinegar is very tangy and can be used in salad dressing or sprinkled on steamed vegetables. One tablespoon can be taken before meals to increase the digestion and absorption of food.

Organic Seasoned Brown Rice Vinegar

Brown rice vinegar is made by an alcohol fermentation of mashed brown rice. It then undergoes another fermentation to produce vinegar. To create seasoned brown rice vinegar, organic grape juice concentrate and sea salt are added. Brown rice vinegar is more acidic than other vinegars. It is delicious added to stir-fries, salad dressings, and marinades. It complements tamari very well and is widely used in Asian cooking.

Organic Red Wine Vinegar

The word "vinegar" is derived from the Old French *vin aigre*, meaning "sour wine." Red wine vinegar is produced by fermenting red wine in wooden barrels. This produces acetic acid, which gives it that distinctive vinegar taste. Red wine vinegar has a characteristic dark red color and red wine flavor. It is delicious used in salad dressings, sauces, soups, and marinades.

Organic White Wine Vinegar

White wine vinegar is a pale and moderately tangy vinegar made from a various blend of white wines. The wine is fermented, aged, and filtered to produce a vinegar with a slightly lower acidity level, making it milder than other vinegars. It is great added to dips to create a little more tang; it can also be used in salad dressings, sauces, and marinades. A dash or two of wine vinegar added at the end of cooking time to soups and stews deepens the flavors.

Organic Balsamic Vinegar

Balsamic vinegar is a thick, aromatic vinegar made from concentrated grape must. Grape must is the freshly pressed juice of the grape, which also contains pulp, skins, stems, and seeds. The must is then boiled down to a sap and aged in wooden barrels for 6 months to 12 years. Some very expensive balsamic vinegars are aged up to 25 years.

Ume Plum Vinegar

Ume plum vinegar is made from ume plums, water, sea salt, and the shiso leaf. Traditionally used in macrobiotic cooking, ume vinegar can be used in salad dressings, miso soup, dips, or sprinkled over sautéed dark leafy greens. Ume plum vinegar is very salty, and therefore can be used as a salt substitute.

Sherry Vinegar

Sherry vinegar has a deep, complex flavor and a dark reddish color. It is made from three different white grape varieties grown in the Jerez region in Spain. Most of the sherry vinegar produced comes from this region making it a popular ingredient in Spanish cooking. Sherry vinegar can be used in salads, sauces, and whole-grain dishes. Balsamic or red wine vinegar can replace sherry.

SALTS AND SALT SEASONINGS

Salt brings depth to the food it is cooked with. Conventional salt production uses chemicals, additives, and heat processing to reach the final end product we call table salt. Unrefined sea salt, on the other hand, contains an abundance of naturally occurring trace minerals. Tamari or coconut aminos are also great salt seasonings that work well as a replacement for traditional soy sauce.

Unrefined Sea Salt

We like to use Redmond Real Salt (www.RealSalt.com) for our sea salt needs, which can be found at your local co-op or health food store. This sea salt comes from a dried ancient seabed that has never been exposed to modern-day pollution, making it one of the purest sea salts available. Real Salt contains over fifty minerals and trace minerals, including calcium, potassium, magnesium, manganese, zinc, and iodine.

Herbamare

Herbamare, which is a flavorful sea salt and herb blend, works great to make flavorful soups and stews. Herbamare is made by steeping fresh organic herbs and vegetables in sea salt for several months before being vacuum-dehydrated.

Coconut Aminos

Coconut aminos are the perfect replacement for soy sauce or tamari for the soy-sensitive individual. Made from fermented raw coconut sap and mineral-rich sea salt, coconut aminos contain 17 amino acids! Use this dark brown sauce anywhere you would use soy sauce—as a dip for sushi, or in stir-fries, salad dressings, and marinades. I find that coconut aminos are not as salty as tamari or soy sauce, so I tend to add an extra pinch of sea salt when I use it in recipes.

Wheat-Free Tamari

Tamari is a natural, aged soy sauce made from soybeans, water, sea salt, and sometimes wheat. If avoiding gluten, look for organic wheat-free tamari. Shoyu is very similar to tamari, except that it contains wheat. Nama Shoyu, which often contains wheat, is a raw, cultured soy sauce rich in enzymes and beneficial bacteria.

Miso

Miso is a sweet, fermented soybean paste usually made with some sort of grain. It comes unpasteurized and in several varieties from robust red to sweet white. It can be made into a soup or a sauce or used as a salt substitute. If you are gluten-sensitive, then be sure to look for miso that says "gluten-free" on the label. This is because miso made with brown rice can have gluten in the koji, which can contain either barley or wheat. Look for a miso that uses rice koji instead. The South River Miso Company produces a gluten-free miso. Check your local health food store or co-op for availability or visit www.SouthRiver Miso.com.

CONDIMENTS

Having a few different healthful, organic condiments available is useful in completing a recipe or rounding out a meal.

Organic Ketchup

Conventional ketchup usually contains highly refined high-fructose corn syrup, which contains mercury and often comes from GMO corn. Look for ketchup that is 100% organic or make your own. See page 343 for our homemade ketchup recipe.

Organic Dijon Mustard

I like to keep a jar of organic Dijon mustard on hand to help create delicious sauces and to use in our salad dressings because it works to emulsify— or to mix together—the oil and vinegar.

Organic Raw Cultured Vegetables and Raw Sauerkraut

Raw cultured vegetables and raw sauerkraut, which provide an abundance of health-promoting friendly bacteria and enzymes to assist with digestion and absorption, are found in the refrigerated section of your local co-op or health food store. Simply place a spoonful or two on your plate along with the rest of your meal. Please refer to "Get Cultured!" (chapter 11) for simple homemade cultured vegetable recipes.

Wasabi

Wasabi is a Japanese horseradish. Wasabi is dried into a pale green powder that, when mixed with water, makes a potent, fiery paste that is typically served with sushi and sashimi. Buy your wasabi as a dry powder and use as needed. Be sure to look for one that does not contain food dyes or extra unnecessary ingredients. Buy pure wasabi powder from your local health food store. Store it in a tightly covered glass jar away from heat or light.

NATURAL SWEETENERS

Natural sweeteners are closer to their whole form than refined sugar and sweeteners. Refined sugar, such as white sugar and brown sugar, has most or all of its natural vitamins and minerals removed during the refining process. These vitamins and minerals are the very nutrients that help to metabolize the sugar you consume, therefore preventing the "sugar blues." Use the following natural sweeteners in place of refined sugar not only for creating delicious wholesome desserts but also to make salad dressing, sauces, and more.

Coconut Nectar

Coconut nectar is the sap from the coconut palm tree. It is very thick and rich with a low glycemic index of about 35, meaning it won't spike blood sugar as quickly as other sweeteners. It contains very little glucose and fructose, a small percentage of sucrose, and a high percentage of fructooligosaccharides (FOS). These indigestible sugars, or prebiotics, feed beneficial bacteria in the gut! Use coconut nectar anywhere a liquid sweetener is called for.

Honey

Honey is a sweet substance made from plant nectar and acid secretions by the honeybee. About 40% of the sugar in honey is fructose. The source of the nectar determines the color, flavor, and texture of honey. Alfalfa and clover honey are the most common types, though other types can be found also. Honey is sold in liquid or crystallized form, and is available raw or pasteurized. Commercial honey is heated to 150 to 160°F to prevent crystallization and yeast formation. Organic or raw honey has not been heat-treated. Honey is sweeter than other liquid sweeteners but can be substituted cup for cup for any of them.

Maple Syrup

Maple syrup is made from the boiled sap of sugar maple trees. Forty gallons of sap is needed to make 1 gallon of syrup. Maple syrup comes in two grades, A and B. Grade A is lighter and more translucent, generally coming from trees tapped early in the season. Grade B is darker and richer, coming from trees tapped later in the season. Maple syrup contains manganese, zinc, calcium, and potassium. We prefer to use Grade B maple syrup because of its rich flavor.

Sorghum Syrup

Sorghum syrup is a thick, dark syrup similar in flavor to molasses. It comes from the sweet sorghum plant, a grain related to millet that is similar in appearance to corn. The juice is extracted from the plant and then boiled down to a syrup.

Blackstrap Molasses

Molasses is a dark, thick syrup made as a by-product of making refined sugar. It contains all of the minerals from the cane juice in a concentrated syrup. Rich in iron and other minerals, molasses has a strong, deep flavor and can be added to breads and muffins or drizzled on top of hot cereal. Look for "unsulphured molasses," which indicates that no sulphur was used in the extraction process.

Brown Rice Syrup

Brown rice syrup is made from brown rice that has been soaked, sprouted, and cooked with an enzyme that breaks the starches into maltose.

Brown rice syrup has a light, mild flavor and a similar appearance to honey, though less sweet. Rice syrup can be substituted 1 for 1 for honey or maple syrup. Lundberg Brown Rice Syrup is gluten-free.

Frozen Fruit Juice Concentrate

Frozen fruit juice concentrate can be used to sweeten fruit pies, crisps, or other desserts. Simply thaw and use. I prefer organic apple juice concentrate because of its mild flavor and neutral color.

Coconut Sugar

Coconut sugar is basically dried and granulated coconut nectar and comes with the same low-glycemic properties. It is light brown in color and the flavor is rich and caramel-like. Use it anywhere a granulated sugar is called for. This is our preferred granulated sweetener; I buy it in 5-pound bags online.

Whole Cane Sugar

Whole cane sugar, also called dried cane juice, is made from the dried juice of the sugar cane plant. Many of the minerals from the plant are still present, which helps you digest the sugars. Dried cane juice resembles brown sugar in appearance and taste, though it is less sweet. It can be substituted for white sugar cup for cup in baked goods. Trade names for this type of sugar are Rapadura and Sucanat.

Date Sugar*

Date sugar is made from ground, dehydrated dates. It has a similar taste and appearance to brown sugar, but the taste is slightly less sweet. It can be substituted cup for cup in baked goods.

*Although dates themselves are gluten-free, oat flour is often added when processing date sugar, making this type of sweetener unsuitable for the gluten-sensitive individual.

Medjool Dates

Dates can be used in combination with other dried fruits and nuts to make nutritious raw desserts or snacks. We like to use the Medjool date, which has a nice moisture content and a very sweet, delicate flavor.

Stevia

Stevia is derived from the leaves of a South American shrub, *Stevia rebaudiana*. Stevia is about 300 times sweeter than cane sugar, or sucrose. Stevia is not absorbed through the digestive tract, and therefore has no calories. Stevia does not affect blood sugar levels and is therefore acceptable for people with diabetes or hyperglycemia. Stevia can be found in either the natural sweetener or dietary supplement section of your local co-op or health food store. It comes in several forms: dried leaf, liquid extract, or a powdered extract.

BASIC HERBS AND SPICES

Herbs and spices are the musical notes that form the orchestra of your meal—essential components to a flavorful and delicious meal. Spices enhance the natural sweetness of foods. Herbs provide color and a diverse array of flavors to foods. If your recipes have not been turning out well, it could be that your spices and herbs are too old and flavorless. Throw away (or compost) the out-of-date ones and begin to stock your kitchen with smaller amounts of fresh spices and herbs. In the following paragraphs, you will find the herbs and spices that appear most frequently in this book.

An herb is the leaf, root, stem, or flower of a plant that usually grows in a temperate climate. Fresh herbs have more flavor and more nutritional value than dried herbs. Use 1 teaspoon of dried herb for 1 tablespoon of fresh herb in a recipe. A spice is the whole or ground bud, fruit, flower, seed, or bark of a plant that usually grows in a tropical climate. Always use your dried herbs and ground spices within 6 months; otherwise, they will lose their color and flavor and become bitter. Whole spices such as cloves, nutmeg, and cinnamon sticks maintain quality for 2 to 3 years if stored properly. Spices and dried herbs should be stored in a glass jar with an airtight lid. Keep the jars in a closed cupboard well out of reach from direct sunlight and heat.

Your local food co-op or health food store is usually a great place to buy organic dried herbs and spices. You can utilize their bulk bins or buy spices in smaller quantities. It may also help to buy spices in their whole form, and then grind them as needed using a mortar and pestle or coffee grinder.

Dried Thyme

Thyme is one of my all time favorite herbs. It is a member of the mint family and its use dates back to at least 3500 BC. Thyme has a strong, aromatic flavor and a bright, sharp taste. It is used in vegetable dishes, soups and stews, and meat dishes. Thyme acts as a digestive aid, stimulating the production of gastric fluids.

Dried Rosemary

Rosemary is an evergreen shrub of the mint family native to the Mediterranean region. It contains the oil of camphor, which gives it that pungent flavor and wonderful aroma. Though I always prefer to use fresh rosemary in recipes, having a jar of dried rosemary stocked in your spice cabinet definitely comes in handy. When using dried rosemary, it is best to crush it with a mortar and pestle before using it in recipes. Rosemary is delicious added to bean soups, stews, or meat dishes, or sprinkled on top of vegetable dishes. The fresh flowering tops can even be added to salads.

Dried Oregano

Oregano is native to Europe and a member of the mint family. Oregano varies in flavor from mild common oregano and the more strongly flavored Greek and Spanish oregano, to the intensely flavored Mexican oregano, which is used in chili powder blends and other dishes. Oregano enhances the flavor of almost anything it is cooked with, from potato dishes and marinara sauces to savory stews and enchiladas.

Bay Leaves

The fragrant bay tree is native to the Mediterranean Basin. Bay leaves are strongly flavored if freshly dried and should be used sparingly. They offer a strong spicy flavor reminiscent of pine, nutmeg, and pepper. The whole leaves are usually added to simmering beans, meat dishes, stews, and soup stocks. The leaves should always be removed from the dish before it is served.

Italian Seasoning

Italian seasoning usually consists of a blend of dried oregano, marjoram, thyme, basil, rosemary, and sage. It is great to have on hand for making Mediterranean-style soups, stews, and sauces.

Black Peppercorns

Pepper is the small berry of a tropical vining shrub from the Malabar Coast of India. It was first cultivated around 1000 BC. It was soon carried to other parts of the world; and in medieval Europe, it was so precious that it was classed with gold, silver, and gems. Black peppercorns are berries that are picked when unripe, but full-size, and allowed to dry in the sun to develop their color and flavor. It is best to use whole black peppercorns and then grind them as needed in a handheld pepper mill. Ground black pepper loses its flavor and volatile oils quickly and turns bitter if ground too far in advance. In addition most preground black pepper is toasted, and once toasted, it acts as an irritant to the gut. Use freshly ground pepper to spice up just about any savory dish. Whole peppercorns can be added to soup stocks, pickles, and marinades.

Cumin Seed and Ground Cumin

Cumin is indigenous to the eastern Mediterranean region, especially near the upper Nile. Cumin, with its strongly aromatic, spicy, yet somewhat earthy flavor, can be toasted in a hot skillet in its whole seed form to deepen its flavor, or it can be used in its ground form. Ground cumin loses its flavor and freshness very quickly, so buy smaller amounts and replace it frequently. The whole seed can be ground with a mortar and pestle when needed. Cumin is used in curry dishes, soups, stews, and Mexican dishes such as beans, rice, and chili. Cumin acts as a natural digestive aid and carminative. It aids in the secretion of digestive juices and helps to relieve pain and cramping in the abdomen.

Ground Coriander

Coriander seeds are the seeds of the cilantro plant. Coriander is indigenous to the Mediterranean regions of Africa and Asia and is one of the most ancient herbs still in use today. Coriander was cultivated in Egyptian gardens thousands of years before the birth of Christ. Freshly ground coriander seeds have a distinctive spicy-sweet aromatic flavor. They are one of the main spices in curries, but can also be used to flavor cakes, desserts, and many types of savory dishes.

Cinnamon

Strongly aromatic and sweet tasting, cinnamon is the dried inner bark of a tropical evergreen laurel tree native to India and Sri Lanka. The flavor of cinnamon becomes stronger once it has been ground, though it quickly becomes stale in its ground state. It is best purchased in small quantities and constantly replaced. Cinnamon adds a warm flavor to many desserts, whole-grain breakfast cereals, curries, sauces, and pilafs.

Cardamom

The cardamom plant is a tropical shrub of the ginger family native to Ceylon and India. Cardamom is a warming spice that acts as a carminative and sweetens the breath. Cardamom is the world's third most expensive spice, behind saffron and vanilla, because each seedpod must be handpicked. It is such an intensely flavored spice that only a small amount is needed in cooking. It is available both in its ground form and in its whole pod form. Because it rapidly loses flavor when ground, it is best purchased in its whole form and then ground as needed. If purchasing the ground spice, be sure to only buy small amounts and then replace as needed.

Ground Ginger

The warm spiciness of ground ginger is a fantastic addition to many desserts. I like to use fresh ginger in most savory soups and stews, but occasionally if I am out of fresh ginger I will replace it with dried.

Garlic Powder

Garlic powder offers a mild garlic flavor to bean dips and other dishes. It can be used to replace fresh garlic when the taste may be too strong for some, like children, breastfeeding moms, or people who simply cannot tolerate a lot of garlic.

Turmeric

Turmeric is an East Indian tropical plant of the ginger family. The bright orange-yellow rhizome is peeled, dried, and ground into a fine powder. Occasionally you may be able to find fresh turmeric at your local market or health food store. The fresh rhizome can be peeled and finely diced and then added to curry dishes. Turmeric powder is one of the main ingredients in curry powder and is what lends curry dishes their bright yellow color. Turmeric is one of the best anti-inflammatory and anticarcinogenic spices.

Cayenne Pepper

A high-quality, fresh cayenne pepper should be used sparingly as its flavor is very intense. It can be used to enliven flavors of almost any dish, but it is most commonly used in soups and stews. Cayenne pepper is a natural stimulant, producing warmth and improving circulation. It aids in digestion and provides a cleansing effect on the bowels.

Chili Powder

Chili powder is a blend of cayenne pepper, cumin, oregano, paprika, garlic powder, and sometimes salt. Chili powder is used in chili and other spicy soups and stews.

Chipotle Chile Powder

Chipotle chile powder is made by first roasting jalapeño peppers, then drying them and grinding them to a powder. Chipotle chile powder imparts a smoky flavor to any dish it is added to.

Curry Powder

Curry powder is a combination of many different spices, from as few as five to as many as fifty different ingredients. The base of most curry powders includes ground red chile peppers, turmeric, and coriander. Other ingredients may be added such as cumin, allspice, caraway, cardamom, cinnamon, cloves, fenugreek, ginger, white or black pepper, saffron, and many others. Curry powder has been shown to increase metabolism, help with breathing difficulties, and reduce cholesterol.

Garam Masala

Garam masala is a sweetly pungent blend of spices common in Indian cuisine. It is usually a mix of cinnamon, cumin, cloves, nutmeg, black pepper, and cardamom, and sometimes coriander and fennel.

Mexican Seasoning

Mexican seasoning is usually a blend of ground chile peppers, dehydrated garlic, dehydrated onion, paprika, cumin, celery seed, oregano, cayenne pepper, and bay leaf. It is a great blend to have on hand for making casseroles and bean dishes, or to simply sprinkle over sautéed vegetables.

RAW NUTS AND SEEDS

Raw nuts can be used as a base to create nutritious desserts or used to accent other dishes, like salads and grain dishes. Raw seeds work well sprinkled over salads and vegetable dishes, and also made into raw pâtes. Both raw nuts and seeds can be used to make a variety of dairy-free milks. Flaxseeds and chia seeds can be used as an egg replacement in baked goods. Store raw, shelled nuts and seeds in either the refrigerator or freezer to prevent them from becoming rancid.

Cashews

Cashews are an excellent source of copper, which is needed for antioxidants and tissue-forming enzymes in the body. Cashews are also high in the heart-healthy monounsaturated fat, oleic acid. Cashews can be blended into a sweet cream and used to top desserts or used as a replacement for dairy in cream soups and ice cream. They can also be lightly roasted in the oven with a little sea salt and used to top curries or stir-fries.

Almonds

Almonds are the seed of a stone fruit, similar to an apricot. Almonds are high in manganese and vitamin E, two nutrients utilized for antioxidant functions in the body. Numerous research studies have shown that eating almonds lowers cholesterol, increases antioxidant levels in the body, assists with weight loss, and regulates blood sugar. Almonds are delicious consumed as a quick snack. They can also be soaked overnight and added to smoothies, or can be ground into a flour to increase nutrients and flavor in baked goods. Look for a source of truly raw organic almonds or sprouted almonds. All raw almonds sold in the United States have been either steam pasteurized or chemically pasteurized unless you purchase them directly from the farm that grew them.

Walnuts

Walnuts are an excellent source of antioxidants and omega-3 fatty acids; in fact, a ¼-cup serving provides over 90% of your daily need for these essential fats. Lightly roasted walnuts are a delicious addition to salads or a topping to whole-grain breakfast cereals. They can also be eaten raw as a snack in combination with organic dried fruit. You can also soak raw walnuts overnight to create creamy salad dressings, pâtes, and raw desserts.

Hazelnuts

Widely grown in the Pacific Northwest, where they are also called filberts, hazelnuts add a delicious nutty flavor to salads, main courses, and desserts; we even like to add them to our whole-grain cereals in the morning. Hazelnuts are high in heart-healthy monounsaturated fats, vitamin E, B vitamins, and a host of phytochemicals that benefit the immune system. Hazelnuts are also high in arginine, an amino acid that relaxes blood vessels, and folic acid. In fact, hazelnuts have the highest concentration of folic acid among all the tree nuts.

Pecans

Pecans are an excellent source of both the gamma- and alpha-tocopherol forms of vitamin E.

Pecans are also an excellent source of plant-based zinc. Zinc is usually found in higher concentrations in animal foods. Pecans are rich in antioxidants, calcium, magnesium, phosphorus, potassium, and B vitamins, including natural folates. Pecans can be used in whole-grain dishes and salads, and to make many decadent raw desserts.

Brazil Nuts

Brazil nuts originated in Brazil and grow wild in the Amazon rainforest of South America. Brazil nuts are an excellent source of selenium; in fact, 6 to 8 nuts provide a whopping 840 micrograms! Brazil nuts are also a good source of magnesium and thiamin. Brazil nuts make a great snack and can be used to top whole-grain breakfast cereals or replace other nuts in raw dessert recipes.

Pine Nuts

Pine nuts are the edible seeds of the pine tree. They are found on the pinecone where they are covered by a hard shell. Most of the pine nuts available today come from Southern Europe, particularly from the Stone Pine, which has been cultivated for over 6,000 years. Pine nuts in the United States, from the Colorado piñon tree, have been harvested by Native Americans for over 10,000 years. Pine nuts contain about 31 grams of protein per 100 grams of nut, the highest of any nuts and seeds. They are also rich in monounsaturated fats. Pine nuts are probably best known for their appearance in pesto, though they can also be used in desserts, whole-grain dishes, or as a garnish for many savory dishes. Pine nuts can become rancid very quickly. Store them in an airtight glass jar in the refrigerator for up to 1 month or freeze for up to a year.

Pumpkin Seeds

Pumpkin seeds, also known as *pepitas*, are flat, dark green seeds. Pumpkin seeds are very rich in minerals, particularly manganese, magnesium, phosphorus, iron, copper, and zinc. They are also high in vitamin K1 and the amino acid tryptophan. Pumpkin seeds are delicious lightly toasted and added to salads. They can also be ground to a powder in a coffee grinder and mixed into whole-grain baby cereals for babies 10 months and older. When purchasing pumpkin seeds, look for the green seeds not encased in the outer white hull.

Sunflower Seeds

Sunflower seeds come from the beautiful sunflower. Sunflower seeds are high in polyunsaturated fat, manganese, magnesium, selenium, and vitamin B1. Sunflower seeds are also a fantastic source of vitamin E, the body's primary fat-soluble antioxidant. Sunflower seeds can be added to salads, combined with whole grains and spices to make vegetarian burgers, used as a garnish for vegetable dishes, soaked and puréed with vegetables for raw pâtes, or used in combination with other nuts to make delicious raw desserts.

Sesame Seeds

The use of sesame seeds as a condiment dates back to as early as 1600 BC. Sesame seeds add a delicious nutty flavor to a variety of Asian dishes, such as stir-fries and noodle dishes. They are also the main ingredient in tahini (sesame seed paste). Sesame seeds are very rich in copper, calcium, and manganese. They are also a great source of magnesium, iron, phosphorus, zinc, and vitamin B1.

Flaxseeds

Flaxseeds are available in two varieties, golden and brown. They are a fantastic source of omega-3 fatty acids, though they need to be ground in order for the body to utilize these fats. Omega-3 fatty acids help to calm inflammation in the body and have been shown to benefit many disease states. Unfortunately, foods that are high in omega-3 fatty acids, like flax, spoil very quickly.

Flaxseeds and flax oil should be stored in the refrigerator or freezer. Flaxseeds can be added to smoothies, or ground and sprinkled on top of just about any food, from whole-grain cereals to vegetable dishes. Flaxseeds also work as an egg replacement in baked goods. Use 1 heaping tablespoon of ground flax mixed with 2 to 3 tablespoons of hot water. This will replace 1 egg in any baked good.

Chia Seeds

Chia seeds can be either blackish-gray or white, and contain a powerhouse of nutrients! They are a concentrated source of omega-3 fatty acids, amino acids, carbohydrates, minerals, fiber, and antioxidants. The fat in chia seeds consists of approximately 55% omega-3's, 18% omega-6's, 10% saturated fat, and 6% omega-9's. Chia seeds come from the plant *Salvia hispanica*. Their use dates back to ancient Mayan and Aztec cultures where they were typically consumed in a drink and used for strength and endurance. We like to add a few tablespoons to nearly all of our smoothies, use the ground seeds as a binder in gluten-free baking, and sprinkle them onto fruit salads. Store them in your freezer or refrigerator.

NUT AND SEED BUTTERS

Nut and seed butters, which are rich in protein, work well to make a quick sandwich or to spread onto whole-grain toast. They are also very useful in making healthy dips and sauces. Store opened jars in the refrigerator. Some more unusual nut and seed butters include pecan, hemp, and pumpkin seed. Check your local co-op or health food store for availability.

Almond Butter

Almond butter, with its sweet taste and smooth texture, is delicious for making sandwiches, can be used to make savory sauces, and can be used as a dip for fruits and vegetables. We like to use raw, organic almond butter for eating or in raw desserts; and use roasted almond butter for baking muffins and grain-free desserts.

Cashew Butter

Cashew butter can be used to make savory sauces, dips, vegan gravy, and raw desserts. It can be found raw or roasted in the nut butter section of your local co-op or health food store. We like to buy Artisana brand raw cashew butter.

Unsalted Peanut Butter

Peanuts, contrary to their name, are not actually true nuts. They are a member of a family of legumes related to peas, lentils, chickpeas, and other beans. Peanut butter is rich in manganese, vitamin E, niacin, folic acid, and protein. Peanut skins also contain the phenolic antioxidant, resveratrol, which is also found in red grapes and red wine. Unsalted peanut butter can be used to make a quick sandwich or a delicious sauce to top steamed greens, noodle dishes, and more. Always purchase organic peanut butter as it does not contain any additives such as hydrogenated vegetable oils.

Sunflower Seed Butter

You can purchase either raw or roasted sunflower seed butter. The latter has a similar flavor and texture to that of peanut butter and can be replaced for it in any recipe that calls for peanut butter. Be sure to purchase organic sunflower seed butter; the nonorganic varieties sometimes have added sugar and other ingredients.

Pumpkin Seed Butter

Raw pumpkin seed butter can be dolloped over whole-grain cereals, used as a dip for fruits and vegetables, used to make raw energy bars, and also used as a base in savory sauces.

Sesame Tahini

Sesame tahini is simply made from ground sesame seeds. It comes salted and unsalted and also roasted or raw. Be sure to always buy organic.

WHOLE GRAINS

Keep a variety of whole grains on hand to create filling yet energizing meals. Only buy what you think you will use within a few months. Whole grains should be stored in airtight containers in a cool dark place. Grains stored this way can be kept for up to 6 to 9 months. It is also helpful to have a variety of whole-grain pastas on hand to make as part of a quick meal. All of the following grains are gluten-free. Check our resource guide in the back of the book for a source of certified gluten-free oats.

Short-Grain Brown Rice

Brown rice is an excellent source of manganese and a good source of selenium, magnesium, and fiber. When cooked, short-grain brown rice tends to stick together, making it an ideal component to vegetarian burgers, croquettes, puddings, risotto, or rice balls.

Sweet Brown Rice

Sweet brown rice, sometimes called glutinous brown rice, has a sweet taste and sticky texture when cooked. It can be ground and cooked into a delicious, creamy breakfast cereal, or used in combination with short-grain brown rice as a filling for nori rolls (sushi).

Brown Jasmine Rice

Brown jasmine rice is an aromatic long-grain rice originally grown in Thailand. When it is being cooked, the delicate, nutty aroma will fill your kitchen. Brown jasmine rice can be used to make pilafs or fried rice, or it can be simply served with flavorful curries and stews.

Brown Basmati Rice

Brown basmati rice is another long-grain aromatic rice. It can be used interchangeably with brown jasmine rice. Brown basmati rice is ideal for making pilafs, fried rice, or stuffing, or it can be served alongside fragrant curries and stews.

Millet

Millet is a small, round, yellow grain with a sweet, earthy taste. Millet is a good source of manganese, phosphorus, magnesium, and fiber. Millet is native to the East Indies and North Africa, though now it is used throughout the world as a staple grain. Millet can be used for making savory grain-based casseroles, breakfast cereals, croquettes, and more.

Quinoa

Quinoa is an ancient Incan grain that comes from the Andes Mountains in South America. Although considered a grain, quinoa is actually a seed from a plant similar to spinach and chard. Quinoa is an excellent source of plant-based protein, containing all nine essential amino acids. It is also a great source of manganese, magnesium, and iron. Quinoa's light, fluffy nature makes it ideal for creating grain-based salads. It is also great in pilafs or breakfast cereals, or served alongside savory stews.

Amaranth

Amaranth, an ancient Aztec grain, is high in protein, calcium, and iron. Amaranth sustained the Aztec culture until 1521, when Cortez arrived and banished the crop. It survived in remote wild areas and was then rediscovered in 1972 by a U.S. botanical research team. Amaranth, like quinoa, is a seed of a broad-leafed plant. The leaves and stems of amaranth are also edible and extremely nutritious, being particularly high in calcium. Amaranth greens can be used as a substitute for spinach in any recipe. The grain can be used to make savory casseroles, puddings, and breakfast cereals.

Buckwheat

Buckwheat, a hardy plant that grows in poor, rocky soil and extreme climates, is native to Manchuria and Siberia. The grain is actually the seed of a plant related to rhubarb. After harvesting, the black, hard, inedible outer shell needs to be removed in order to access the inner kernel. The kernel is then split into pieces, called groats, which are sold either roasted or raw. The roasted groats, also called kasha, have a robust flavor. The raw groats are much milder in flavor. Buckwheat can be made into a cereal or a pilaf, or it can be ground into flour and made into a noodle, which is very popular in Japan. Buckwheat is especially famous for its blood sugar–regulating properties, and is therefore very useful for diabetics.

Teff

Teff is a very tiny grain that is available in three colors—white, red, and brown—each with its own distinct flavor. Teff originated in Africa where it was once a foraged wild grass before it was cultivated as a staple grain for the Ethiopians. Teff is very high in protein and iron. Teff can be cooked into a delicious nutty breakfast porridge, used to make casseroles, or used as an alternative to corn in polenta.

Rolled Oats

Oats, originally from Western Europe, help to regulate both blood sugar and the thyroid. Oats also support the nervous system and improve resistance to stress. Rolled oats are made from hulled oats that have been steamed and rolled flat. Instant or quick-cooking oats have been precooked in water, dried, and then rolled super thin. Although they cook faster than thick rolled oats, they have much less nutritional value due to the high heat processing. Be sure to always purchase organic oats! Conventional oats are typically sprayed with herbicides, which are large contributors to the decline in digestive health and rise in food allergies we are seeing today. Rolled oats are subject to rancidity within 1 to 3 months after milling; it is therefore advisable to store large quantities in the refrigerator to prevent rancidity. Rolled oats can be cooked into a delicious, warming breakfast cereal, ground into flour to make pancakes, or used to make many decadent desserts.

Polenta

Polenta is made by coarsely grinding dried corn kernels. It is then cooked with water and sea salt and baked in the oven to make a warming casserole. It is often served with chicken or fish stews and is also delicious topped with a fresh marinara sauce. It is easy and quick to cook, making it a great component to any evening meal. Corn is high in thiamin, folic acid, and fiber. It is also a great source of the antioxidant carotenoid, beta-cyrptoxanthin. Always remember to buy organic corn products to keep your family safe and healthy. Over 90% of the corn grown today is genetically modified. New research has shown that GMOs cause cancer, tumor growth, and may be a large contributor to the increase in food allergies.

Popcorn Kernels

Popcorn kernels are great to have stocked in your pantry. Popcorn cooks easily and quickly on the stovetop, making it a great, healthful snack. Look for organic popcorn kernels in the bulk section of your local co-op or health food store.

Brown Rice Noodles

Brown rice noodles are great to have stocked in your pantry. They can be part of a very quick meal, be used in broth-based soups, or be used to make more complex noodle dishes. Look for a brand that says "gluten-free" on the label. We like to purchase Jovial brand brown rice noodles.

Quinoa Noodles

Quinoa noodles are gluten-free and come in different shapes and sizes. Quinoa noodles can be added to soups at the end of cooking time, made into noodle vegetable salads, or used to make homemade macaroni and cheese.

GLUTEN-FREE FLOURS

Go through your pantry and cabinets and discard any old whole-grain flours (over a year old) as they can spoil easily. The oils found in the germ and bran of whole grains can go rancid quite easily when ground into flours. Store your whole-grain flours in the refrigerator or freezer if you will not be using them right away. Brown rice flour, buckwheat flour, teff flour, millet flour, quinoa flour, amaranth flour, sorghum flour, and tapioca flour are naturally gluten-free. Be sure to look for a gluten-free symbol on the label as some flours may be processed in the same facility as gluten-containing flours and therefore cross contaminated.

Blanched Almond Flour

This sweet-tasting grain-free flour is high in protein and typically very easy to digest. It is made by first blanching raw almonds to remove the skins, and then grinding to a very fine consistency. Use almond flour to make healthy cookies, cakes, pancakes, brownies, and more! You can find organic blanched almond flour online from www.Nuts.com.

Brown Rice Flour

Brown rice flour is a staple gluten-free baking flour in our house. Its subtle flavor makes an ideal base for cakes, breads, muffins, and desserts. For a more nutritious baked good, use sprouted brown rice flour anywhere brown rice flour is called for in a recipe.

Buckwheat Flour

The packaged buckwheat flour you buy in the store is ground from roasted buckwheat groats, so it has a very robust flavor. I prefer to grind my own from raw buckwheat groats. They grind up very quickly to a fine powder in a coffee grinder and even faster if you own a grain grinder. Buckwheat flour makes a delicious pancake, and can also be used to make muffins, quick breads, and some desserts.

Coconut Flour

Coconut flour is made by grinding dried, defatted coconut meat. It is a grain-free flour very high in fiber; in fact, 1 tablespoon contains 5 grams of fiber! It is also very low in carbohydrates—1 tablespoon contains 8 grams. Because of its high-fiber content, baking with coconut flour can be tricky at first. You do not need as much coconut flour as you would grain flours in recipes. In fact, it is best to have an equal ratio of flour to liquid when using 100% coconut flour in a recipe. Coconut flour offers a slightly sweet coconut flavor to your baked goods. Store it in a glass jar in your freezer or refrigerator for the best shelf life.

Teff Flour

Teff's tiny size makes it impractical to hull or degerm, so the entire grain is milled, leaving all of the nutrients intact. Teff flour is highly nutritious, being particularly high in iron, protein, fiber, and complex carbohydrates. It comes in two varieties, ivory or brown. The rich, buttery flavor of teff flour makes an ideal addition to most baked goods. Use it to make pancakes, brownies, cookies, yeast breads, quick breads, and more. You can replace half of the brown rice flour in our recipes with teff flour with good results. Teff flour can also be mixed with water and fermented to make the popular Ethiopian flatbread called *injera*.

Millet Flour

Millet flour's light yellow color and sweet flavor works well in cakes, quick breads, and muffins. It can be substituted for brown rice flour in most recipes. Be sure to purchase organic millet flour that is certified gluten-free. Millet can often be cross contaminated with wheat berries in the field.

Quinoa Flour

Quinoa flour has a strong flavor and should be used in combination with other mild flours such as brown rice flour. Quinoa flour is very high in protein, making it a great addition to quick breads and muffins.

Amaranth Flour

Amaranth flour has a distinct, sweet, nutty flavor, though it can sometimes leave a bitter aftertaste. It is high in protein and iron and should be used in combination with other flours in baking.

Sorghum Flour

Sorghum flour adds delicious flavor and texture to gluten-free baked goods. It is a good substitute for whole wheat flour, as it has a similar taste and texture.

Arrowroot Powder

Arrowroot powder is the pure starch extracted from the rhizome of several different perennial herbs that grow in rainforest habitats. It can be used in combination with other gluten-free flours to replace wheat flour in baking; or used to thicken sauces, soups, puddings, gravies, and desserts. Use it where cornstarch is called for in a recipe, making sure that you mix it with cold water before adding it to a hot liquid, such as in making gravy. Two teaspoons of arrowroot can be substituted for 1 tablespoon of cornstarch.

Tapioca Flour

Tapioca flour comes from the ground starch of the cassava root. A small part of tapioca flour is used in combination with other gluten-free flours in baked goods to help them stick together. Gluten-free and egg-free baked goods made without the addition of a small amount of starch may crumble and fall apart once baked.

BEANS

Beans need to be fresh in order to cook properly. Discard dry beans that are older than 9 months, and restock your pantry with small amounts of your favorite beans. Buy organic dry beans in bulk from your local health food store or food co-op. Store dry beans in the coolest and driest place in your kitchen. This will preserve their freshness and make them last longer. Beans stored in this way can be kept for 6 to 9 months. Mark the date of purchase on your bean containers so you will know to discard them if they are older than 9 months. Organic canned beans are an acceptable substitute for dry beans, especially if you are not accustomed to planning ahead for your meals. Keep a few cans of each of your favorite beans stocked in your pantry. Be sure to buy from a company, such as Eden Foods, that uses BPA-free cans.

Dried Kidney Beans

Kidney beans are great for making chili or spicy Cajun dishes, or they can be used in bean salads. As with most beans, kidney beans are very high in molybdenum, folates, tryptophan, fiber, manganese, and protein.

Dried Black Beans

Black beans are so versatile; they can be used to make spicy soups and stews, used in enchiladas or grain and bean salads, or used for breakfast with eggs and salsa. Black beans are rich in antioxidant compounds called anthocyanins, which work to protect against cancer.

Dried Chickpeas

Chickpeas, also called garbanzo beans, are used in a wide variety of ethnic cuisine from Mediterranean to Indian cooking. They can be used to make soups, stews, curries, grain and bean salads, bean dips, such as hummus, and more.

Dried White Beans

Small white beans, such as navy or Great Northern, are delicious in savory soups and stews or vegetable and bean salads.

Dried Pink Beans

Pink beans can be used to make Mexican dishes and are delicious in savory vegetable-bean soups. They can be used interchangeably with pinto beans.

Dried Pinto Beans

Pinto beans can be used in combination with kidney beans and black beans to make fabulous chili, or they can be used in a variety of soups and stews.

Dried Red, Green, and French Lentils

Lentils are so versatile and quick to cook that they are a staple in our house. Very high in protein, iron, and other minerals, they are essential to the well-stocked pantry. Lentils can be made into delicious Indian stews, called *dal*, or can be made into savory soups, or grain and bean salads.

Lentils sprout easily, making a great addition to a garden salad!

Yellow and Green Split Peas

Yellow and green split peas, like lentils, cook up rather quickly. They can be used to make savory split pea soups, and are often used in Ethiopian cooking to make spicy stews.

Tempeh

Tempeh, pronounced "TEM-pay," is a traditional Indonesian food. It is made from fully cooked soybeans that have been fermented with a mold called rhizopus and formed into cakes. Tempeh needs to be refrigerated or frozen. Tempeh takes on the flavor of whatever it is marinated with. Lime, lemon, vinegar, tamari, herbs, and spices can be combined in varying combinations to make fabulous marinades. After the tempeh has been marinated, we sauté it in olive oil or coconut oil.

Tofu

Tofu, or bean curd, is made from soybeans that have been cooked, made into milk, and then coagulated. Different types of coagulants may be used for making tofu, including calcium sulfate, nigari, and magnesium chloride. The soy milk curdles when heated and the curds are then skimmed off and pressed into blocks. Tofu can be found extra-firm, firm, or soft in the refrigerated section of your local co-op or health food store. Tofu can be marinated and sautéed like tempeh, crumbled into enchiladas and lasagna, or made into tofu scramble.

MEAT, POULTRY, FISH, AND EGGS

If you find that adding animal products benefits your health, then it is of utmost importance to choose the cleanest and most sustainable forms available. The labeling of these products can be deceiving and it is important to understand how to read them so you can remain in good health. Finding sources of the highest-quality meat, poultry, and eggs just takes a willingness to search a little and talk with your local farmers. The more demand for humanely treated and sustainably raised meat, the more farmers will produce it.

Eggs

Eggs in the grocery store come with all sorts of different labels that can be confusing, such as pastured, cage-free, vegetarian-fed, organic, and free-range. But what do these mean? Basically, unless a label says pastured and organic, the chickens could be fed GMO grains, have their beaks clipped, and be packed tightly in large barns. The conventional eggs you buy from the grocery store generally come from chickens with clipped beaks kept in horrific conditions, packed by the tens of thousands in large poultry barns. These eggs should be avoided at all times—remember if you are eating out or eating baked goods made with eggs, this is usually the variety being used unless stated otherwise. The label "vegetarian-fed" only means that the chickens were not fed any animal by-products in their feed, but they are still usually fed GMO grains. The label "cage-free" only means that the chickens were not kept in small wire cages but instead packed in open poultry barns, which can be just as horrific; and they are still fed nonorganic feed as well as possible antibiotics. The "organic" label means the chickens were fed organic, GMO-free grains and had access to the outdoors. "Pastured" eggs mean the chickens were raised on open land (usually surrounded by large wire cages to protect them from predators) and allowed to eat their natural diet of bugs and grasses. Sometimes they are still fed a small amount of grains in the winter. It is up to the farmer to determine the type and quality of the feed since there is no certification at this time for "pastured." We suggest you purchase only local, organic, pastured eggs, or raise your own egg-laying chickens.

Chicken and Turkey

Chickens and turkeys come with similar labels as those found on eggs. It is very important to choose the highest-quality poultry available. If you can't find a source locally, check the resource guide at the back of this book for online ordering sources. Though, chances are, you probably have a local farm in your area raising organic, pastured chickens that may not be available at your local health food store. If you can't find pastured chickens, the next best thing is to buy organic. The term "free-range" doesn't mean much as the chickens are usually fed nonorganic, GMO grains and can still be given antibiotics. You can purchase organic, pastured chickens from a local farmer and then freeze them whole for up to a year. Pastured heritage turkeys are usually available for preorder from local farms in early autumn to be picked up at Thanksgiving.

Beef and Pork

Most beef and pork you buy in the grocery store or eat in a restaurant comes from something called a concentrated animal feeding operation (CAFO). These facilities concentrate thousands of animals into very tight spaces, feeding them GMO grains that are laced with toxic herbicide residues and antibiotics. "Grass-fed" beef is the better option, but the cows may still be grazing on grasses sprayed with herbicides and they may be given antibiotics, though grass-fed cows typically don't need them when raised on their natural diet. The best option is to find a source of organic, pastured beef. This means that the cows ate a diet of organic grasses for their entire lives. Check the freezer section of your local health food store, talk with small local farmers about buying quarters or halves of cows (you will get all of the meat cut and packed to freeze), or buy it frozen online, such as from U.S. Wellness Meats. When purchasing pork, look for a small local farm raising "pastured, organic" pigs and buy directly from them.

Fish

We don't recommend eating a diet high in seafood. Our oceans, lakes, and rivers have become too polluted to rely on fish and shellfish as mainstays in the diet. The high levels of mercury, PCBs, and other toxins are stored in the tissues and fat of fish. Generally, species higher up on the food chain have the most concentrated toxins and should always be avoided, such as tuna, shark, swordfish, orange roughy, king mackerel, marlin, tilefish, and ahi. Seafood with the lowest levels of toxins can be eaten no more than twice a week. These include wild Alaskan salmon, herring, anchovies, pollock, tilapia, and domestic crab. Wild Alaskan halibut should be consumed no more than 6 times a month because it contains a moderate amount of mercury. We suggest purchasing fresh fish from your local fish market and reducing overall consumption. If buying canned fish, look for it packed and sold in glass jars as the cans used are usually lined with BPA—a hormone-disrupting chemical.

ORGANIC TOMATO PRODUCTS

Tomatoes can add depth and flavor to your meals, especially in bean soups and stews. It will be helpful to have the following tomato products on hand to use for some of the recipes in this book. Choose organic whenever possible as they will be lower in sodium and residual chemicals. I like to buy fresh plum tomatoes in the summertime from my local organic farmers and freeze them whole. Then, in the wintertime when I am making soups and stews that call for diced tomatoes I will take a few out of the freezer and run them under hot water to remove their skins, then chop while still frozen— it's the perfect replacement to canned diced tomatoes! Fresh tomatoes can also be cut in half and dehydrated, and then stored in glass jars in your pantry.

Strained Tomatoes

Bionaturae makes a wonderful tomato purée that is sold in glass jars. You can use it in place of tomato sauce in any recipe.

Tomato Paste

Small amounts of tomato paste can be added to dull-tasting bean or vegetable stews and soups to enliven the flavors. Tomato paste can also be used to make savory sauces. We like to use the brand Bionaturae because it comes in glass jars.

FROZEN FOODS

Frozen foods offer variety to your diet when fresh foods are not in season. We like to buy from our local farmers' market, or harvest our own fruits and vegetables when they are in season and freeze them. Please see page 81 for freezing tips.

Organic Peas

Frozen peas are nice to have on hand to cook up for a quick side dish, especially for hungry children. They are also delicious added to split pea and other soups, curries, grain salads, and more.

Organic Spinach

Frozen organic spinach can be added to many different soups and stews for color, texture, and a host of valuable nutrients, such as vitamin K1, beta-carotene, manganese, folates, magnesium, iron, and calcium.

Organic Cherries

Frozen cherries provide a delicious, quick frozen snack. They can also be added to smoothies, used to make dairy-free sorbets, or puréed to be used as a baby food. We like to harvest our own cherries in July or buy them from organic farms by the case, pit them, and stock our freezer full for the winter!

Organic Blueberries

Frozen blueberries are another healthful frozen snack. In fact, our children have been eating them that way since they were about 9 months old. Frozen blueberries can be added to whole-grain cereals in the morning, used to make smoothies or jams, or blended up with other fruits and frozen into Popsicle molds for a delicious snack.

Organic Peaches

Frozen peaches are a fantastic addition to smoothies and homemade ice cream. They can also be thawed and puréed and be used in muffins. We buy organic peaches by the case from organic farms in the summertime, cut them in half, pit them, and store in containers in our freezer.

SEA VEGETABLES

The use of sea vegetables helps to round out the flavors and add extra minerals to your recipes. Sea vegetables lend a natural saltiness to foods. Seaweed can be used as a snack or added to soups, salads, stews, and grain and bean dishes. The naturally occurring glutamic acid in seaweeds also acts as a flavor enhancer in your recipes. Sea vegetables can be found in the dried form either in the bulk section or in packages in the macrobiotic section of your local co-op or health food store. Store your sea vegetables in glass jars or sealed containers in your pantry away from heat and light.

Kombu

The use of the seaweed kombu, or kelp, is essential in cooking beans, as it contains glutamic acid, which helps to break down the indigestible, gas-producing sugars, raffinose and stacchiose, in beans. Kombu is also one of the main ingredients used in Japanese soup stocks and broths. Kombu reduces blood cholesterol and lowers hypertension.

Wakame

Wakame is a brown Japanese seaweed that grows in long, ribbon-like strands. It can be soaked in water, cut up, and then added to salads, vegetable dishes, nut pâtes, and more. The Japanese use it to flavor fish stock (dashi). It is also delicious in miso soup.

Hijiki

Hijiki has been used for hundreds of years in Japan where it is known as "the bearer of wealth and beauty." The harvested plants are cut and sun-dried, boiled until soft, and then dried again. Hijiki is very rich in minerals, especially calcium and iron. It should be soaked before use because it will quadruple in volume. Hijiki makes an excellent addition to Asian noodle salads, grain dishes, and tofu dishes.

Arame

Arame, which is one of the richest sources of iodine, is a member of the kelp family closely related to kombu and wakame. Arame is harvested not only in Japan, but also Peru and the Pacific North American coast. Arame grows in wide leaves up to a foot in length. After harvesting, the leaves are cut into long strands, cooked for 7 hours, sun-dried, and packaged. Arame has a mild, sweet flavor that many people enjoy. Arame is best when soaked before use. It can be added to stir-fries, soups, stews, or even tofu scramble.

Nori

Nori comes in thin sheets and is used to make sushi. It can also be wrapped around rice balls, cut into strips and used for a garnish, or broken into pieces and added to salads or soups. We also love to eat plain nori as a snack. Nori has the highest protein content of all the seaweeds and is the most easily digested. Nori contains an enzyme that helps to break down cholesterol deposits in the body.

Dulse Flakes

Dulse flakes, which are rich in iron, can be used much like sea salt to enhance the flavor and saltiness of your dishes. Dulse grows in temperate to frigid zones of the Atlantic and Pacific. The use of dulse as a food dates back to the eighteenth century in the British Isles where it was commonly eaten with fish, potatoes, and butter.

DRIED FRUIT

Dried organic fruit is essential to a well-stocked pantry. It is wonderful eaten as a quick, nutritious snack when away from home. Dried fruit can also be added to desserts, whole-grain dishes, stews, and salads. Look for dried fruit that is darker in color than the fresh fruit of the same kind. Dried fruit that is the same color as the fresh fruit means that it has been preserved with sulfur dioxide. Fresh, in-season fruit can be harvested yourself or purchased from your local farmers' market and then dried in a food dehydrator. It typically takes about 5 pounds of fresh fruit to equal 1 pound of dried fruit. Living in the Pacific Northwest, we have access to an abundance of fresh local fruit that is excellent for drying. Our favorite fruit to dry is the Italian plum—it grows in abundance everywhere here! We cut the ripe plums into quarters and dry them in our food dehydrator. Unfortunately, they don't even last until winter because they are such a delicious treat! When purchasing dried fruit, always choose organic. Store dried fruit in tightly covered glass jars in your pantry.

Raisins

Raisins are made by dehydrating grapes. Look for sun-dried raisins as some companies use a higher heat mechanical process that destroys nutrients. Raisins are one of the top sources of the trace mineral boron, which is important for bone health and converting vitamin D to its active form. Raisins are rich in antioxidants, which prevent free radical damage in the body. The phytochemicals in raisins, particularly oleanolic acid, are effective in killing bacteria that cause cavities and gum disease. Raisins can be eaten as a delicious, sweet snack, used to top salads, or used in spicy stews.

Currants

Currants, which are actually dried Corinth grapes (also called Zante currants), are very similar to raisins in their antioxidant values and nutrient content. Currants are delicious added to salads, stews, grain pilafs, quick breads, and trail mixes.

Dried Cranberries

The cranberry plant is a small evergreen shrub related to the blueberry. It grows in open bogs and swampy marshes from Alaska to Tennessee. Dried cranberries, which have been fruit juice sweetened, are so versatile they can be used in whole-grain pilafs, sprinkled atop whole-grain breakfast cereals, used in many desserts and quick breads, or eaten as a sweet snack. When buying dried cranberries, look for the organic, fruit juice–sweetened variety.

Dried Cherries

Dried cherries can be used to top breakfast cereals in the morning, used to make dried fruit compotes, or used in trail mixes, whole-grain pilafs, and stuffing. Look for organic, unsweetened dried cherries when purchasing from the store. Cherries are on the list for the top 12 fruits and vegetables to have the highest levels of chemical pesticides used on them. Always buy organic dried cherries.

Dried Apricots

Dried apricots are a superconcentrated source of nutrients. They are high in iron, potassium, beta-carotene, phosphorus, and fiber. Dried apricots are also an amazing source of fructooligosaccharides—long-chain fruit sugars that feed beneficial bacteria in our guts. Dried apricots can be cooked with meats or fish, added to quick breads, muffins, and desserts, or eaten as a delicious snack. You can easily dehydrate them yourself by buying a case of organic apricots from your local farm or health food store in the summertime. Slice them in half, remove the pits, and place in a single layer in your food dehydrator; dehydrate at or below 115°F until leathery. Then store in a sealed glass jar in your pantry. When purchasing at the store, look for organic, unsulphured apricots.

Dried Apples

Dried apples are fun to make in autumn when there is an overabundance of fresh apples. Simply cut them into slices with their peels intact, and spread them out onto a food dehydrator. Dehydrate at a low temperature until dry. Dried apples make a great snack in the wintertime; they can also be added to trail mixes and desserts, such as our Dried Fruit Compote, page 377.

Dried Pears

We dehydrate pears in autumn with the same method used on apples as described above. Dried pears make an excellent sweet snack and can be added to desserts, trail mixes, and stews.

Dried Figs

Dried figs make a superb snack. They can also be chopped up and sprinkled on top of stews, fish dishes, or vegetables. We like to use fresh figs when they are in season, though dried figs can replace fresh in any recipe.

Dried Plums

Both the fresh and dried version of plums (prunes) are nutritional powerhouses. High in beta-carotene, potassium, fiber, copper, and antioxidants, they make a great addition to the whole foods pantry. Plums, both dried and fresh, are high in special phytochemicals called neochlorogenic and chlorogenic acid. These compounds act as antioxidants in the body, scavenging free radicals and helping to prevent oxygen-based damage to fats. Dried plums make an exquisite, sweet-tasting snack and can also be made into delicious desserts, or chopped and added to quick breads and muffins.

Goji Berries

Goji berries, native to Tibet and Mongolia, contain more protein than whole wheat, more beta-carotene than carrots, and 500 times more vitamin C by weight than oranges. Goji berries are packed with numerous antioxidants, trace minerals, and essential vitamins, including vitamins B1 and B6. Goji berries can be eaten as a snack, soaked in water, and added to smoothies, and are great as part of a trail mix. Goji berries can be found at your local health food store or co-op and can also be ordered online.

SPECIALTY ITEMS

Olives

Olives are a fruit that must be cured before they are edible. A brine made from salt and water is typically used, though Kalamata olives are cured in a salted vinegar brine. Look for olives that are made with sea salt and avoid brands that have been treated with preservatives. Olives are an essential part of a well-stocked pantry. They can be used to make dips, spreads, salads, or main dishes, or simply eaten as a nutritious snack. Olives come in green and black varieties and can be found flavored with many things such as garlic, lemon, and chile peppers. Green olives are younger and tend to be lighter and fruitier in flavor. Black olives are ripe and more mature. Olives can be stored in their brine in the refrigerator for several months.

Capers

Capers are the unopened green flower buds of the *Capparis spinosa* bush. Manual labor is required to gather capers because the buds must be picked each morning just as they reach the proper size. After the buds are picked, they are usually sun-dried, then pickled in a salted vinegar brine. Capers are a delicious addition to sauces, dips, or vegetables dishes, or they can be used as a garnish for meat or fish. Look for organic capers or a preservative-free variety.

Sun-Dried Tomatoes

Sun-dried tomatoes are a flavorful and nutritious way to add an extra bit of zest to your recipes. Look for organic sun-dried tomatoes. Most commercial varieties of sun-dried tomatoes are processed at high temperatures, which destroys precious nutrients. Some companies also add sulfur dioxide as a preservative. Store dry pieces in a glass jar in your pantry. Sun-dried tomatoes also come packed in extra-virgin olive oil. These are found in glass jars at your local co-op or health food store. A good company to buy from is Mediterranean Organic. Olive oil packed sun-dried tomatoes do not need to be soaked in water before using, ultimately making them more convenient.

OTHER ITEMS

The following list of foods will be helpful to have stocked in your pantry to make many of the recipes in this book.

Vanilla Extract

Vanilla extract can be made with either alcohol or glycerine (nonalcoholic). We typically like to use the nonalcoholic variety for dishes that are not cooked, such as raw desserts. The alcohol in traditional vanilla extract will evaporate with heat in cooked desserts. Vanilla extract enhances the sweetness of whatever it is added to.

Almond Extract

Almond extract comes from the bitter almond, an unpalatable relative of the sweet almond. The highly valued oil is extracted by heating the almond and then pressing the oil. The bitterness is destroyed with the heat. Almond extract can be made with alcohol or glycerin (nonalcoholic). We usually use organic almond flavoring, which is nonalcoholic.

Lemon Flavoring

Lemon flavoring is the essential oil extract of the lemon peel combined with a carrier oil. It can replace lemon zest in baked goods or be used in sauces and soups to create a hint of lemon flavor. The brand Simply Organic makes a great lemon flavoring, which can be found at your local food co-op or health food store.

Organic Dark Chocolate Chips

Chocolate chips are only as good as the chocolate from which they are made. Look for a high-quality, organic dark chocolate chip, such as Dagoba's Chocodrops. Antioxidant-rich dark chocolate chips can be added to cookies or chocolate cakes, or melted to create a decadent frosting.

Organic Cocoa Powder

The cacao tree is native to tropical America and can grow up to 30 feet tall. The ripe pods that grow on the tree are 7 to 12 inches long and dark reddish brown or purple in color. The pods are split open and the pulp and seeds are removed and then piled in heaps and laid out on grates for several days. During this time, the seeds and pulp undergo "sweating," where the thick pulp liquefies as it ferments. The fermented pulp drains away, leaving cacao seeds behind. The cacao seeds are then roasted or left raw and cracked. Now called cocoa nibs, they are ground into a thick, oily paste called chocolate liquor. The cocoa fat is rendered into a yellowish cocoa butter and the remaining powder is cocoa powder. Cocoa powder can be found raw or roasted. Raw cacao powder has about seven times as many antioxidants as roasted cocoa powder! They can both be used interchangeably in recipes where cocoa or cacao powder is called for, though we use raw cacao powder exclusively in baking and in raw desserts. Always purchase organic cocoa powder as the conventional varieties are treated with numerous chemicals and usually employ child labor.

Raw Carob Powder

The carob tree is native to southwestern Europe and western Asia and is widely cultivated in the Mediterranean region. In the United

States, carob is grown mostly in California. The carob tree bears pods that are harvested in September. After the pods are sun-dried, the seeds are removed and the pulp is ground into carob powder. Carob powder can be found roasted or raw; we prefer to use raw. It can be used in place of cocoa powder in most recipes.

Kudzu

Kudzu is a coarse, high-climbing, twining, trailing, perennial vine that grows in Asia and the southeastern United States. Kudzu powder is a starch from the kudzu root. The powder comes in crumbly white chunks and is used to thicken sauces or create a gel when cooked with a liquid and then cooled.

Agar Flakes and Powder

Agar flakes or powder are the products of the mucilage of several species of red algae. The flavorless mucilage is formed into bars and then flakes or powder. Agar will gel a liquid much like gelatin does, though it will have a firmer texture. Two tablespoons of flakes equals 1 teaspoon of powder. One tablespoon of flakes will gel 1 cup of liquid. Agar flakes can be used to make healthful gelled desserts.

Tapioca Pearls

Tapioca pearls are made from the starch obtained from the tuberous root of the cassava plant. They make a delicious pudding when combined with other ingredients such as nut milks and fruit. Tapioca pearls usually need to be soaked for a few hours before using.

Canned Coconut Milk

We like to keep a few cans of organic coconut milk on hand for making curries, creamy soups, desserts, and dairy-free ice cream. Look for a brand that uses BPA-free cans and is organic.

9

ESSENTIAL COOKING EQUIPMENT

And in the end it's not the years in your life that count. It's the life in your years.
—Abraham Lincoln

Now that your pantry is stocked and you are ready to prepare a meal, we thought you might like to know what types of cooking equipment you will need. Having the proper cooking equipment is essential to making the time you spend cooking easy and enjoyable! Some of these items will cut down on preparation time considerably. If you are new to cooking and do not own many kitchen items, then simply begin by adding one item at a time.

POTS AND PANS

Stocking your kitchen with a high-quality set of stainless steel pots and pans is essential to your cooking and to your health. Recent research on nonstick cookware reveals that it is made using the chemical perfluorooctanic acid (PFOA). The Environmental Protection Agency advisory panel

calls PFOA "a likely human carcinogen." According to research from Johns Hopkins Hospital in 2004, PFOA was found in the umbilical cord blood of 99% of 300 babies born there. When these nonstick pots and pans are heated they release at least six different toxic gases, some of which have been found to be carcinogenic. We recommend that you take all of your nonstick cookware out of your house and replace them with some high-quality alternatives.

Look for 18/10 stainless steel pots and pans with a thick aluminum core. The 18/10 refers to the proportion of chromium to nickel in the stainless steel alloy. The aluminum core maintains and distributes heat evenly which helps to prevent burning and sticking and is essential for cooking whole grains. If you cannot afford to buy a set of new cookware then we recommend buying one 11-inch stainless steel skillet, one 3-quart stainless steel saucepan, and one 8-quart stainless steel stockpot. These three pots and pans will get you through most of the recipes in this book. I like to use stainless steel pots and pans that have a glass lid so you can easily see how the food is cooking without disturbing it. You may also choose to use a totally nonreactive, enamel-lined, cast-iron cookware such as Le Creuset for all of your cooking needs. This cookware is typically more expensive than stainless steel, so you can decide what works best for you. Cast-iron skillets are my favorite alternative to nonstick pans as they are naturally nonstick as long as they are cared for properly. I like to use cast-iron skillets for cooking pancakes or making fried rice dishes.

- ✓ 8-inch stainless steel skillet
- ✓ 10-inch stainless steel skillet
- ✓ 11- or 12-inch deep stainless steel skillet with lid
- ✓ 1 stainless steel wok
- ✓ 1.5-quart stainless steel saucepan with lid
- ✓ 2-quart stainless steel pot with lid
- ✓ 3- or 3½-quart stainless steel pot with lid
- ✓ 6-quart stainless steel pot with lid
- ✓ 8-quart stainless steel stockpot with lid
- ✓ 10- to 12-inch cast-iron deep skillet
- ✓ 10-inch enamel-lined, cast-iron Dutch oven, at least 4 inches deep

BAKING DISHES

Stocking your kitchen with a few pieces of high-quality baking equipment will be essential for creating many of the baked goods and other recipes in this book. Having a variety of glass bakeware, stoneware, and other items instead of aluminum and nonstick bakeware, will not only create better tasting dishes but will also benefit your health. We realize it is not always possible to have the highest-quality bakeware. Favor glass or stone baking dishes and avoid aluminum and nonstick to the best of your ability.

- ✓ 10 x 14-inch glass or stone baking dish
- ✓ 1 or 2 glass or stone 9 x 5-inch bread pans
- ✓ 1 or 2 glass or stone 9 x 13-inch baking dishes
- ✓ 1 square glass 8 x 8-inch baking dish
- ✓ 1 stone or stainless steel muffin pan
- ✓ 1 stone or stainless steel Bundt pan
- ✓ 2 stone or stainless steel cookie sheets
- ✓ 9-inch glass pie plate
- ✓ 9.5- or 10-inch stone or glass deep-dish pie plate
- ✓ A variety of sizes of glass or stone casserole dishes with lids

ELECTRIC EQUIPMENT

The following pieces of kitchen tools are essential to making many of the recipes in this book. A food processor is used to make raw nut pâtes and raw desserts, as well as for grating and chopping large amounts of vegetables and fruits. We use our Vitamix every day for blending green smoothies and making sauces, jams, soups, grain-free pancakes, etc. I use my stainless steel immersion blender to purée soups in the pot, or to purée a creamy dressing in the jar. Coffee grinders can be used to grind small amounts of grains, such as raw buckwheat groats, or flaxseeds and chia seeds for baking, as well as nuts and seeds. If you own a high-powered blender you shouldn't need to use a coffee grinder—the blender can handle all of these tasks!

- ✓ 10- to 14-cup food processor
- ✓ High-powered blender such as a Vitamix or Blendtec
- ✓ Stainless steel immersion blender
- ✓ Coffee grinder

KITCHEN GADGETS AND MORE

The following items will be useful to have in your kitchen to make many of the recipes in this book. Having a few high-quality, sharp knifes that feel good to work with will keep cutting and chopping fun and easy.

- ✓ 1 paring knife
- ✓ 1 serrated knife
- ✓ 1 chef's knife
- ✓ 1 mandoline
- ✓ 1 high-quality garlic press
- ✓ 1 ginger grater
- ✓ 1 rasp grater
- ✓ 1 citrus juicer
- ✓ 1 fine-mesh strainer with handle
- ✓ 1 long, stainless steel spoon and 1 slotted spoon
- ✓ 1 thin, wide stainless steel spatula
- ✓ A variety of wooden spoons
- ✓ A variety of sizes of silicone spatulas
- ✓ 4-, 2-, and 1-cup liquid glass measuring cups
- ✓ Dry measuring cup set
- ✓ Measuring spoon set
- ✓ 1 large wooden cutting board for cutting vegetables and fruits
- ✓ 1 small wooden cutting board for cutting meat and fish

FOOD STORAGE CONTAINERS

When you cook your own food, instead of eating packaged meals from the supermarket or eating out, you will need containers for storing leftover food. Most of the recipes in this book make large batches. This makes it easier to stick to a healthy diet because you will have ready-made meals in your fridge at most times.

We prefer to use glass storage containers to store our leftovers. Be sure to have a few different sizes on hand to store everything from large batches of soup to small amounts of ground grains or seeds.

Stainless steel containers work well for freezing meals in. You can also use glass jars to freeze beans, soups, stews, and stocks. Make sure to leave at least an inch of space from the top of the jars when filling them to allow for expansion. I like to also completely cool the food before placing the jar in the freezer. And then I keep the lid off until it has frozen. These three steps should ensure that your jars don't crack when in the freezer.

We like to store our homemade salad dressing in used glass nut butter jars. After you are done with your nut butter, simply rinse out the jar and run it through the dishwasher. When you are ready to make a dressing, just add all the ingredients to the jar, shake well, and store unused portions in the refrigerator.

- ✓ Glass storage containers in a variety of shapes and sizes
- ✓ Stainless steel containers in a variety of shapes and sizes
- ✓ Clean, used nut butter glass jars
- ✓ Widemouthed pint and quart jars

10

DEFINITION OF COOKING TECHNIQUES

Joy is a return to the deep harmony of body, mind, and spirit that was yours at birth and that can be yours again. That openness to love, that capacity for wholeness with the world around you, is still within you.

—*Deepak Chopra*

Cooking and preparing meals is an art of intuition and a science of basic cooking knowledge. Blending the two together will help to create fabulous meals. Below is a list of basic cooking techniques that are used throughout this cookbook. It will be helpful to familiarize yourself with them before moving on to the recipes. When making a recipe, use your intuition as to whether you should add more or less of certain ingredients, and how long to cook some dishes. No recipe can ever be perfect because of the incredible variations in ingredients, cooking equipment, and the person preparing the recipe.

CUTTING TECHNIQUES

Chiffonade: This cutting technique can be used for leafy greens, such as chard, kale, and collards, and fresh herbs, such as basil and mint. Stack the leaves one on top of another and roll tightly lengthwise. Then slice with a sharp knife crosswise to make long, thin strips or ribbons.

Chopping: A chef's knife is typically used for chopping. This general technique involves cutting the food into pieces when no specific size or shape is called for.

Dicing: Dicing food produces small, even squares or cubes. Diced vegetables are typically ⅛- to ¼-inch cubes. Slice the food item into long strips, and then cut across the slices to make cubes. This technique can be used for onions, tomatoes, bell peppers, cucumbers, yams, and squash, as well as many other vegetables and fruits.

Julienne Cut (Matchsticks): The julienne cut creates small matchstick pieces. This technique is particularly useful for cutting vegetables that go into sushi rolls, as well as for many other recipes. Simply take your vegetable, a carrot, for example, and cut it diagonally into ⅛-inch slices. Then take each slice and cut lengthwise into thin strips.

Mincing: Mincing is a technique used for cutting food into very small pieces. Strong-flavored foods such as garlic, shallots, onions, fresh ginger, and hot peppers are typically minced to incorporate flavors evenly. Use a chef's knife and start by slicing the food, then chop back and forth in a rocking motion until the food is in small, fine pieces.

Shredding: Shredded vegetables add a juicy, delicate flavor to salads and can also be used to add extra nutrients to baked goods. Food can be shredded by hand with a handheld stainless steel grater or in a food processor with the grating disk in place. For vegetables, the finer the shred, the sweeter the flavor.

Slicing: Slicing is a broad term used for cutting food into various shapes, such as disks, wedges, or strips. Recipes typically will explain the nature of the slice. Green onions and carrots can be sliced into rounds. A bell pepper can be sliced lengthwise into long strips or sliced horizontally into rings. Apples can be sliced into thin wedges and potatoes can be sliced into rounds or wedges.

Zesting: Zesting is used to remove the outer portion of citrus skin where all of the delicate oils hide. You can zest a citrus fruit with a specialized zesting tool or with a fine rasp grater. The key is to just remove the outer skin and not the bitter white pith beneath. Always zest citrus before juicing.

PREPARATION TECHNIQUES

Marinating: Marinating is pouring a liquid that contains an acidic and/or salty substance, such as vinegar, citrus, or tamari, over the food and allow-ing it sit for a period of time so that the flavors will penetrate the food.

Soaking: Soaking is placing a food in a bowl and covering it with a liquid, usually filtered water, so that the food can rehydrate as it absorbs the liquid. Keep the bowl on your kitchen counter at room temperature. This technique is used for soaking nuts, seeds, beans, whole grains, and dried fruit.

Sprouting: Any raw seeds, nuts, or beans can be sprouted. Sprouting "wakes up" the seed for germination, leading to much more nutritious food. Sprouted foods have higher levels of amino acids, minerals, and vitamins. In the wintertime when fresh, local produce is not as widely available, sprouting is a good alternative for eating live, raw, nutrient-dense plant foods. To sprout, soak your nuts, seeds, or beans in a bowl of filtered water overnight, or for about 12 hours. Then drain and place into a quart jar with a sprouting lid. Every morning and evening, rinse the seeds with fresh water and drain. Make sure they never dry out. Keep doing this until the seeds have sprouted and have reached a desired length or age. For large beans like pinto, black, or kidney that I plan to cook, I place a few cups of dry beans into a large bowl, cover with 3 inches of water, and soak for approximately 24 hours. Then I drain and rinse the beans with fresh water several times and leave the soaked beans in the bowl, uncovered, to sprout. Be sure to drain and rinse them twice daily to keep them moist. I only sprout them until there is a very small tail, 1 to 2 days. Then they are ready to cook! If you are new to sprouting, try green lentils—they are one of the easiest things to sprout! Other foods that we like to sprout are broccoli seeds, radish seeds, sunflower seeds, pumpkin seeds, truly raw almonds, and mung beans.

Puréeing: Puréeing food turns it into a thick, smooth liquid. A blender works best to purée foods, though a

QUICK TIPS FOR FREEZING FOODS

Bananas: Remove the peel, cut into 2-inch slices, and place into a container in your freezer.

Berries: Freeze berries spread out on baking sheets; then when frozen transfer to storage containers and place them back into freezer.

Stone Fruit: Slice in half, remove the pits, and place into layers in reusable plastic or stainless steel containers, using unbleached parchment paper in between each layer. Freeze for up to a year. For cherries, we use a cherry pitter to remove the pits, and then place them all into a large container.

Beans: Cook beans according to directions on pages 180–183, then place into 2- to 3-cup storage containers or quart jars; add bean cooking liquid to cover the beans completely, and store into freezer for up to a year.

Whole Grains: Place cooked and cooled whole grains, such as brown rice, quinoa, and millet into serving-size containers or widemouthed pint jars. This makes it easy to create a whole foods meal when you are cooking for one or two.

Muffins: Cool your freshly cooked muffins to room temperature then place into a plastic bag in a single layer. Store in your freezer.

Meat: Wrap fresh meat in paper (your local meat market would do this) and then place into a plastic freezer bag. Store in a deep freezer for up to a year.

Leftovers: In general, foods that have a higher liquid content, such as soups, casseroles, bean dips, and puréed vegetables and fruits, freeze well. Place cooled food into glass storage containers or widemouthed 1-quart jars and freeze. To use, run the container under hot water to release food. Transfer the frozen food to a pot to reheat.

food processor or handheld immersion blender may also be used. Place foods such as steamed squash, frozen or fresh fruit, or cooked soups into a blender. To blend hot foods, fill the blender no more than halfway, then remove the center cap on the lid to release the steam, place a towel over the lid, and hold it firmly in place. Start on the lowest speed and gradually increase as food is blending.

Freezing: Freezing your own fruits and vegetables that you have either harvested yourself or bought from the farmers' market is a great way to preserve food. Also, freezing your leftovers will

make it easy to have healthy homemade meals on nights you may not want to, or have time to cook. Be sure to label and date your food and use it within 6 to 12 months.

COOKING TECHNIQUES

Baking: Food is placed in a baking dish or pan and into a preheated oven. Moisture is released from the food while it is baking and circulates in the oven. When you are baking more than one dish at a time, be sure to stagger the dishes so that the air can circulate in the oven. All oven temperatures will vary slightly, so you may need to adjust your temperature and/or cooking time to your oven. It is best to purchase a small oven thermometer to measure the actual baking temperature of your oven and then adjust it accordingly.

Blanching: Vegetables are quickly boiled, usually for only a few minutes, and then plunged into a cold-water bath to stop the cooking. This technique works to preserve colors and nutrients in food.

Boiling: Food is placed into water or a cooking liquid, such as stock, in an uncovered pot that has reached a temperature of about 212°F, or when bubbles are visible on the surface. The food is cooked by the rapidly moving liquid. The boiling point can be defined as the temperature at which the vapor pressure of a substance is equal to the external, or atmospheric, pressure. When cooking at higher elevations, the boiling point of a liquid will be lower due to the drop in atmospheric pressure. For each 1,000 feet above sea level the boiling point drops by about 2°F. Water-soluble substances, such as salt and sugar, raise the boiling point of water.

Braising: Food is lightly sautéed, then a small amount of a flavored liquid is added and the pan is covered while the food cooks and absorbs part of the liquid.

Broiling: Turn your oven dial to "broil" and place the food in an oven-safe dish on the rack level indicated in your recipe.

Parboil: Food is partially cooked in boiling water; the cooking is then completed by some other method.

Poaching: Food is cooked by submerging it into a liquid that is just barely simmering. Be sure the food is covered in the cooking liquid by ½ to 1 inch. The cooking liquid is usually stock or water with an acid added to it, such as lemon juice or vinegar. Fresh or dried herbs and a salt or salt seasoning are also added (except for eggs—do not add salt while poaching eggs). This technique works to retain the original shape of the food.

Pressure Cooking: Cooking with a pressure cooker decreases cooking times tremendously. Temperatures inside a pressure cooker can reach 250°F, much higher than boiling temperature. Never fill a pressure cooker more than half full and be sure to use the recommended amount of liquid.

Roasting: Food is cooked by dry heat in an oven, usually with some kind of fat added.

Sautéing: Add a small amount of oil or fat to a heated skillet or sauté pan, then add your cut food. Keep the food moving in the pan to prevent burning and sticking. Sautéing is a quick-moving process that necessitates having all of the ingredients within arm's reach and ready for use. If your food begins to stick to the pan during cooking then add extra fat, water, wine, or stock to the pan.

WATER-OIL SAUTÉ: If you would like to lessen the amount of oil in a dish, you can replace half of it with water. Continue to sauté as directed above.

NO-OIL SAUTÉ: It is not always necessary to sauté in oil. Instead, you may add a small amount of water, broth, or white wine to the pan and sauté as directed above.

Simmering: Cooking food in a liquid on the stovetop where bubbles are barely breaking the surface is simmering. This is usually done by bringing the liquid and food to a boil first and then reducing the heat to low to medium-low and cooking with a lid on the pot.

Steaming: Steaming is a great way to barely cook vegetables until they are crisp-tender. This method of cooking retains more nutrients than other methods. Place about 2 inches of water in a pot, then place a steamer basket in the pot and add your food. Place a lid on the pot and cook for a certain amount of time. You can test doneness with a fork—food should pierce easily, but the fork should not easily go all the way through the piece of food.

Steeping: Steeping extracts color, flavor, and nutrients from the substance being steeped. Place food or herbs into a ceramic or glass dish and pour boiling water over them. Cover the dish and steep for the directed amount of time. Herbs or food are then strained out of the liquid.

Stir-frying: Place the cut food in piles on your cutting board or in separate dishes and line up from longest to shortest cooking time. You may use a wok or a large skillet, but be sure to use stainless steel, not nonstick. Heat your pan over medium-high heat and add some fat—usually coconut oil. Begin by placing the food with the longest cooking time in first, then move up to the food with the shortest cooking time. Keep the food moving in the pan constantly to prevent burning—this process usually only takes a few minutes. Then add a small amount of liquid to the pan and cover with a lid to quickly finish the cooking by steaming.

Toasting: Raw seeds can be toasted to improve flavor and digestibility. To toast seeds, heat a thick-bottomed stainless steel skillet over medium heat. Add enough seeds to the pan to create one layer. Keep the pan moving over the heat source to prevent burning. When the seeds are lightly golden or you have heard popping sounds, then the seeds are done. Immediately transfer them to a plate to cool. Seeds that can be toasted include pumpkin, sunflower, and sesame.

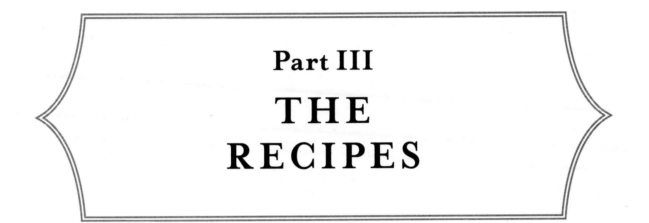

Part III
THE
RECIPES

11

GET CULTURED!

Humankind has not woven the web of life. We are but one thread within it. Whatever we do to the web, we do to ourselves. All things are bound together. All things connect.

—Chief Seattle

Cultured food essentially means fermented—the process of preserving and enriching food using beneficial bacteria.

All life has evolved in the presence of bacteria and depends on them for survival. In roots, bacteria fix minerals from the soil so plants can use them. In animals, they assist with digestion of food, protection from disease, and providing essential nutrients. Likewise, our daily diets should consist of foods containing beneficial bacteria.

Think of kimchi in Korea, sauerkraut in Germany, cucumber pickles in the Middle East, and pickled umeboshi plums in Japan.

For thousands and thousands of years people have been preserving food with the help of bacteria—called lacto-fermentation. When pickling vegetables, *lactobacillus*, a species of bacteria normally present on fresh food, is allowed to flourish. This enables food to break down and become more digestible while providing live enzymes and beneficial bacteria that help with the entire digestive process. This type of anaerobic fermentation uses a salt brine to inhibit harmful microbes as the beneficial species take over and multiply. These beneficial bacteria produce lactic acid as they eat up some of the starches and sugars in the food, lowering the pH, thus inhibiting harmful microorganisms from surviving.

We know now from reading "Digestive Health," chapter 3 in this book, that the world we live in today causes harm to the beneficial bacteria in our guts. There are so many social and environmental actions against them—herbicides, antibiotics, chlorine in our water, and mercury in fish and in dental fillings—that we need to take extra care in maintaining our inner ecology. Having a healthy balance of bacteria in our intestines reduces food allergies and sensitivities, builds a strong immune system, and keeps inflammation in check. Eating cultured foods daily is one thing you can do to help maintain the health of your intestinal flora!

Tips for lacto-fermenting vegetables:

✓ Always use the freshest organic vegetables you can find. If your vegetables have small spots of mold or slime, don't use them.

✓ Only wash your vegetables if necessary. If I see visible dirt on my vegetables I will rinse them off; otherwise I leave them as they are. Friendly bacteria reside on the vegetables and you don't want to wash them all down the drain!

✓ If you see mold on your fermenting vegetables it means oxygen has crept into your jar. Lacto-fermentation is meant to be an anaerobic process—an environment where the *lactobacilli* bacteria can thrive and grow. When fermenting in quart jars there is a possibility of some oxygen creeping in, though I have never had any visible mold in my ferments using this system. Alternatively, you can use a Fido latch-lid jar or an airlock system installed on top of a quart or gallon jar. The latter lets the gases escape, but it doesn't allow oxygen to get in. If you want to spend the money, you can also invest in Harsch ceramic fermenting crocks. These crocks use a rim filled with water to keep oxygen out while still allowing carbon dioxide gases to release. My suggestion is to start fermenting in quart jars and then once you get accustomed to the regular preparation and consumption of cultured foods, you move up to one of the other methods mentioned previously.

✓ If using quart jars, be sure to screw the lids on tightly and then "burp" the jars daily once gases start to form, around day 2. Do this by barely unscrewing the lid and then screwing it back down. You should see extra bubbles rise to the top and hear a slight release of gases.

✓ If some of the brine leaks out during the fermentation process, pour extra in so the vegetables are covered. Use a ratio of 1½ teaspoons sea salt mixed with 1 cup of filtered water.

CULTURED VEGETABLES

If you are new to making sauerkraut, this is one of the easiest recipes to begin with. The food processor does all the work for you—no pounding necessary! Serve a scoop of cultured vegetables with your breakfast, lunch, and dinner! The flavor is very tangy and delicious. Cultured vegetables are rich in beneficial *lactobacilli* bacteria and enzymes, are alkaline-forming, and are full of vitamins—especially vitamin C. Cultured vegetables help to reestablish a healthy inner ecosystem of gut bacteria, improve digestion, control cravings for sweets, and stimulate the liver.

1 medium head green or red cabbage (about 3 pounds), plus 2 small cabbage leaves reserved

2 medium beets, peeled and quartered

4 medium carrots, cut into large chunks

4 to 6 garlic cloves, peeled

freshly squeezed juice of 1 lemon

4 to 6 teaspoons sea salt

1 tablespoon dried dill

Set out two clean, widemouthed, 1-quart jars. Cut the cabbage, except for the 2 reserved cabbage leaves, into chunks and place some of it into a food processor fitted with the "s" blade. Process until finely ground, being careful not to overprocess, then transfer to a large bowl. Repeat until all the cabbage has been processed. Place the beets, carrots, and garlic into the food processor and process until finely ground; add to the bowl with the cabbage.

Add the lemon juice, salt, and dill to the bowl and mix all the ingredients together with a wooden spoon; let rest for about 10 minutes and then stir again.

Spoon the mixture into the two jars until about 1 inch from the top, pressing the vegetables down firmly as you fill them. Fold one of the reserved small cabbage leaves and place it into one jar of the vegetables so that the juices rise above it; repeat with the second jar. Screw the lids on tightly.

Place the jars into another container or baking dish to catch any leaking juices, then place in a spot in your house away from direct sunlight. After about day 2, or when you begin to see tiny bubbles form, slightly unscrew the lids once a day to let any trapped gases escape, and then screw them back down tightly. Let the vegetables ferment for 5 to 10 days.

You can eat them at this point, but it is even better to store the jars in a cool spot, such as a root cellar where the temperature remains around 55°F. You can also store them on one of the shelves on the door of your refrigerator. Then let them continue to ferment for 6 to 12 weeks.

Yield: 2 quarts

GARLIC KALE KRAUT

When you have too much kale growing in your garden and don't know what to do with it . . . make sauerkraut! The word "sauerkraut" comes from the German words *sauer* (sour) and *kraut* (greens or plants). Serve a few scoops of this probiotic and enzyme-rich vegetable dish with any meal!

½ head green cabbage, shredded (about 1½ pounds total), plus 1 small cabbage leaf reserved

6 cups thinly sliced kale

6 garlic cloves, crushed

1 tablespoon sea salt

OPTIONAL ADDITIONS

crushed red chili flakes

chopped green onions

grated carrots

Place all the ingredients, except for the reserved cabbage leaf, into a large bowl and pound with a wooden kraut pounder or other blunt object until the vegetables have softened and released their juices. This usually takes about 5 minutes of continuous pounding.

Scoop the vegetables and juices into a clean, widemouthed, 1-quart jar, pressing them down firmly with the kraut pounder as you add them. Fill to about 1 inch below the top of the jar. Fold the reserved small cabbage leaf and press it into the vegetables, making sure the juices rise above them. Screw the lid on tightly and place the jar into another container to catch any leaking juices. Place the container, undisturbed, in a spot in your house away from direct sunlight.

Let the kraut ferment for 5 to 10 days. Make sure to "burp" the jar every day once bubbles start forming, usually by day 2. You can do this by slightly unscrewing the lid to release the gases and then screwing it back down.

After fermentation it will be ready to eat, but it gets even better with age. If your house is cooler, you can continue to let it ferment for another 2 to 3 weeks. Then place the jar into the refrigerator or a cool place, such as a root cellar, where it will continue to ferment at a much slower rate. You can store your kraut this way for 6 to 8 months.

Yield: 1 quart

ZUCCHINI DILL KRAUT

This recipe is a great way to preserve the summer abundance of garden zucchinis! Serve a scoop with grilled chicken and vegetables for a balanced summer meal.

1 small head cabbage, shredded, plus 1 small cabbage leaf reserved

2 medium zucchini, grated

1 tablespoon sea salt

½ cup chopped fresh dill

2 to 4 garlic cloves, crushed (optional)

Place all the ingredients, except for the reserved cabbage leaf, into a large bowl and pound with a wooden kraut pounder or another blunt object until the juices from the vegetables are released. This usually takes 5 minutes of continuous pounding.

Spoon into a clean, widemouthed, 1-quart jar, pressing down with the kraut pounder until the juices rise above the vegetables. Fold the small cabbage leaf and press it down into the juices; this helps hold the kraut underneath the brine. Make sure to leave about 1 inch of space from the top of the jar. Screw the lid on tightly.

Place the jar into another container or baking dish to catch any leaking juices, then place in a spot in your house away from direct sunlight. Let the kraut ferment for 5 to 10 days. After tiny bubbles begin to form, around day 2, you will need to "burp" the jar every day to let trapped gases escape. You can do this by slightly unscrewing the lid and then screwing it back down.

You can begin to serve the kraut after 5 to 10 days of fermentation, but it is even better to store the jar in a cool spot, such as a root cellar where the temperature remains at around 55°F. You can also store it on one of the shelves on the door of your refrigerator. Then let it continue to ferment for 6 to 12 weeks.

Yield: 1 quart

Tip: Make sure your head of cabbage is no more than 2 pounds. It should preferably weigh about 1½ pounds. When shopping at the grocery store or farmers' market, weigh the cabbage heads to find the right size.

SEA VEGETABLE KRAUT

Sea vegetables are one of the richest sources of iodine—a mineral needed for proper thyroid function. We keep a container of dulse flakes and a container of kelp granules on our dining room table to add to our meals. Having a jar of this sea vegetable kraut in the fridge is also handy! Serve a few spoonfuls with any meal, but it is especially delicious when serving with an Asian-inspired meal.

1 medium head green cabbage, shredded, plus 1 small cabbage leaf reserved

1 tablespoon sea salt

1 bunch green onions, chopped

¼ cup arame, soaked in warm water for 15 minutes

1 tablespoon dulse flakes

one 3-inch piece fresh ginger, grated

Place the shredded cabbage (reserve the cabbage leaf) and sea salt into a large bowl and pound with a wooden kraut pounder or other blunt object until the cabbage has softened and released its juices. This usually takes about 5 minutes of continuous pounding. Then add the green onions, soaked and drained arame, dulse flakes, and ginger, mix together with the cabbage, and pound again for another minute.

Scoop the vegetables and juices into a clean, widemouthed, 1-quart jar, pressing them down firmly as you add them. Fill to about 1 inch below the top of the jar. Fold the reserved small cabbage leaf and press it into the vegetables, making sure the juices rise above them. Screw the lid on tightly and place the jar into another container to catch any leaking juices. Place the container, undisturbed, in a spot in your house away from direct sunlight.

Let the kraut ferment for 5 to 10 days. Make sure to "burp" the jar every day once bubbles start forming, usually by day 2. You can do this by slightly unscrewing the lid to release the gases and then screwing it back down.

After fermentation it will be ready to eat, but it gets even better with age. If your house is cooler, you can continue to let it ferment for another 2 to 3 weeks. Then place the jar into the refrigerator where it will continue to ferment at a much slower rate. You can store your kraut this way for 6 to 8 months.

Yield: 1 quart

CURTIDO

Curtido is a South American vegetable dish traditionally made with vinegar. I've altered it to use lacto-fermentation instead. Serve it with meat, fish, or beans to aid in the digestion of these foods. Though not traditional, I prefer to add crushed red chili flakes for a spicy flare.

---

1 small head cabbage, shredded (about 1½ pounds)

2 to 3 large carrots, grated

1 small onion, thinly sliced

2 tablespoons freshly squeezed lime juice

1 tablespoon dried oregano or ¼ cup chopped fresh

1 to 2 teaspoons crushed red chili flakes (optional)

1 tablespoon sea salt

Place all the ingredients into a large bowl and pound with a wooden kraut pounder or another blunt object until the juices from the vegetables are released. This usually takes 5 minutes of continuous pounding.

Spoon the curtido into a clean, widemouthed, 1-quart jar, pressing down with the kraut pounder until the juices rise above the vegetables. Make sure to leave about 1 inch of space from the top of the jar. Fold a cabbage leaf and press it into the vegetables so the juices rise above it. Screw the lid on tightly.

Place the jar into another container or baking dish to catch any leaking juices, then place in a spot in your house away from direct sunlight.

Let the curtido ferment for 5 to 10 days. Make sure to "burp" the jar every day once bubbles start forming, usually by day 2. You can do this by slightly unscrewing the lid to release the gases and then screwing it back down.

After fermentation it will be ready to eat, but it is even better to store the jar in a cool spot, such as a root cellar where the temperature remains at around 55°F. You can also store it on one of the shelves on the door of your refrigerator. Then let it continue to ferment for 6 to 12 weeks.

> **Tip:** Make sure your head of cabbage is no more than 2 pounds. It should preferably weigh about 1½ pounds. When shopping at the grocery store or farmers' market, weigh the cabbage heads to find the right size.

Yield: 1 quart

DILL PICKLES

I make a few gallon jars of lacto-fermented pickles every summer. They keep in my refrigerator for up to 6 months! When making pickles, it is important to buy pickling cucumbers, often called gherkins, which have thinner skins and fewer seeds. Larger ones will need to be cut into spears, but smaller ones can be left whole. I like to separate them by size and make one jar of small ones and another jar with spears.

1 to 1½ pounds pickling cucumbers
½ bunch fresh flowering dill
3 to 4 garlic cloves, chopped
1 tablespoon pickling spice

1 grape leaf or sour cherry leaf (optional)
2 cups water
1 tablespoon sea salt
1 small cabbage leaf or boiled rock

Rinse the cucumbers. If they are large, cut the ends off and then cut them into quarters lengthwise, forming spears. Place the dill, garlic, and pickling spice into the bottom of a clean, widemouthed, 1-quart jar. Add the pickles, packing them into the jar. Add the grape or sour cherry leaf, if desired; this helps to keep the pickles crisp.

In a 2-cup liquid glass, measure the water and whisk together with the sea salt and then pour over the pickles until the liquid rises above them by ½ inch. Fold the reserved small cabbage leaf and place it, or the boiled rock, over the pickles so they stay beneath the brine. Screw a tight-fitting lid onto the jar. Place it in a spot in your house away from direct sunlight and let ferment for 5 to 10 days. Make sure to "burp" the jar every day once bubbles start forming, usually by day 2. You can do this by slightly unscrewing the lid to release the gases and then screwing it back down. When it is soured to your liking, then transfer to your refrigerator and store for up to 6 months.

Yield: 1 quart

DILLY CARROTS AND GREEN BEANS

This is our children's favorite lacto-fermented recipe. Once fermentation is complete, the five of them can go through two jars in a day if we let them! Needless to say, I have to make large batches of this recipe! Sometimes I like to add hot chile peppers to one jar and black peppercorns to another. I've also used pickling spice, which is quite delicious as well.

---

2 to 3 sprigs fresh flowering dill

3 to 4 garlic cloves, chopped

4 to 5 carrots, cut into spears

¼ pound green beans, ends trimmed

1 tablespoon sea salt

2 cups water

1 small cabbage leaf or boiled rock

Place the dill and garlic at the bottom of a clean, widemouthed, 1-quart jar. Add the carrots and green beans, making sure that the ends stay 1 inch below the top of the jar. If you need to, take a green bean or carrot out and cut it to fit. Pack them in tightly.

Mix the sea salt and water together in a 2-cup liquid glass measuring cup and pour over the vegetables until they are submerged with at least a ½ inch of brine on top. Fold the small cabbage leaf and place it, or the boiled rock, on top and push it down to submerge the vegetables; they need to stay below the brine to properly ferment.

Cover the jar tightly with the lid and store in a dark place to ferment. It should take 5 to 10 days depending on the temperature of your house. The warmer it is, the shorter it takes to ferment. You can check them after 5 days; they should be sour and crispy. Make sure to "burp" the jar every day once bubbles start forming, usually by day 2. You can do this by slightly unscrewing the lid to release the gases and then screwing it back down.

Once the vegetables have fermented to your liking, transfer the jar to the refrigerator and store for up to 6 months. They will keep fermenting while in the refrigerator, just at a much slower rate.

Yield: 1 quart

GINGERED DAIKON AND CARROT STICKS

When you are looking for something crunchy and spicy to eat, try these! I like to keep a jar in my refrigerator at all times. My children sneak the carrot sticks as soon as I put the jar into the refrigerator. You can add other flavors if you wish—try chopped garlic and chile peppers!

---

1 medium daikon radish

3 medium carrots

one 2-inch piece fresh ginger, peeled and thinly sliced

1 tablespoon sea salt

2 cups water

1 small cabbage leaf or boiled rock

Peel the daikon radish and cut it into sticks a little shorter than the length of a quart jar. Cut the carrots into sticks of a similar length.

Put the sliced ginger into the bottom of a clean, widemouthed, 1-quart jar. Add the carrot and daikon sticks, packing them in tightly.

Mix the sea salt and water together in a 2-cup liquid glass measuring cup and pour over the vegetables until they are submerged with at least a ½ inch of brine on top. Fold the small cabbage leaf and place it, or the boiled rock, on top and push it down to submerge the vegetables; they need to stay below the brine to properly ferment.

Cover the jar tightly with the lid and store in a dark place to ferment. It should take 5 to 10 days depending on the temperature of your house. The warmer it is, the shorter it takes to ferment. You can check them after 5 days; they should be sour and crispy. Make sure to "burp" the jar every day once bubbles start forming, usually by day 2. You can do this by slightly unscrewing the lid to release the gases and then screwing it back down.

Once the vegetables have fermented to your liking, transfer the jar to the refrigerator and store for up to 6 months. They will keep fermenting while in the refrigerator, just at a much slower rate.

Yield: 1 quart

PICKLED BASIL BEETS

Serve these probiotic-rich beets with scrambled eggs in the morning or on top of a green salad for lunch. You can use the flavorful purple brine in place of vinegar in a salad dressing. Generally I use 3 tablespoons of brine to 4 tablespoons of extra-virgin olive oil.

---

3 medium beets, peeled and sliced into thin rounds

1 small red onion, sliced into thin rounds

½ cup fresh basil leaves

1 tablespoon sea salt

2 cups water

1 small cabbage leaf or boiled rock

Layer the sliced beets, onion, and basil in a clean, widemouthed, 1-quart jar, packing them down.

Mix the sea salt and water together in a 2-cup liquid glass measuring cup and pour over the vegetables until they are submerged with at least a ½ inch of brine on top. Fold the small cabbage leaf and place it, or the boiled rock, on top and push it down to submerge the vegetables; they need to stay below the brine to properly ferment.

Cover the jar tightly with the lid and store it in a dark place to ferment. It should take 5 to 10 days depending on the temperature of your house. The warmer it is, the shorter it takes to ferment. You can check them after 5 days; they should be sour and crispy. Make sure to "burp" the jar every day once bubbles start forming, usually by day 2. You can do this by slightly unscrewing the lid to release the gases and then screwing it back down.

Once the beets have fermented to your liking, transfer the jar to the refrigerator and store for up to 6 months. They will keep fermenting while in the refrigerator, just at a much slower rate.

Yield: 1 quart

PICKLED LEMON-ROSEMARY CAULIFLOWER

Lacto-fermentation is a great way to preserve some of the cauliflower harvest. After trying this version, create your own. Some other flavors we like to add to cauliflower are garlic, peppercorns, dill, and hot peppers. Serve a few spoonfuls of this recipe with a Mediterranean-style main dish.

1 small head cauliflower, chopped into small pieces

1 lemon, cut into quarters

2 large sprigs fresh rosemary

1 tablespoon sea salt

2 cups water

1 small cabbage leaf or boiled rock

Place the cauliflower, lemon quarters, and rosemary into a clean, widemouthed, 1-quart jar and pack down so they are about 1 inch from the top of the jar.

Mix the sea salt and water together in a 2-cup liquid glass measuring cup and pour over vegetables until they are submerged with at least a ½ inch of brine on top. Fold the small cabbage leaf and place it, or the boiled rock, on top and push it down to submerge the vegetables; they need to stay below the brine to properly ferment.

Cover the jar tightly with the lid and store it in a dark place to ferment. It should take 5 to 10 days depending on the temperature of your house. The warmer it is, the shorter it takes to ferment. You can check them after 5 days; they should be sour and crispy. Make sure to "burp" the jar every day once bubbles start forming, usually by day 2. You can do this by slightly unscrewing the lid to release the gases and then screwing it back down.

Once the cauliflower has fermented to your liking, transfer the jar to the refrigerator and store for up to 6 months. It will keep fermenting while in the refrigerator, just at a much slower rate.

Yield: 1 quart

PICKLED GARLIC SCAPES

Garlic scapes are available in the spring and early summer. They are the long, flowering stalks of the garlic bulb and are trimmed off to help the garlic grow larger. They have a potent garlicky flavor and can be used in stir-fries, pesto, soups, and stews. I like to ferment garlic scapes and then add them to a meal as a garnish. You can add other vegetables to the jar if desired. Try carrot sticks, radishes, turnips, or hot chile peppers!

---

2 bunches fresh garlic scapes
1 tablespoon sea salt
2 cups water
1 small cabbage leaf or boiled rock

OPTIONAL ADDITIONS

carrot sticks
radishes
dried hot peppers
whole black peppercorns

Cut the garlic scapes into 3- to 5-inch pieces. Pack them into a clean, widemouthed, 1-quart jar. Add any optional additions now.

Mix the sea salt and water together in a 2-cup liquid glass measuring cup and pour over the vegetables until they are submerged with at least a ½ inch of brine on top. Fold the small cabbage leaf and place it, or the boiled rock, on top and push it down to submerge the vegetables; they need to stay below the brine to properly ferment.

Cover the jar tightly with the lid and store in a dark place to ferment. It should take 5 to 10 days depending on the temperature of your house. The warmer it is, the shorter it takes to ferment. You can check them after 5 days; they should be sour and crispy. Make sure to "burp" the jar every day once bubbles start forming, usually by day 2. You can do this by slightly unscrewing the lid to release the gases and then screwing it back down.

Once the garlic scapes have fermented to your liking, transfer the jar to the refrigerator and store for up to 6 months. They will keep fermenting while in the refrigerator, just at a much slower rate.

Yield: 1 quart

PICKLED RADISHES

Lacto-fermented radishes are one of our children's favorite foods! Reach for a jar of these instead of a bag of potato chips when you are craving something salty and crunchy—your body will thank you.

---

2 to 3 bunches radishes

3 to 4 garlic cloves, chopped

1 tablespoon whole pink peppercorns

1 tablespoon sea salt

2 cups water

1 small cabbage leaf or boiled rock

Trim the ends off the radishes. If they are large, cut them into quarters. Place the garlic and peppercorns into a clean, widemouthed, 1-quart jar. Add the radishes, packing them in, until they are about 1 inch from the top of the jar.

Mix the sea salt and water together in a 2-cup liquid glass measuring cup and pour over the vegetables until they are submerged with at least a ½ inch of brine on top. Fold the small cabbage leaf and place it, or the boiled rock, on top and push it down to submerge the vegetables; they need to stay below the brine to properly ferment.

Cover the jar tightly with the lid and store in a dark place to ferment. It should take 5 to 10 days depending on the temperature of your house. The warmer it is, the shorter it takes to ferment. You can check them after 5 days; they should be sour and crispy. Make sure to "burp" the jar every day once bubbles start forming, usually by day 2. You can do this by slightly unscrewing the lid to release the gases and then screwing it back down.

Once the radishes have fermented to your liking, transfer the jar to the refrigerator and store for up to 6 months. They will keep fermenting while in the refrigerator, just at a much slower rate.

Yield: 1 quart

PICKLED TURNIPS

Turnips often get passed by in the market more than other vegetables because most of us don't know what to do with them. Try this alternative to cucumber pickles and you might just fall in love with turnips! I prefer to use smaller size turnips for pickling, but if you can only find large turnips then cut them into chunks or quarters.

---

2 bunches turnips

½ small red onion, cut into thick slices

1 tablespoon pickling spice

1 tablespoon sea salt

2 cups water

1 small cabbage leaf or boiled rock

Cut the greens off the turnips and rinse them. Cut larger turnips into smaller chunks. Set aside. Place the onion slices and pickling spice at the bottom of a clean, widemouthed, 1-quart jar. Add the turnips, making sure that they are packed in and at least 1 inch from the top of the jar.

Mix the sea salt and water together in a 2-cup liquid glass measuring cup and pour over the vegetables until they are submerged with at least a ½ inch of brine on top. Fold the small cabbage leaf and place it, or the boiled rock, on top and push it down to submerge the turnips; they need to stay below the brine to properly ferment.

Cover the jar tightly with the lid and store in a dark place to ferment. It should take 5 to 10 days depending on the temperature of your house. The warmer it is, the shorter it takes to ferment. You can check them after 5 days; they should be sour and crispy. Make sure to "burp" the jar every day once bubbles start forming, usually by day 2. You can do this by slightly unscrewing the lid to release the gases and then screwing it back down.

Once the turnips have fermented to your liking, transfer the jar to the refrigerator and store for up to 6 months. They will keep fermenting while in the refrigerator, just at a much slower rate.

Yield: 1 quart

LIVE HOT PEPPER RELISH

Use this enzyme-rich, raw hot pepper relish to top scrambled eggs, chicken fajitas, or quinoa and beans. I use a food processor to quickly chop all of the ingredients so I don't have to cut so many hot peppers! Make sure you don't over process them or they will turn to mush.

---

1 small red onion, coarsely chopped

1 large red bell pepper, coarsely chopped

10 large or 20 small jalapeño peppers, stemmed

3 to 4 garlic cloves

1 tablespoon sea salt

water, as needed

1 small cabbage leaf

Place the onion, bell and jalapeño peppers, and garlic into a food processor fitted with the "s" blade and pulse until the vegetables are chopped finely, being careful not to overprocess them.

Spoon the chopped vegetables into a clean, widemouthed, 1-quart jar until they are 1 inch from the top. Add the sea salt and enough water to cover them; stir. Fold the cabbage leaf and press it on top of the vegetables until the liquid rises above it. Screw the lid on tightly.

Place the jar in a spot in your house away from direct sunlight. Let it ferment for 5 to 10 days. Make sure to "burp" the jar every day once bubbles start forming, usually by day 2. You can do this by slightly unscrewing the lid to release the gases and then screwing it back down. You can taste the relish after 5 days to see if it is done to your liking. It should be sour and spicy, with visible tiny bubbles in the brine.

Store the jar into your refrigerator for up to 6 months.

Yield: 1 quart

COCONUT MILK YOGURT

Enjoy this nutritious dairy-free yogurt in place of cow's milk yogurt. Serve it topped with fresh berries, figs, or peaches, and a sprinkling of chopped nuts for dessert. Be sure to use the full-fat canned coconut milk for this recipe. The agar and gelatin powders serve as thickeners; you can purchase them online (see Resources, page 429). For the probiotic powder, we use Ther-Biotic Complete from Klaire Labs.

---

3 cups full-fat coconut milk (about two 14-ounce cans)

1 cup nut milk

1 tablespoon pure maple syrup

2 tablespoons arrowroot powder

½ teaspoon agar powder or 2 teaspoons gelatin

pinch sea salt

1 to 2 teaspoons probiotic powder

Place all the ingredients except for the probiotic powder into a blender and blend on high for about 30 seconds to combine. Pour into a pot and place on the stovetop. Bring to a simmer over medium to medium-low heat and cook for 5 to 6 minutes, whisking constantly, until thickened (if you are using gelatin, it won't thicken until chilled). Remove the pot from the heat and let cool to about 98°F; this will take 45 minutes to 1 hour.

Once the mixture has cooled, whisk in the probiotic powder. Pour the yogurt into a 1-quart jar or four to five 8-ounce mason jars. Screw on the lid(s) and place into a yogurt maker or a cooler surrounded by a heating pad or jars filled with hot water and towels. Let the yogurt culture for 8 to 15 hours. You can taste it after 8 hours to see how soured it is. If you are using the cooler method, I would suggest refilling the jars with fresh hot water and letting the yogurt culture for 5 to 7 more hours, and then refrigerate to set.

Yield: 1 quart

> **Tip:** I like to use cashew milk for the nut milk called for in this recipe. I make it by adding 2 tablespoons raw cashew butter to a blender and then filling it with water to the 1-cup mark and blending until smooth. It's so easy! You can do this with raw almond butter to make almond milk, or add 2 tablespoons hemp seeds to make hemp milk.

SOURED COCONUT CREAM

This is a great replacement for dairy sour cream, and it's so simple to make! Use it to top bean soups, enchiladas, or tacos—basically anywhere sour cream is called for. Be sure to use the full-fat coconut milk, not the light variety. For the probiotic powder, we use Ther-Biotic Complete by Klaire Labs.

two 14-ounce cans coconut milk, chilled
1 teaspoon probiotic powder

pinch sea salt

Place the two cans of coconut milk in the refrigerator for about 24 hours.

Open the cans of coconut milk and scoop off the thick white cream at the top. Pour off the water into a jar (reserve it to use for smoothies).

Heat the coconut cream in a small saucepan over the lowest heat to about 97° to 98°F. Remove the pan from the stovetop and whisk in the probiotic powder. Pour into a clean 1-quart jar, cover with a clean dishtowel, and secure with a rubber band.

Let the jar sit out for 24 to 48 hours on your kitchen counter to culture. Then stir in a pinch or two of sea salt, cover the jar with a lid, and place into the refrigerator to solidify. Use as desired. The cream will last in the refrigerator for up to 2 weeks.

Yield: 1 to 2 cups (varies depending on how much cream is in each can)

COCONUT WATER KEFIR

You can use the juice from cracked fresh, young coconuts, or young coconut water from the can. Serve this probiotic-rich drink in lieu of soda. You can also add freshly grated ginger to the coconut water if you would like to make a warming digestive tonic. Water kefir grains can be purchased from Cultures for Health (www.CulturesForHealth.com). This brand is dairy-free and is designed for use with water and coconut water. You may also use a kefir starter powder from Body Ecology (www.BodyEcology .com).

1 quart coconut water

one 1-liter glass bottle with a latch lid

1 packet kefir grains or starter powder

Heat the coconut water to 92°F in a pot on the stovetop over the lowest heat.

Use a funnel to assist with pouring the coconut water into the glass bottle. Add the kefir grains or powder. Latch the lid on and shake gently. Place on the countertop in your kitchen away from direct sunlight for 1 to 4 days, depending on the temperature in your house. It should be quite fizzy when it's ready. Be careful when opening the bottle, pressure from gases might build up inside the bottle. Strain out the grains and reuse for another batch. Refrigerate until ready to serve.

Yield: 1 liter (32 ounces)

Variation: You can make live ginger soda by adding 2 tablespoons of grated fresh ginger to the bottle on day 1. Then strain when the fermentation is complete. Add liquid stevia to sweeten it.

Tip: If you use the Body Ecology Kefir starter packs you won't have kefir grains to strain out once culturing is complete. You'll need a new package each time you want to make a batch. If you use water kefir grains, you can use them over again for a new batch after straining.

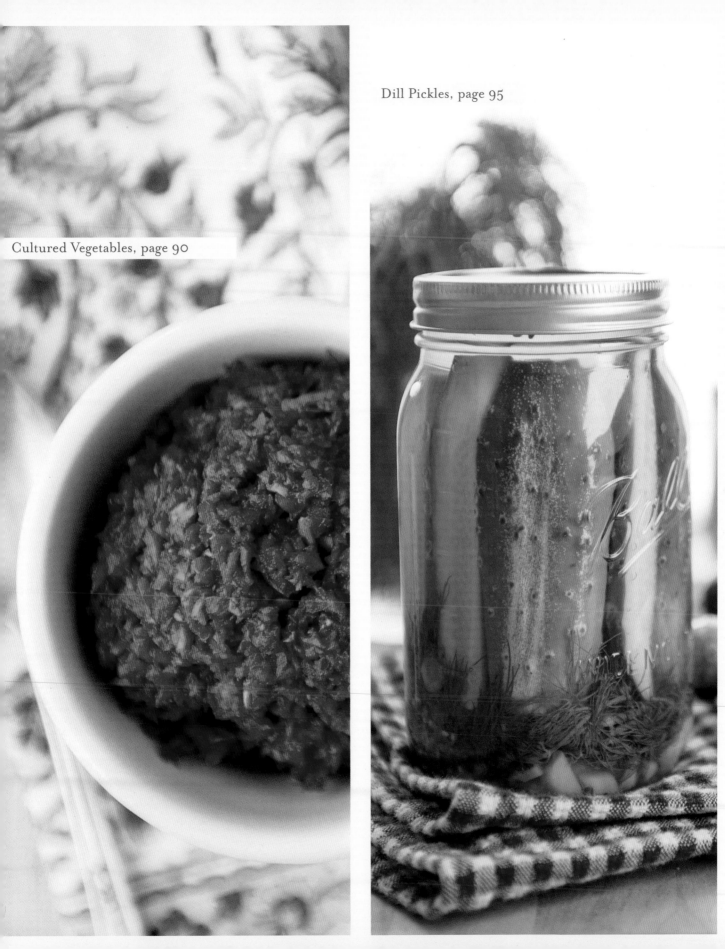

Cultured Vegetables, page 90

Dill Pickles, page 95

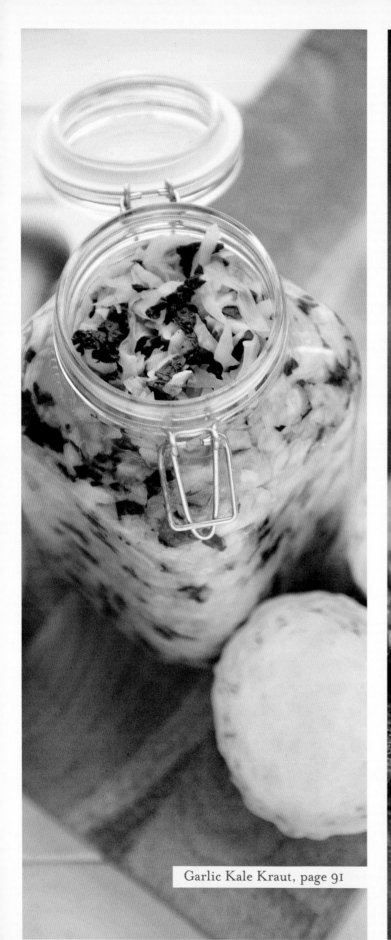

Garlic Kale Kraut, page 91

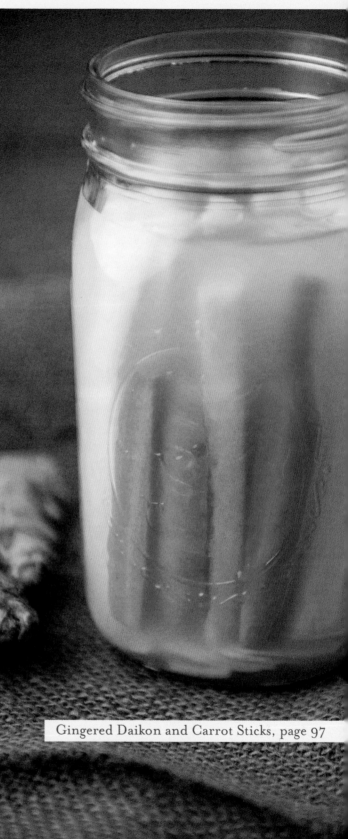

Gingered Daikon and Carrot Sticks, page 97

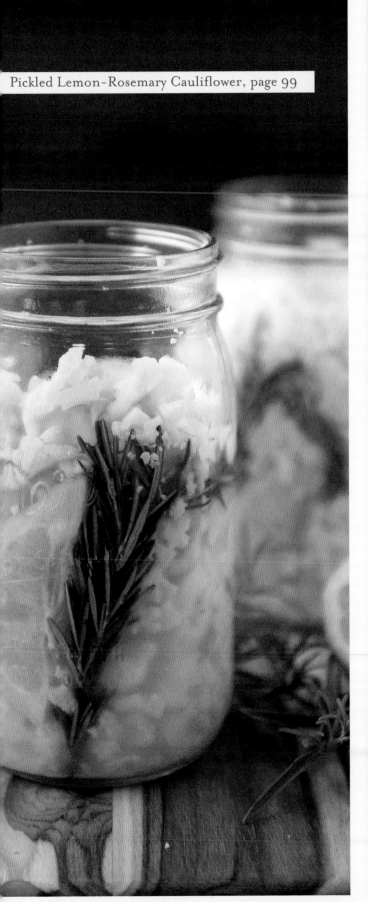

Pickled Lemon–Rosemary Cauliflower, page 99

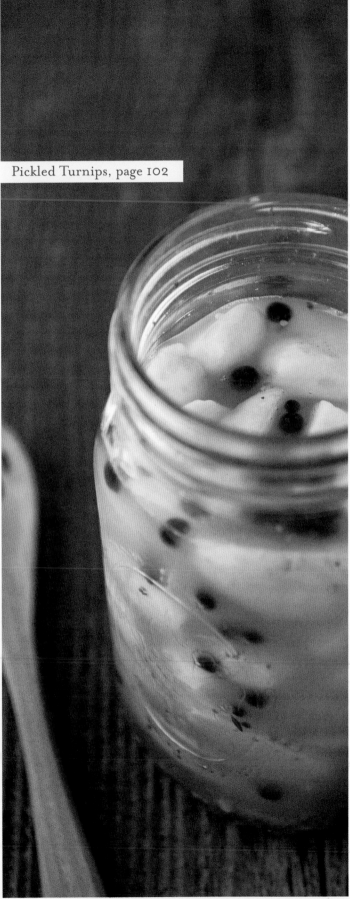

Pickled Turnips, page 102

Live Hot Pepper Relish, page 103

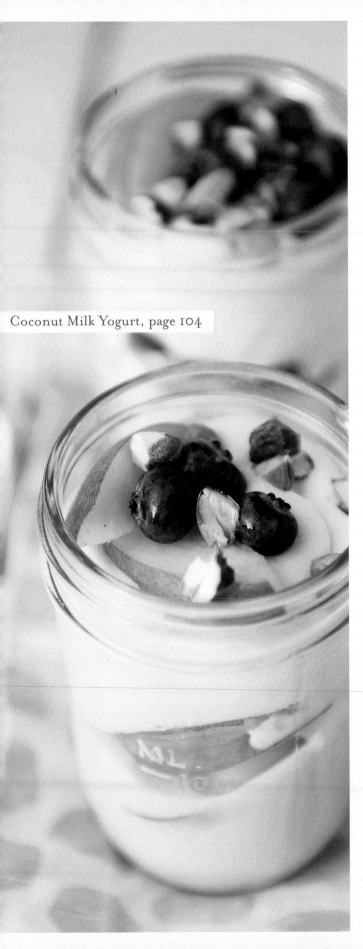

Coconut Milk Yogurt, page 104

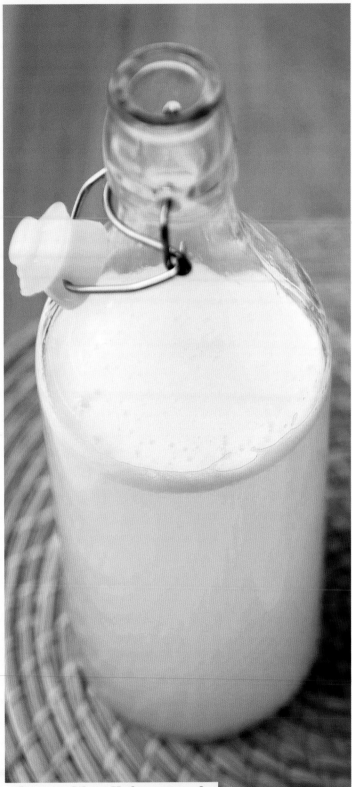

Coconut Water Kefir, page 106

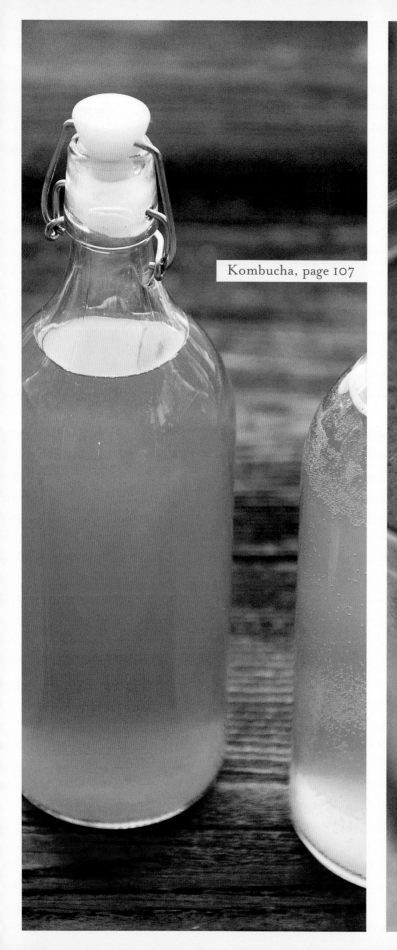

Kombucha, page 107

Berry Antioxidant Smoothie, page 112

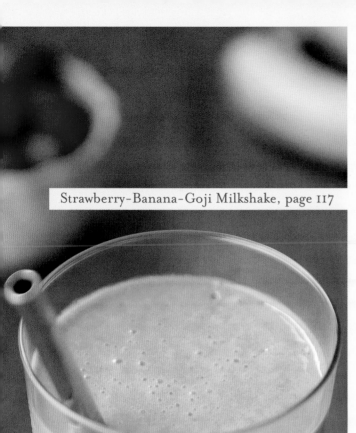

Strawberry-Banana-Goji Milkshake, page 117

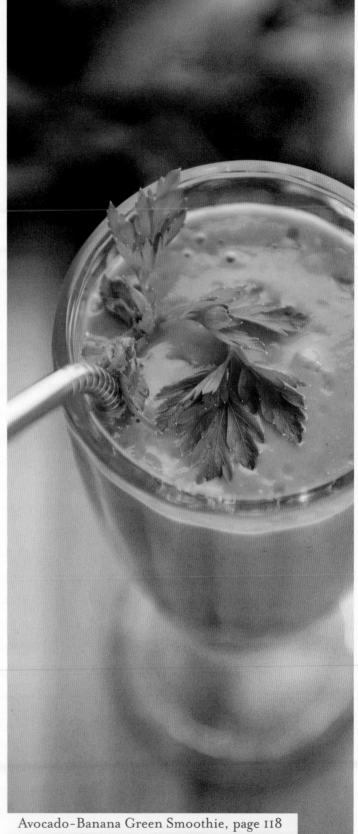

Avocado-Banana Green Smoothie, page 118

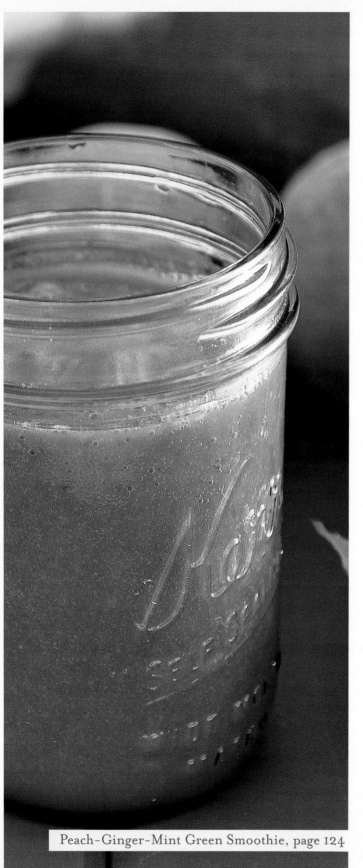

Peach-Ginger-Mint Green Smoothie, page 124

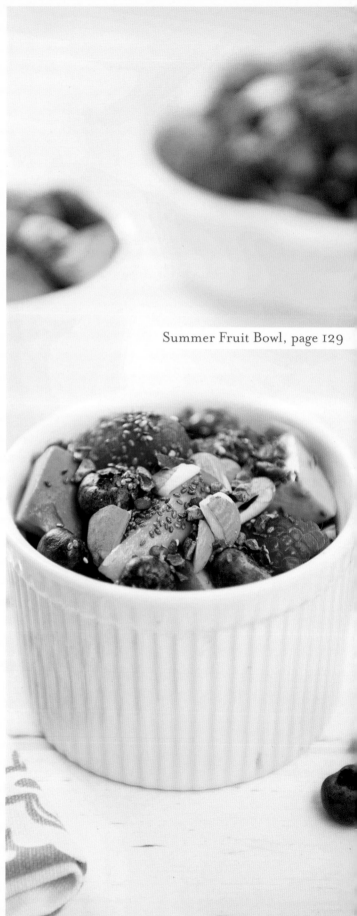

Summer Fruit Bowl, page 129

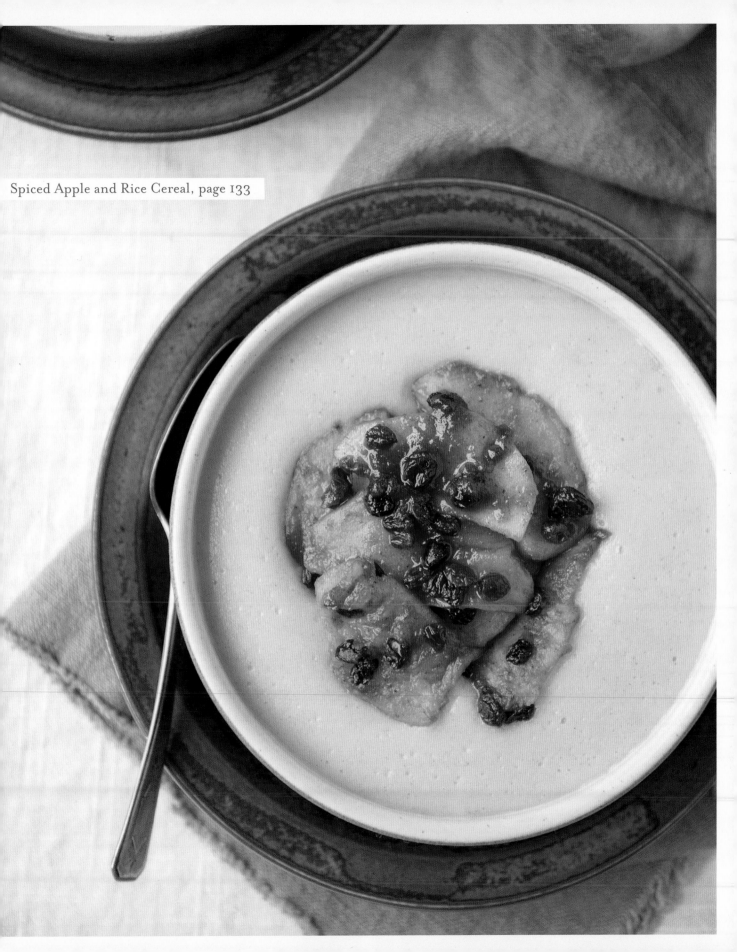

Spiced Apple and Rice Cereal, page 133

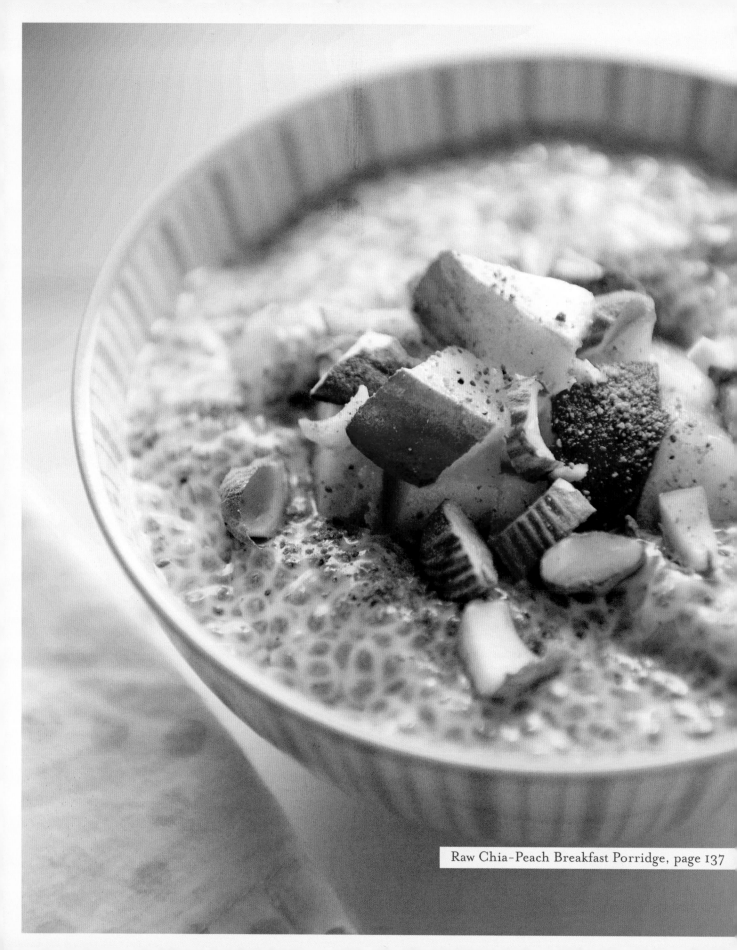

Raw Chia-Peach Breakfast Porridge, page 137

Banana-Almond Pancakes, page 138

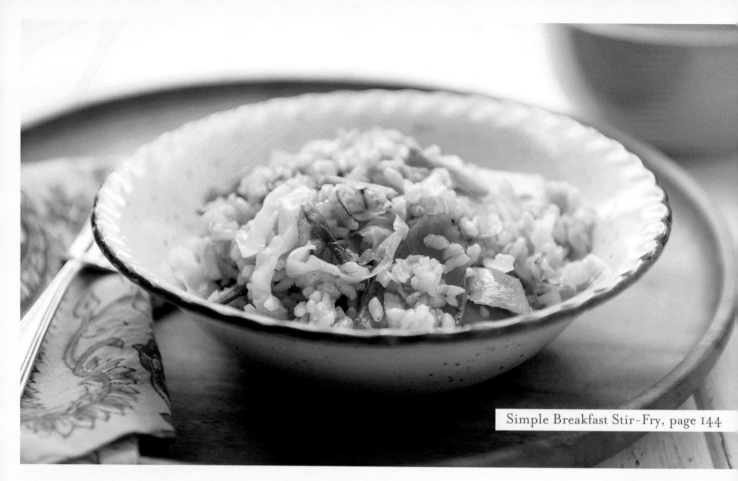

Simple Breakfast Stir-Fry, page 144

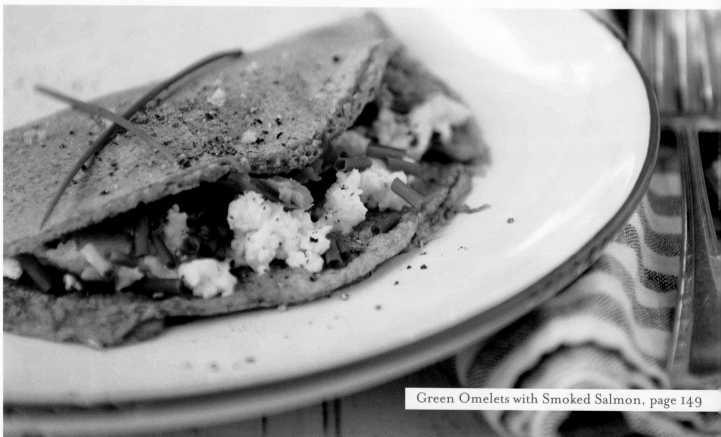

Green Omelets with Smoked Salmon, page 149

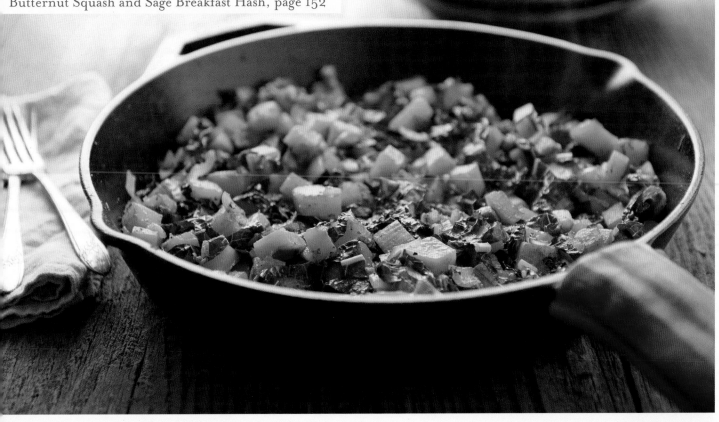

Butternut Squash and Sage Breakfast Hash, page 152

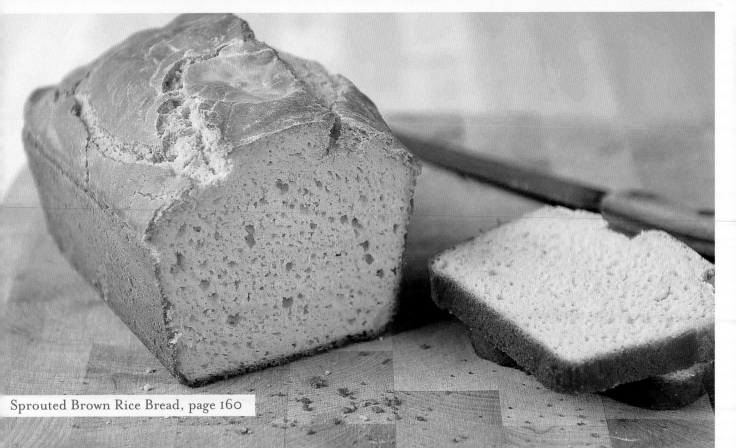

Sprouted Brown Rice Bread, page 160

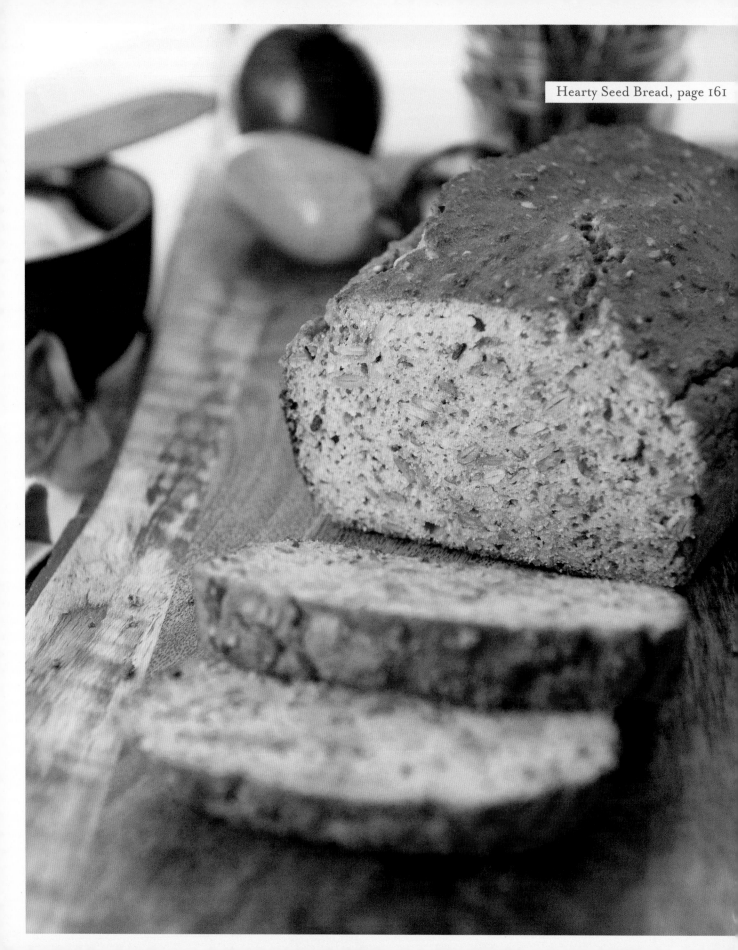

Hearty Seed Bread, page 161

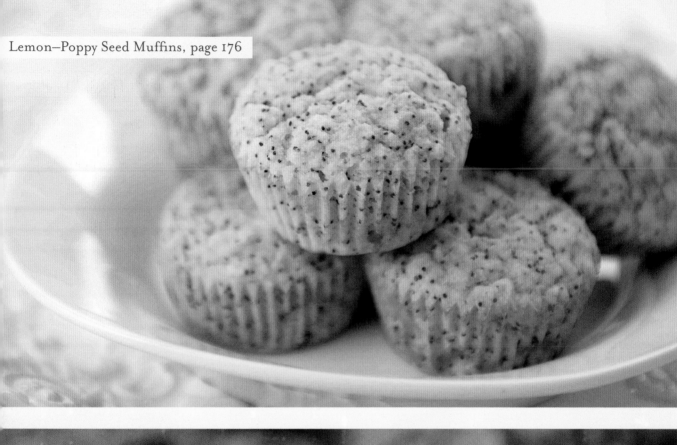

Lemon–Poppy Seed Muffins, page 176

Apple-Cranberry Oatmeal Muffins, page 172

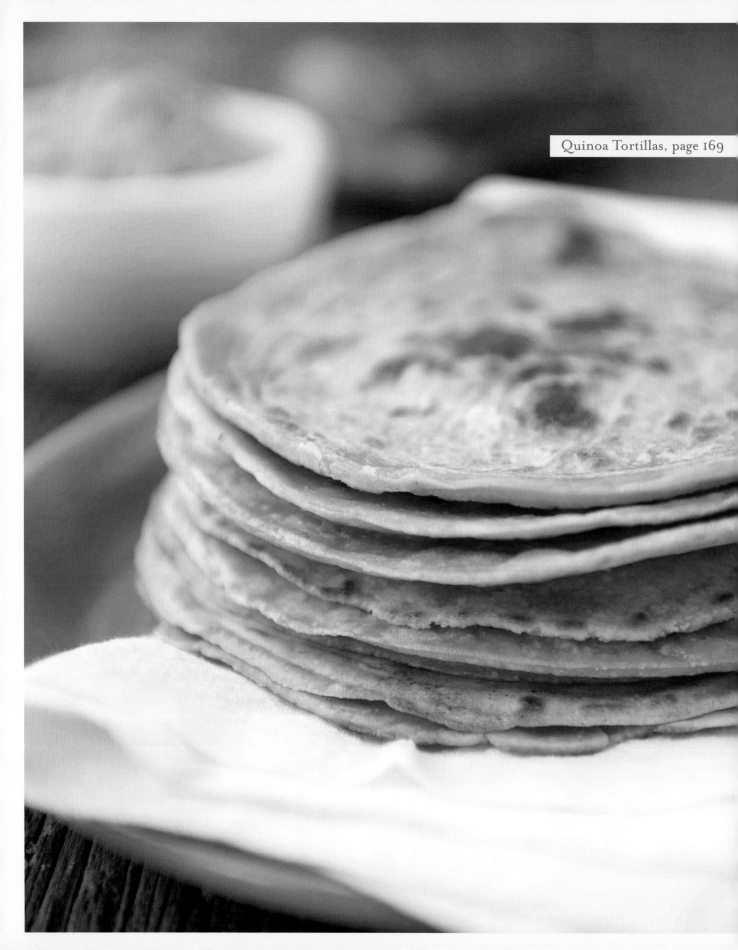

Quinoa Tortillas, page 169

KOMBUCHA

Kombucha, pronounced "kum-BOO-sha," is a drink made from tea, sugar, and a special kombucha culture. A kombucha culture looks sort of like a large pancake, though it conforms to fit the shape of the container it is in. The culture itself is a living relationship of different beneficial bacteria and special yeast cultures. The sugar is a simple carbohydrate that provides food for the yeast and bacteria. The tea provides substances that aid in the brewing process: caffeine, oxygen, nitrogen, tannic acid, vitamins, and some minerals. The yeasts break down the sugar and the bacteria then digest the yeast by-products, which create your kombucha brew. After the fermentation process is complete you are left with probiotics (beneficial bacteria), enzymes, acids (acetic, lactic, ascorbic, glucuronic), alcohol (0.5%), carbon dioxide and carbonic acid, glucose and other simple sugars (about 5%, depending on how much sugar used), B vitamins, and amino acids. You can order a healthy kombucha culture from www.CulturesForHealth.com. Though, if you ask around, you are sure to find someone who is willing to give you one.

12 cups water

¾ cup organic cane sugar

6 organic black tea bags

1 healthy kombucha culture

1½ cups plain kombucha brew as starter

Clean a large 1-gallon glass jar and set it on the countertop. Boil 12 cups of water. Place the sugar into your jar. Then pour the boiling water over the sugar and stir with a clean wooden spoon. Add the tea bags and let steep 15 to 20 minutes. Remove the tea bags and cool to room temperature.

Add your kombucha culture and 1½ cups starter brew (you can used some reserved from your last batch or buy a bottle of plain kombucha from the store). Cover the jar with a clean cloth or paper towel and secure with a rubber band.

Let the jar sit in a spot away from direct sunlight for 7 to 15 days. Begin tasting it after 7 days; if you let it ferment too long it will begin to turn into vinegar and will be too acidic to drink (you can still use it to make salad dressings though). Fermentation will happen faster in the warmer summer months, and slower in the cooler winter months. You can use pH strips to test the acidity of your brew. It should be between 2.5 to 4.

Strain your brew into a clean container and store in the refrigerator, reserving 1 cup for your next batch. Start the process again with your kombucha culture.

Each time you brew, your culture will "birth" another culture. You can give these away, plant them in your garden for compost, or use them to have a few batches of kombucha brewing at once.

Yield: about 3 quarts

Herbal Variations: Add these herbs to the boiled water in the pot along with the sugar; steep for 20 minutes. Then strain into the 1-gallon glass jar using a fine-mesh strainer lined with a coffee filter or cheesecloth.

ROOIBOS ROSE

4 tablespoons dried rose petals	3 oolong tea bags
2 to 3 tablespoons loose rooibos tea	

TULSI-GREEN

3 green tea bags	3 holy basil (tulsi) tea bags

NETTLE-DANDELION

3 white tea bags	1 tablespoon dried dandelion leaf
2 tablespoons dried nettle leaf	

Flavored Variations: Adding juice, citrus, or ginger to your brewing kombucha can damage the scoby or "mother." To make flavored kombucha you can do a second ferment, adding the flavorings after your plain kombucha has fermented for 7 to 15 days. This will also add more carbonation, creating a fizzier drink! You will need a few 1-liter glass bottles with a latch lid or you can use 1-quart jars with a lid. Using a funnel, strain your brewed kombucha into your clean glass bottles or jars about three-quarters of the way full. Add in your flavorings and put the lid on. Let ferment for 2 to 3 more days away from direct sunlight. I don't recommend doing a second ferment for longer than 3 days as pressure can build up inside the glass bottle. Be careful when you open the lid. Then strain through a fine-mesh strainer if necessary and store in the refrigerator.

GINGER-CITRUS

1 tablespoon grated fresh ginger	1 tablespoon freshly squeezed lemon juice
¼ cup freshly squeezed orange juice	

BLACKBERRY-ACAI

2 teaspoons acai powder	¼ cup mashed fresh blackberries

GRAPE SODA

¼ cup organic grape juice

CHERRY-LIME

¼ cup organic cherry juice	1 tablespoon freshly squeezed lime juice

KOMBUCHA SOURDOUGH BREAD STARTER

I normally use water and flour to make my sourdough starter. The wild yeasts present on the grains and in the air get it going quite quickly. I've heard reports that some people have a difficult time creating an active gluten-free sourdough culture this way. Using kombucha, which is full of yeasts and beneficial bacteria, is a way to ensure an active starter. Just make sure to feed your starter with equal parts water and flour every time you see a dark liquid form on top—called hooch. Use your starter to make Injera (page 168), Sourdough Pancakes (page 141), or Gluten-Free Sourdough Bread (page 159).

1 cup gluten-free, whole-grain flour
1 cup plain kombucha

more flour and water, for feeding

Place 1 cup of any gluten-free, whole-grain flour (brown rice, millet, sorghum, quinoa, amaranth, buckwheat, teff) and 1 cup of plain kombucha into a widemouthed, 1-quart jar and whisk together. Place a clean dishtowel over the jar and secure with a rubber band. Let the jar rest on your kitchen countertop away from direct sunlight for about 24 hours.

After 24 hours, add ¼ cup of gluten-free flour and ¼ cup of water and whisk together. You will keep feeding your starter like this about twice a day, or every time you see a dark layer of liquid form at the top of the starter. This layer means that your starter is starving and needs to be fed.

As your starter grows, you will need to start adding more flour and water at each feeding. By day 3 or 4 begin using ½ cup of flour and ½ cup of water. You will need to transfer your starter to a larger jar. I like to use a 2½-quart mason jar or a 1-gallon glass jar. By day 5 or 6 you should have an active bubbly starter. You can use it at this point to make injera or pancakes, but wait until it is more mature for bread baking. I like to wait until mine is at least 2 to 3 weeks old before baking bread. If you don't begin using it, you will need to increase the amount of flour and water at each feeding to 1 cup of each—your growing starter requires more food to keep it alive!

If you go on vacation, or don't plan on using your starter for a while, place it your refrigerator with a lid and feed it every 2 to 3 weeks.

Yield: 1 sourdough bread starter

12

SMOOTHIES

It is health that is the real wealth and not pieces of gold and silver.
—Mahatma Gandhi

It is indisputable that increasing the amounts of fruits and vegetables in your diet will bring you health and longevity. One of the best ways to do this is through drinking smoothies! Blenders break down food like greens, seeds, and nuts into easier-to-digest particles. In fact, a blender breaks open the cell walls of plants, freeing up vital nutrients for your body to soak up. These vital nutrients found in plants, such as antioxidants, minerals, vitamins, and amino acids, are what you build every aspect of your cells with—your health. Over 10,000 miraculous plant chemicals have been researched in the last decade, and estimates are that over four times that amount will be discovered in the next decade. Want to be fit and healthy? Eat more vegetables and fruits...and drink smoothies!

All of the recipes in this chapter are designed for a high-powered blender, such as a Vitamix or Blendtec. If you don't own one, we suggest cutting the recipe in half and making sure your blender blade is very sharp. If you are making a green smoothie with kale or collard greens, remove the tough stems that run down the center of the green leaves and tear the leaves into pieces. A high-powered blender will blend the tough stems to a fine purée but a regular blender won't. Also, if you plan on adding chia or flaxseeds to your smoothie, make sure you grind them first in a coffee grinder. A regular blender will not be able to break them down and blend them into the smoothie like a high-powered blender can.

Store your smoothies in a glass jar in your refrigerator for up to 2 days. We like to turn leftover fruit smoothies into Popsicles. I even do this with a fruity-tasting green smoothie on occasion. They make the perfect healthy afternoon treat!

BERRY ANTIOXIDANT SMOOTHIE

The beautiful dark purple and blue hues you see on berries are actually powerful antioxidants that protect against macular degeneration, reduce cardiovascular disease, decrease cancer risk, and protect brain cells! This smoothie combines blackberries, blueberries, and cherries but you can add whatever frozen berries you have on hand. Since we freeze the black currants growing in our garden during the summer, I like to add a small handful of them to this smoothie as well. Acai powder is a purple superfood powder from a berry growing in the Amazon. It is concentrated in antioxidants, amino acids, and essential fats.

2 cups Raw Almond Milk (page 417)
3 to 4 Medjool dates, pitted
1 cup frozen blackberries
1 cup frozen blueberries

1 cup frozen cherries
2 tablespoons acai powder
1 tablespoon chia seeds

Place the almond milk and dates into a high-powered blender and blend on high for about 30 seconds. Add the remaining ingredients and blend until smooth and creamy. Serve immediately.

Yield: 2 to 4 servings

Variation: Use cashew milk (see page 419) or hemp milk in place of the almond milk.

CHERRY-ALMOND SMOOTHIE

This nutrient-dense smoothie can protect your arteries and help lower your blood pressure. Almonds are a rich source of magnesium; in fact, ½ cup provides almost 200 milligrams, which is about 50% of the daily value for this mineral. Magnesium helps your blood vessels relax, which improves the flow of blood and oxygen throughout the body.

½ cup raw almonds (soaked overnight)

½ cup water

1 ripe pear, cored and cut into wedges

1 cup pitted frozen cherries

The night before you plan to make this smoothie, soak the almonds by placing them in a small dish or jar. Cover them with water and set them on the countertop to soak overnight or for at least 8 hours.

In the morning drain off the soaking water and rinse the almonds. Place them in the blender with the water and blend on high until thick and creamy. Add the pear and cherries and blend for another minute until very creamy.

Yield: 1 to 2 servings

CHILLED CHAI SMOOTHIE

Chai tea is one of my favorite beverages, but during the summertime a hot cup of tea just won't do. We make this smoothie to help beat the heat, plus it makes a nourishing and filling snack!

2 cups Raw Almond Milk (page 417)

4 to 5 Medjool dates, pitted

1 tablespoon chia seeds

1 to 1½ teaspoons ground cinnamon

1 teaspoon ground ginger

¼ teaspoon ground cardamom

3 cups ice cubes

Place all the ingredients into a high-powered blender and blend until smooth and creamy. Taste and add more spices or sweetener if desired. Add the ice cubes and blend until smooth and frothy. Serve immediately.

Yield: 4 servings

Variation: Replace the raw almond milk with cashew milk (see page 419) or with a blend of coconut milk and homemade hemp milk.

COCOA MOLE SMOOTHIE

This smoothie can be served as a dessert beverage after any Mexican-style meal. The cinnamon is the secret ingredient to this great-tasting drink!

½ cup raw cashews

1 cup water

1 large frozen banana, broken into chunks

1 to 2 tablespoons raw cacao powder

1 to 2 tablespoons honey or coconut nectar

½ to 1 teaspoon ground cinnamon

¼ teaspoon chili powder, or to taste

Place the cashews and water into a high-powered blender and blend on high until smooth and creamy. Add the banana chunks, cacao, honey, cinnamon, and chili powder and blend well. Serve immediately.

Yield: 2 to 4 servings

Tip: To freeze your ripe bananas, simply remove the peels, put them into storage containers, and place in the freezer.

ENERGIZING BERRY-NUT SMOOTHIE

This smoothie makes for a quick breakfast on the go or a nourishing afternoon snack. You can even add a few handfuls of fresh spinach or lettuce while blending for a more nutrient-packed drink.

1 cup raw cashews

1 cup water

1 large frozen banana, broken into chunks

½ cup frozen blueberries

½ cup frozen cherries

Place the raw cashews and water in a high-powered blender and blend on high until smooth and creamy. Add the frozen banana chunks, blueberries, and cherries and blend until smooth. Serve immediately.

Yield: 2 servings

FRESH COCONUT-BERRY SLUSHY

This special treat is what our children consider ice cream. When it first comes out of the blender it is very thick, but as it sits, it begins to thaw. You will need a very strong knife to crack open the coconut.

1 young coconut

2 frozen peaches or 2 cups diced frozen mango

2 cups frozen berries (raspberries, strawberries, or cherries)

1 teaspoon organic vanilla powder

Crack open the top of the young coconut and pour the coconut water into a blender. Then crack open the entire coconut, scrape out all of the meat, and place it into the blender with the water. Blend until smooth and creamy; add the remaining ingredients and blend until creamy. Serve immediately.

Yield: 4 servings

MORNING MACA POWER SMOOTHIE

We like to make this as an energizing pre-workout drink. Served about 2 hours before yoga, hiking, or running, this smoothie provides clean-burning, sustained energy that won't weigh you down. We order truly raw organic almonds online since most raw almonds sold in the store have been pasteurized. We like to buy large bunches of bananas, peel them, and freeze them whole to have on hand for recipes like this one! This recipe works best if you are using a high-powered blender.

---

1 cup raw almonds

3 cups water

3 medium frozen bananas, broken into chunks

1 cup frozen blueberries or cherries

1 to 2 tablespoons whole chia seeds

1 to 2 tablespoons maca powder

2 to 4 tablespoons hemp protein powder (optional)

The night before you plan to make this smoothie, place the almonds in a bowl and cover with about 2 inches of water. Let them soak for at least 8 hours; they will plump up and become soft during soaking. Drain and rinse.

Add the soaked almonds to the blender along with the water and blend on high until smooth and creamy. Add the remaining ingredients and any optional superfood powders and blend again until smooth and creamy. Serve immediately.

Yield: 2 to 4 servings

STRAWBERRY-BANANA-GOJI MILKSHAKE

Who doesn't love a good milkshake! This smoothie makes a great after-school snack for children or a refreshing summertime treat. I like to add a tablespoon of hemp protein powder to add more protein, but it isn't necessary. Goji berries are bright orange-red berries that come from a shrub that's native to China. They contain a powerhouse of antioxidants, minerals, trace minerals, and amino acids. They have been used medicinally in Asia for thousands of years.

2 cups Raw Almond Milk (page 417)
½ cup dried goji berries
2 medium frozen bananas, broken into chunks

2 cups frozen strawberries
1 tablespoon hemp protein powder (optional)
½ teaspoon organic vanilla powder (optional)

Place the almond milk and goji berries into a high-powered blender and blend until smooth. Add the remaining ingredients and blend until smooth and creamy. For a thinner smoothie, add more milk. Serve immediately.

> **Tip:** Make sure your bananas are very ripe when you freeze them. Underripe bananas will produce a sour-tasting smoothie.

Yield: 2 to 4 servings

Variation: Use cashew milk (see page 419) or hemp milk in place of the almond milk.

STRAWBERRY-MINT SLUSHY

During the summertime heat, there is nothing more refreshing and nourishing for the body than a frozen fruit smoothie. Try this one out to bathe your cells in antioxidants, vitamin C, and anti-inflammatory compounds.

3 cups frozen strawberries
freshly squeezed juice of 2 lemons

½ cup packed fresh mint leaves
2 to 3 cups water

Place all the ingredients into a high-powered blender and blend until smooth. Serve immediately.

Yield: 4 servings

SUMMER PEACH AND GINGER SMOOTHIE

This smoothie is a great way to use extra peaches from the summer harvest. The sweetness of the peaches and the spiciness of the ginger provide a wonderful combination.

---

2 ripe peaches, halved
one 1½-inch piece fresh ginger
½ cup coconut milk

1 tablespoon raw honey or coconut nectar
1 to 2 cups ice cubes

Place the peach halves, ginger, coconut milk, and honey into a blender and blend on high until very smooth. Add the ice cubes and blend to the desired consistency. Serve immediately.

Yield: 2 to 4 servings

AVOCADO-BANANA GREEN SMOOTHIE

I like to make this smoothie as an afternoon snack for my children when they come home from school. If there is any leftover smoothie, I pour it into Popsicle molds and freeze. The Popsicles are a brilliant, beautiful green! Did you know that eating a diet rich in raw plant foods lowers systemic inflammation in the body, which reduces the likelihood of developing food and environmental allergies? So drink up!

---

1 medium banana
1 small avocado
2 cups packed fresh spinach

one 1-inch piece fresh ginger
one 1-inch piece fresh turmeric
2 to 2½ cups coconut water

Place all the ingredients into a blender and blend until smooth. Serve immediately, or pour into glass jars and store in the refrigerator for up to 2 days, or freeze Popsicle molds.

Yield: 2 to 4 servings

CREAMY ALMOND-KALE SMOOTHIE

This smoothie recipe makes a great after-school snack for your children. Serve it with carrot sticks and apple slices. I also like to make it for breakfast and serve it along with scrambled eggs.

---

2 cups Raw Almond Milk (page 417)
½ bunch kale

1 to 2 pears, cored and chopped

Place the almond milk and kale into a high-powered blender and blend until smooth and creamy. Start by adding 1 pear and, if you need the smoothie a little sweeter, add part or all of the second pear and blend again until smooth and creamy. Drink immediately, or store in a covered glass jar in your refrigerator for up to 2 days.

Yield: 4 cups

GREEN GRAPE SMOOTHIE

This smoothie is both refreshing and cleansing. I like to make it on a warm summer afternoon to help rehydrate and cool down. For maximum cleansing benefits, drink this smoothie at least 2 hours after or 1 hour before a meal. When organic grapes are in season, I take them off the vine and store them in my freezer to be able to have them on hand for smoothies like this one.

---

2 cups frozen green grapes

1 small cucumber, chopped

freshly squeezed juice of 1 lime

2 cups water

4 cups chopped green leaf lettuce, rinsed

3 to 4 dandelion greens (optional)

1 tablespoon chia seeds

Place the grapes, cucumber, lime juice, and water into a blender and blend until smooth. Add the lettuce, dandelion greens, and chia seeds and blend again until smooth. Serve immediately. Store any leftover smoothie in a glass jar in the refrigerator for up to 2 days, or pour into Popsicle molds for green fruit pops!

Yield: 2 to 4 servings

Variation: Replace the lettuce with kale, collard greens, or any other green that is fresh and in season.

GREEN TEA ANTIOXIDANT SMOOTHIE

This is one of my favorite smoothies to drink for breakfast before I go to yoga. I love the kick from the green tea, plus the smoothie is so easy to digest that I can get into those twisting poses without feeling like I'm still trying to digest breakfast! Change up the greens based on what you have on hand. I've used kale, lettuce, broccoli leaves, and collards—they all work.

2 cups chilled green tea

2 pears, cored

2 cups chopped bok choy

1 cup spinach leaves

one 1-inch piece fresh ginger

2 tablespoons hemp seeds

1 tablespoon chia seeds

a few ice cubes

Place all the ingredients into a high-powered blender and blend until smooth. Add a few ice cubes for a cold smoothie, and blend again. Serve immediately, or pour into a tightly sealed glass jar and store in your refrigerator for up to a day.

Yield: 2 to 4 servings

Tip: To make green tea, pour 2 cups of boiling water over 2 organic green tea bags (I use a 2-cup liquid glass measure). Then steep for about 3 minutes, remove the tea bags and transfer the tea to the refrigerator to chill.

LEMONY CABBAGE AND CRANBERRY SMOOTHIE

This smoothie has a beautiful pink hue from the cranberries and is as medicinal as it is delicious. Cabbage is a rich source of cancer-fighting phytochemicals called glucosinolates. Cranberries are also a rich source of phytochemicals including proanthocyanidins, which work in the body to prevent and treat urinary tract infections; quinic acid, which helps to prevent kidney stones; and anthocyanidins, which have been shown to inhibit the development of atherosclerosis, cancer, and other degenerative diseases. Fresh cranberries have the highest antioxidant levels compared to dried cranberries or processed juices.

2 medium apples, cored and cut into chunks

2 ripe pears, cored and cut into chunks

1 cup water

freshly squeezed juice of 2 lemons

½ cup fresh or frozen cranberries

5 Napa or Savoy cabbage leaves

one 1- to 2-inch piece fresh ginger

Place the apple and pear chunks, water, and lemon juice into a high-powered blender and blend until smooth and creamy. Add the cranberries, cabbage leaves, and ginger and blend again on high until very smooth. Serve immediately, or store in a glass jar in the refrigerator for up to 2 days.

Yield: 2 to 4 servings

MINTY GREEN SMOOTHIE

Drinking your greens in a smoothie is an easy and digestible way to get many of the green vegetables we need daily to support and recharge our bodies. Kale is a powerful, medicinal food providing ample protective phytochemicals. This recipe is very adaptable to what you have on hand; try substituting the banana for another pear and add the juice of a lime.

---

1 ripe banana, peeled and broken into chunks

1 medium apple, cored and cut into chunks

1 ripe pear, cored and cut into chunks

freshly squeezed juice of 1 lemon

2 to 3 cups water

3 to 4 large spinach leaves

3 to 4 kale leaves

¼ cup fresh parsley leaves

1 small handful fresh mint leaves

Place the banana, apple, and pear chunks, lemon juice, and water into the blender. Blend on high, stopping as needed to push the fruit down.

Add the spinach leaves, kale, parsley, and mint and blend again until very smooth, adding more water if needed and blending until completely smooth and a brilliant green.

Yield: 2 to 4 servings

MINTY AVOCADO-KALE SMOOTHIE

The fat from the avocados in this smoothie helps to absorb the carotenoids in the greens! Enjoy this tasty smoothie as a snack or as an energizing breakfast.

---

2 ripe pears, cored
2 small avocados
freshly squeezed juice of 2 lemons
one 1-inch piece fresh ginger

5 to 6 large kale leaves
1 handful fresh mint leaves
3 to 4 cups water

Place all the ingredients into a high-powered blender and blend until smooth. Serve immediately, or pour into quart jars and store in the refrigerator for up to 2 days.

Yield: 2 to 4 servings

PEACH-GINGER-MINT GREEN SMOOTHIE

If you don't have peaches use plums, apples, pears, or a mixture of frozen blueberries and cherries instead. If you want to make this more refreshing on a hot summer afternoon, add a few handfuls of ice cubes to the blender and blend again. I like to use this smoothie as a late afternoon pick-me-up— green smoothies are a natural energizing drink! Add a squeeze of fresh lime juice to each serving if desired.

---

3 large peaches, pitted
one 2-inch piece fresh ginger
1 small bunch bok choy
½ bunch kale

1 medium cucumber, cut into large pieces
1 large handful fresh mint leaves
2 to 3 cups water

Place all the ingredients into a high-powered blender and blend until smooth. For a thinner smoothie, add more water. If it is too bitter, add another piece of fruit or liquid stevia to taste.

Yield: 2 quarts

REFRESHING APPLE-CILANTRO GREEN SMOOTHIE

My mother-in-law taught me how to make this amazing green drink! I would have never thought to add cilantro to a smoothie before she showed me. The avocado adds some fat, which slows down the digestion of the smoothie. Sometimes I will drink a quart of this for breakfast, or will enjoy a glass late in the afternoon for an energy boost!

2 apples, cored	1 bunch fresh cilantro, leaves and stems
2 small avocados	freshly squeezed juice of 2 limes
4 to 5 collard greens	3 cups water

Place all the ingredients into a high-powered blender and blend until smooth. Add more water for a thinner consistency. This smoothie will keep in the refrigerator for up to 2 days.

Yield: 2 to 4 servings

TOM'S FRUITY MEDICINE CHEST SMOOTHIE

Tom makes a large batch of this smoothie nearly every morning. The fruit in it changes according to the seasons. In the summer we use peaches and nectarines instead of pears and apples. The fruit is a rich source of soluble fiber and a host of vitamins and antioxidants. The greens offer powerful phytochemicals. Cabbage is a potent food that affects many pathways in the body. Ginger is a powerful anti-inflammatory. The lemon offers vitamin C and bioflavonoids. And yes, it tastes great, as many of the people in our cooking classes will tell you. This smoothie makes enough to fill a Vitamix so divide the recipe in half if you are using a regular blender.

2 apples, cored and cut into chunks
2 ripe pears, cored and cut into chunks
2 to 3 cups water
freshly squeezed juice of 2 lemons
one 1- to 2-inch piece fresh ginger
5 kale leaves
5 romaine lettuce leaves, spinach leaves, or collard greens

1 cup coarsely chopped green cabbage (optional)

OPTIONAL ADDITIONS
1 kiwi fruit
1 handful fresh parsley or mint leaves
2 tablespoons chia seeds
½ cup soaked goji berries

Place the apple and pear chunks, water, and lemon juice into a high-powered blender and blend until smooth and creamy. Add any optional additions you would like; blend again.

Add the ginger, kale, lettuce, and cabbage and blend again until very smooth. For a thinner smoothie, add more water. If the taste is too "lettucy" for you, add another pear and blend again.

Yield: 2 to 4 servings

13

BREAKFAST

Wisdom begins in wonder.

—*Socrates*

The word *breakfast* literally means "to break the fast." This is a time of the day when your body is ready to receive nourishment after a night of fasting. The mind and body function much better throughout the day if they are fed upon awakening.

Skipping breakfast may lead to overeating at later meals. This is because you will be hungrier and will tend to eat faster and larger portions to relieve the hunger and desire for food. When you are very hungry it is easier to eat too much as well as to eat foods that have a high fat and sugar content.

One of the fastest ways to boost your metabolism is to simply eat a nutritious breakfast every morning. Choose foods such as whole-grain cereals, any combination of nuts and fruits, organic eggs, tofu, or even miso soup with fish added to it. All of these foods eaten first thing in the morning readily give your metabolism a boost for the entire day and provide your body with the nutrients you need to function properly. If you are unaccustomed to consuming food in the morning, then it may take a little more planning until you get in the habit of morning meals. Plan your breakfast before you go to bed the night before. Set out any items to be used to prepare your breakfast and be sure your kitchen is clean.

QUICK NUTRITIOUS BREAKFAST IDEAS

- ✓ Plain cooked millet or quinoa with chopped raw nuts and fresh or dried fruit on top. (See pages 262–264 for how to cook whole grains.)
- ✓ 2 organic hard-boiled eggs, steamed kale, cooked quinoa, and a spoonful of raw cultured vegetables on the side
- ✓ A bowl of your favorite seasonal organic fruit topped with soaked raw almonds
- ✓ Leftover beans and grains wrapped up in a lettuce or cabbage leaf with your favorite fixings
- ✓ Leftover cooked salmon over Breakfast Greens (page 155)
- ✓ Gluten-free muffin and a fresh green smoothie
- ✓ Leftover cooked brown rice stir-fried with vegetables and eggs
- ✓ Sautéed organic sausages and a green smoothie

GLORIOUS MORNING FRUIT BOWL

Fruit bowls provide a light breakfast for those days when you feel a little sluggish in the morning. Soaking the almonds overnight helps them to become more digestible and allows for their nutrients to become more bioavailable. You could use raw sprouted almonds instead of soaking your own. These can sometimes be found at your local health food store.

½ cup raw organic almonds

1 ripe mango, peeled and cut into chunks

1 ripe banana, peeled and sliced

2 kiwis, peeled and diced

1 ripe pear, cut into chunks

2 tablespoons freshly squeezed lime juice

2 to 4 tablespoons organic shredded coconut

Soak the almonds in a bowl filled with 1½ cups filtered water, at room temperature, for 8 to 10 hours or overnight.

In the morning drain off the soaking water and rinse the almonds well. Transfer the almonds to a cutting board and chop.

Transfer the chopped almonds to a bowl and gently mix with the remaining ingredients.

Yield: 2 to 4 servings

SUMMER FRUIT BOWL

I like to make some variation of this recipe at least twice a week for breakfast in the summertime. We pile on the chopped almonds, chia seeds, and raw cacao nibs to help stay satisfied longer.

2 peaches, chopped

1 to 2 small avocados, diced

1 cup fresh blueberries

1 cup fresh raspberries

freshly squeezed juice of 1 lime

½ cup raw sprouted almonds, chopped

¼ cup raw cacao nibs

2 tablespoons chia seeds

Place the peaches, avocados, blueberries, raspberries, and lime juice into a serving bowl and gently toss together. Sprinkle with the almonds, cacao nibs, and chia seeds. Serve immediately.

Yield: 2 to 4 servings

CINNAMON-SPICED GRANOLA

This easy-to-make granola is perfect to have on hand for busy mornings. It can be topped with fresh fruit, served with a dollop of organic yogurt, or served as a breakfast cereal with raw almond milk or homemade Coconut Milk Yogurt (page 104). You can add any dried fruit after it has been cooked. If you have a nut allergy, then substitute sunflower seeds and pumpkin seeds for the nuts.

3 cups rolled oats
1 cup coarsely chopped raw walnuts
1 cup coarsely chopped raw almonds
1 tablespoon ground cinnamon
½ teaspoon ground nutmeg
¼ teaspoon ground cloves
¼ teaspoon ground ginger
¼ teaspoon sea salt
½ cup pure maple syrup
½ cup melted virgin coconut oil
1 teaspoon vanilla extract

OPTIONAL ADDITIONS
chopped dried apple
raisins
dried cranberries
dried cherries
shredded coconut
sunflower seeds
pumpkin seeds

Preheat the oven to 300°F. Place the rolled oats, chopped nuts, spices, and sea salt into a medium bowl and mix well.

Add the maple syrup, melted coconut oil, and vanilla to the oat mixture and toss together using two spoons.

Spread the mixture out on a large baking sheet and bake for 35 to 40 minutes, turning occasionally with a spatula.

Remove from the oven and stir in dried fruit if using. Let cool completely before transferring to a large glass jar. Granola will keep in a tightly sealed jar in your pantry for about 2 to 3 weeks.

Yield: 5 cups

MORNING MILLET CEREAL

This delicious breakfast cereal is wonderful by itself or it can be topped with chopped dates and nuts. My favorite way to serve this is to top each bowl with diced fresh peaches, raw almond milk, and a dash of ground nutmeg. Millet is a good source of manganese, phosphorus, and magnesium.

1 cup millet (soaked overnight)
1 tablespoon raw apple cider vinegar

3 to 4 cups water
pinch sea salt

Place the millet in a bowl and cover with at least 1 inch of water; add the vinegar. Let the mixture soak on your countertop for 8 to 12 hours, or overnight.

In the morning, drain and rinse the millet in a fine-mesh strainer. Place the millet, water, and sea salt into a blender and blend on high until smooth. Pour the mixture into a medium saucepan and bring to a boil, whisking constantly. Reduce the heat to low and continue to cook, stirring occasionally, until the cereal has thickened and the millet is cooked, about 15 minutes. Serve hot.

Yield: 4 small servings

SWEET RICE CEREAL

This creamy, warming cereal can be served as a light breakfast or bedtime snack. I used to cook this at night when I was pregnant with my twins—it would stave off late-night hunger and help me sleep. It is best topped with a little maple syrup and a spoonful of virgin coconut oil or pastured butter. Brown rice is an excellent source of manganese and a good source of selenium and magnesium.

---

1 cup sweet brown rice (soaked overnight)
1 tablespoon raw apple cider vinegar

3 cups water
pinch sea salt

Place the sweet rice in a bowl and cover with at least 1 inch of water; add the vinegar. Let the mixture soak on your countertop for 8 to 12 hours, or overnight.

In the morning, drain and rinse the rice in a fine-mesh strainer. Place the rice, water, and sea salt into a blender and blend on high until smooth. Pour the mixture into a medium saucepan and bring to a boil, whisking constantly. Reduce the heat to low and continue to cook, stirring occasionally, until the cereal has thickened and rice is cooked, about 15 minutes. Serve hot.

Yield: 3 to 4 servings

SPICED APPLE AND RICE CEREAL

Serve this warming cereal on a cool fall morning before work or school. In the summertime, we like to use fresh peaches instead of apples for the topping and freshly ground raw almonds instead of walnuts for the garnish.

CEREAL

1 cup brown basmati rice (soaked overnight)

1 tablespoon raw apple cider vinegar

3 to 4 cups water

½ teaspoon ground cinnamon

¼ teaspoon ground cardamom

pinch sea salt

APPLE TOPPING

2 teaspoons virgin coconut oil or organic butter

2 to 3 tart apples, cored and thinly sliced

¼ cup dried currants (optional)

2 tablespoons pure maple syrup

1 teaspoon ground cinnamon

¼ teaspoon ground nutmeg

4 to 6 tablespoons water

GARNISH

chopped raw walnuts (optional)

To make the cereal, place the rice in a bowl and cover with at least 1 inch of water; add the vinegar. Let the mixture soak on your countertop for 8 to 12 hours, or overnight.

In the morning, drain and rinse the rice in a fine-mesh strainer. Place the rice, water, spices, and sea salt into a blender and blend on high until smooth. Pour the mixture into a medium saucepan and bring to a boil, whisking constantly. Reduce the heat to low and continue to cook, stirring occasionally, until the cereal has thickened and the rice is cooked, about 10 minutes. For a thinner consistency, add more water. When cooked, remove from the heat.

To make the topping, heat the coconut oil in a 10-inch skillet over medium heat. Add the apples, currants, maple syrup, cinnamon, and nutmeg and sauté for about 2 minutes. Add the water and simmer, uncovered, for about 5 minutes, stirring frequently.

Fill individual serving bowls with the hot cereal and spoon the apple mixture over each. Garnish with chopped walnuts if desired.

Yield: 4 small servings

TEFF BREAKFAST PORRIDGE

Teff, an ancient Ethiopian grain, is very high in protein and iron. It cooks quickly and easily, making it an ideal quick breakfast. Try topping the porridge with dried cranberries or cherries and finely chopped nuts. In the summertime, we top this with sliced peaches or nectarines, ground raw almonds, and a drizzle of honey.

3 cups water	1 cup teff grain
pinch sea salt	

In a medium pot, bring the water and sea salt to a boil. Add the teff and stir a little. Cook, covered, for 15 to 20 minutes, stirring occasionally toward the end of the cooking time.

Ladle into serving bowls and top with dried or fresh fruit and chopped nuts if desired.

Yield: 2 to 3 servings

WARMING THREE-GRAIN MORNING CEREAL

The combination of the quinoa, millet, and amaranth make this morning porridge especially nutritious and very high in protein. The nutty flavor of the three grains lends some heartiness to your morning meal. Try adding some ground toasted pumpkin seeds on top with sliced apples and a dash of honey or maple syrup.

¾ cup quinoa

¾ cup millet

¾ cup amaranth

5 cups water

pinch sea salt

Rinse the all the grains in a very fine-mesh strainer. Let warm water run through them while you move them around with your hand. Rinsing is a very important step to remove the bitter saponin coating on the outside of the grains.

Place the washed grains into a 2- or 3-quart pot with the water and sea salt, cover, and bring to a boil. Reduce the heat to low and simmer for about 25 minutes. Remove from the heat and serve with your favorite toppings.

Yield: 3 to 4 servings

> **Tip:** For increased digestibility, soak the grains overnight in a bowl of filtered water and 1 tablespoon raw apple cider vinegar. Then rinse and drain in a fine-mesh strainer and proceed with the recipe as directed.

NUTTY GRAIN-FREE BREAKFAST PORRIDGE

I like to make this as a quick high-protein breakfast for my children before school. They like it sprinkled with cinnamon and frozen blueberries. You can use different nuts and seeds in place of the ones I use here. I prefer using the small native pecans as the base in this porridge for their mild flavor and sweetness. For better digestion and nutrient absorption, use soaked and dehydrated nuts. Alternatively, you can soak the nuts called for in this recipe overnight, drain, and then use as directed below.

1 cup raw pecans

½ cup raw almonds

2 tablespoons flaxseeds

1 tablespoon chia seeds

2 Medjool dates, pitted

2 cups water

Place all the ingredients into a high-powered blender and blend until smooth. Pour into a medium saucepan over low heat, and cook, stirring frequently, until thickened and warmed, about 5 minutes. Serve immediately with your favorite toppings.

Yield: 4 servings

RAW CHIA-PEACH BREAKFAST PORRIDGE

When soaked, chia seeds expand and thicken the liquid they are in. You can also make a raw pudding using this method by adding a few more tablespoons of sweetener. I love the combination of peaches, almond milk, and freshly grated nutmeg, but you can play around with the ingredients. Try mashed banana in place of the peach, and add a sprinkling of raw cacao nibs on top of the pudding. You can also stir in fresh berries and ground cinnamon for another variation.

This porridge requires overnight soaking and refrigeration.

2 cups Raw Almond Milk (page 417)	**OPTIONAL TOPPINGS**
6 tablespoons whole chia seeds	chopped raw almonds
1 tablespoon pure maple syrup	diced peaches
¼ teaspoon organic vanilla powder	fresh blueberries
1 large peach, diced	freshly grated nutmeg

Place the raw almond milk, chia seeds, maple syrup, and vanilla powder into a 1-quart glass jar. Screw on the lid and shake well. Let the mixture sit on the countertop for about 30 minutes, then shake again. Transfer the jar to the refrigerator to sit overnight, or for about 8 hours.

In the morning, shake the jar again. If you have time, it is best to bring the porridge to room temperature before serving. Pour the chia porridge into a serving bowl, stir in the peaches, and serve with optional toppings if using. Store any leftover porridge in a covered glass container in the refrigerator for up to 3 days.

Yield: 3 to 4 servings

BANANA-ALMOND PANCAKES

I love making these high-protein, grain-free pancakes for my children in the morning. They like them drizzled with maple syrup; I like them topped with fresh berries and sliced bananas.

---

4 large organic eggs

1 medium ripe banana

½ cup water

2 cups blanched almond flour

⅓ cup arrowroot powder

½ teaspoon baking soda

¼ teaspoon sea salt

organic butter or virgin coconut oil, for cooking

Heat a 10-inch cast-iron or stainless steel skillet over medium-low heat. I like to make sure my skillet has preheated completely before making the first pancake.

Place all the ingredients except for the butter or coconut oil into a blender and blend until smooth. Add a few teaspoons of butter or coconut oil to the hot skillet. Pour in the batter, using about ⅓ cup per pancake, and cook for 60 to 90 seconds on the first side; then flip and cook for about 60 seconds on the opposite side. Continue making pancakes until all of the batter has been used, adding more butter as needed in between batches to prevent sticking. Transfer to a warm plate and serve.

Yield: 8 to 10 pancakes

BUCKWHEAT PANCAKES

These rich yet light pancakes are always a crowd-pleaser. Try serving them with pure maple syrup, fresh plum or apricot slices, and a sprinkling of cinnamon. They are also delicious served with the Warm Berry Sauce (page 359). I prefer to grind my own buckwheat flour from raw buckwheat groats in a coffee grinder just prior to making these. I find the flavor superior to packaged buckwheat flour. Many people who dislike the strong flavor of buckwheat will enjoy these when made with the freshly ground flour.

DRY INGREDIENTS

1 heaping cup freshly ground buckwheat flour

¼ cup tapioca flour

1 teaspoon baking powder

½ teaspoon baking soda

¼ teaspoon sea salt

WET INGREDIENTS

1 to 1½ cups milk (dairy or nondairy)

1 large organic egg

2 tablespoons melted virgin coconut oil or organic butter

1 tablespoon pure maple syrup

virgin coconut oil or organic butter for cooking

In a medium bowl, mix together the dry ingredients. In a separate bowl, whisk together the wet ingredients. Add the wet ingredients to the dry and gently mix until all the ingredients are combined. Let the batter rest a few minutes to thicken up.

Heat a heavy-bottomed stainless steel skillet over medium heat. Add a few teaspoons of coconut oil. When the skillet has heated, add about ½ cup of the batter per pancake and cook for 1 to 2 minutes, or until the tops begin to bubble; flip and cook for a minute or so more on the opposite side. Repeat making pancakes until all of the batter has been used, adding a little coconut oil in between batches to prevent sticking. Transfer the pancakes to a warm plate and serve.

> **Tip:** To grind fresh buckwheat flour, add 2 cups raw buckwheat groats to a high-powered blender and blend to a fine flour. You can do this in a coffee grinder as well, ½ cup at a time. I buy raw, organic buckwheat groats from Bob's Red Mill, which are also certified gluten-free.

Yield: 5 to 7 pancakes

Egg-Free Variation: Replace the egg with 1 tablespoon ground chia seeds, whisked with ¼ cup warm water.

OATMEAL-BLUEBERRY-BANANA PANCAKES

Serve these little gems alongside sautéed zucchini and sausages for a balanced breakfast.

1½ cups gluten-free rolled oats
¾ teaspoon baking powder
¼ teaspoon baking soda
pinch sea salt
¼ cup water

2 tablespoons melted virgin coconut oil
1 tablespoon pure maple syrup
1 small banana, lightly mashed
½ cup blueberries
virgin coconut oil, for cooking

Grind the oats to a fine powder in an electric mixer or coffee grinder. Place the ground oats, baking powder, baking soda, and sea salt into a medium mixing bowl and stir to combine.

In a separate bowl, combine the water, melted coconut oil, maple syrup, and mashed banana and stir together. Pour the wet ingredients into the dry and mix to combine. Gently fold in the blueberries. If the batter is too thick, add more water.

Heat a heavy-bottomed skillet over medium-low heat. Add a little coconut oil and drop the batter into the skillet, using ½ cup per pancake. Cook for about 2 minutes on each side. Watch the temperature very carefully to avoid burning. Add more coconut oil to the skillet before cooking the next pancake. Repeat this process until all the batter has been used.

Yield: 5 to 7 small pancakes

SOURDOUGH PANCAKES

Serve these nourishing pancakes with a green smoothie and a poached egg for breakfast. Sometimes my children will pack leftover pancakes for their school lunch! Be sure to use your sourdough starter when it is active and bubbly, within a few hours after feeding it.

1 cup sourdough starter (page 109)

1 cup gluten-free, whole-grain flour

2 large organic eggs

½ cup water

2 tablespoons melted organic butter or virgin coconut oil, plus more for cooking

2 tablespoons coconut sugar

½ teaspoon baking soda

½ teaspoon sea salt

Heat a large heavy-bottomed skillet over medium-low heat. I use a 12-inch cast-iron skillet so I can cook two pancakes at once.

Add all the ingredients except for the maple syrup to a medium mixing bowl and whisk together. Drop the batter onto the hot skillet using ¼ cup per pancake. Cook for 60 seconds on each side. Repeat the process with the remaining batter.

Serve with pure maple syrup or jam, if desired.

Yield: about twelve 4-inch pancakes

GERMAN BANANA-CINNAMON PANCAKES

My German grandmother passed a recipe down to my mom called "onguspinoncus"—another name for a German pancake made with eggs, milk, flour, butter, and sugar that's baked in the oven. We used to have it for breakfast a few times a month and it was always a favorite treat! I've created a new grain-free version that's much healthier. I highly recommend using a cast-iron skillet, but if you don't own one you can use a baking dish instead. Serve with sliced bananas, a sprinkling of cinnamon, and a dollop of homemade Coconut Milk Yogurt (page 104).

5 large organic eggs
1 cup coconut milk
1 large ripe banana
½ cup blanched almond flour, packed
¼ cup arrowroot powder

2 to 3 teaspoons ground cinnamon
pinch sea salt
2 to 3 tablespoons virgin coconut oil or organic butter

Preheat the oven to 425°F.

Put all the ingredients except the coconut oil into a blender and blend on high until smooth and creamy. Heat a 10-inch cast-iron skillet over low heat. Add the coconut oil or butter to the skillet and let it melt.

Pour in the pancake batter. Place the skillet into the oven and bake the pancake for 20 to 25 minutes. It should puff up by the end of baking time and then sink down as it cools. Remove the skillet from the oven, slice the pancake into wedges, and serve with desired toppings.

Yield: 4 to 6 servings

ROOT VEGETABLE PANCAKES

Serve these hearty pancakes with scrambled organic eggs or tofu and a spoonful of Cultured Vegetables (page 90). I like to use my food processor for these; first I mince the onion with the "s" blade, then I put in the grating disk and grate the vegetables. It only takes a minute or two to do all this. To get the pancakes on the table faster, try cooking them in two or three skillets at once.

1 small onion, minced

1 small yam, peeled and grated

2 medium yellow or red potatoes, grated

1 carrot, grated

¼ to ½ cup brown rice flour or sorghum flour

1 tablespoon dulse flakes

1 teaspoon dried thyme

½ teaspoon sea salt or Herbamare

extra-virgin olive oil, for cooking

Place the minced onion and grated vegetables into a large bowl. Add the flour, dulse flakes, thyme, and sea salt or Herbamare and mix well.

Heat a 10-inch cast-iron skillet over medium heat. Form the vegetable mixture into thin patties with your hands. They will fall apart when raw, but when cooked the starches will be released and they will hold together.

Add a few teaspoons olive oil and one or two patties to the heated skillet. Cover the skillet with a lid and cook for approximately 5 minutes. Flip the patties, cover, and cook for another 5 minutes. Transfer to a serving platter. Add a little more olive oil to the skillet for each batch of patties you cook, adjusting the temperature as needed to prevent burning.

Yield: 5 to 7 pancakes

Variation: Add 1 large organic egg to the grated root vegetable mixture and stir well. This helps the pancakes cook up easier, though the egg-free version works great too.

SIMPLE BREAKFAST STIR-FRY

We often have leftover rice from the previous night's dinner. By using it for breakfast you can create a very quick and healthy meal. I serve this simple stir-fry along with fried organic eggs and a spoonful of Cultured Vegetables (page 90).

---

1 tablespoon toasted sesame oil

4 to 5 green onions, cut into 1-inch pieces

2 to 3 carrots, sliced

2 cups sliced green cabbage

3 cups cooked brown rice

sea salt

freshly ground black pepper

Heat the sesame oil in an 11- or 12-inch cast-iron skillet over medium heat. Add the green onions, carrots, and cabbage and sauté 5 to 10 minutes, or until they reach the desired tenderness. Add the cooked brown rice and stir-fry it with the vegetables for another minute or two, adding more oil if necessary so that the rice doesn't stick to the skillet. Season to taste with sea salt and pepper. Serve immediately.

Yield: 2 to 4 servings

Variation: Use leftover quinoa or millet in place of the rice.

> **Tip:** Instead of black pepper, I like to use a spice called *Pippali*, which is a close relative of black pepper. It stimulates the metabolism and digestion, as well as promotes healthy blood circulation. It has a warming, mildly spicy flavor. In fact, you can use it anywhere black pepper is called for in a recipe; however, this recipe seems to benefit most from the addition of Pippali.

TOFU SCRAMBLE

Serve this egg-free scramble recipe with the Minty Green Smoothie (page 123), or the Breakfast Greens (page 155) for a balanced meal.

1 tablespoon extra-virgin olive oil or coconut oil
5 green onions, sliced into rounds
1½ cups chopped mushrooms
1 small red bell pepper, diced
1 teaspoon dried thyme

1 garlic clove, crushed
½ to 1 teaspoon ground turmeric
1 teaspoon sea salt or Herbamare
1 pound organic firm tofu, crumbled

Heat the oil in a 10- or 11-inch skillet over medium heat. Add the green onions, mushrooms, and bell pepper and sauté until tender, 5 to 7 minutes.

Add the thyme, garlic, turmeric, and sea salt and sauté a minute more, stirring to coat.

Add the crumbled tofu, mixing it into the vegetables, and sauté 2 minutes more. If the mixture seems dry, add a few tablespoons of water.

Yield: 3 to 4 servings

TOFU AND ARAME SCRAMBLE

Arame is a sea vegetable that is harvested off the coast of Ise, Japan. With its sweet mild flavor, arame is a good sea vegetable to start with if you are unfamiliar with the flavors of seaweeds. It is rich in iodine, magnesium, calcium, and carotenoids. It is also a source of potassium, iron, vitamin B2, zinc, and many essential trace minerals. Serve with Root Vegetable Pancakes (page 143) and Breakfast Greens (page 155) for a meal that will keep you going all morning long.

¼ cup arame, soaked in water for 10 minutes

1 cup water

1 tablespoon extra-virgin olive oil or virgin coconut oil

1 bunch green onions, sliced into rounds

1 small red bell pepper, diced

3 garlic cloves, crushed

1½ teaspoons ground coriander

1 teaspoon ground turmeric

1 pound organic firm tofu, crumbled

1 to 2 tablespoons wheat-free tamari

¼ cup chopped fresh cilantro

Drain the arame, place it into a small pot with a cup of water, and simmer for 10 minutes; drain and set aside.

Heat the olive oil in a 10- or 11-inch skillet over medium heat. Add the green onions, bell pepper, and garlic and sauté for about 5 minutes, or until the bell pepper is tender.

Add the coriander, turmeric, tofu, and arame and cook for 5 to 7 minutes, stirring occasionally. Remove from the heat, add the tamari, and mix well. Sprinkle with the cilantro and serve.

Yield: 3 to 4 servings

SIMPLE SCRAMBLED EGGS

This is a tasty way to add more flavor and nutrients to plain scrambled eggs. When buying eggs, look for organic, pastured eggs. This means the chickens had plenty of room to roam outside on pastureland, eating their natural diet of grasses and bugs. Avoid "free-range" eggs, which just means the chickens were raised indoors in large hen houses and fed a diet of nonorganic grains (often genetically modified).

4 large organic, pastured eggs

2 tablespoons water

organic butter or virgin coconut oil, for cooking

½ cup chopped cherry tomatoes

¼ cup chopped fresh cilantro

4 green onions, thinly sliced

organic hot sauce

sea salt or Herbamare

Crack the eggs into a small mixing bowl, add the water, and whisk together.

Heat a 10-inch cast-iron or stainless steel skillet over medium-low heat. Add 2 to 3 teaspoons of organic butter or coconut oil and heat until melted. Add the eggs and scramble them with a silicone spatula, being very careful not to brown them.

Remove the skillet from the heat, add the tomatoes, cilantro, and green onions, and stir in gently. Season with hot sauce and sea salt or Herbamare to taste.

Yield: 2 servings

> **Tip:** The trick to making scrambled eggs that don't stick to the pan is to make sure the pan has preheated for at least 5 minutes over medium-low heat. Then add the butter or coconut oil and let it heat up for about 30 seconds before adding the eggs.

FRIED EGGS AND RAPINI

Rapini, also called broccoli rabe or broccoli rape, is a pungent, slightly bitter green. It is best sautéed lightly and then sprinkled with a little vinegar to balance the flavors. It's so addicting—I'll eat a whole bunch myself! This recipe is what we consider "fast food" in our house. I make it for an easy breakfast or dinner and serve with Injera (page 168) and a few spoonfuls of my Live Hot Pepper Relish (page 103) or Cultured Vegetables (page 90).

2 to 3 teaspoons extra-virgin olive oil or organic butter, plus more for cooking the eggs

1 large bunch rapini, trimmed and chopped

2 garlic cloves, crushed

2 large organic eggs

2 teaspoons raw apple cider vinegar

sea salt

freshly ground black pepper

Heat the olive oil in a 10-inch cast-iron skillet over medium heat. Add the rapini and garlic and sauté for about 2 minutes. Push the rapini to the side of the skillet into a pile. Add a few more teaspoons of oil to the skillet, crack in the eggs, and cook for 60 seconds on each side.

Sprinkle the rapini with the vinegar, season with sea salt and pepper, and serve.

Yield: 1 to 2 servings

Variation: If you can't find rapini, substitute mustard greens, spinach, or kale.

GREEN OMELETS WITH SMOKED SALMON

This recipe is a fun twist to regular omelets. Here in the Pacific Northwest we have access to high-quality smoked wild salmon. If you can't find it you can use leftover cooked salmon instead. I like to add fresh organic cheese from my local farmers' market. Use organic feta cheese if you don't have access to fresh cheese, or omit it altogether. Other vegetables you can add to the filling include sautéed zucchini, cooked chanterelle mushrooms, or sautéed spinach.

OMELETS

4 large organic eggs

1 cup packed fresh spinach leaves

1 to 2 teaspoons butter or virgin coconut oil, for cooking

FILLING

¼ cup smoked salmon, crumbled

¼ cup crumbled fresh organic cheese

2 tablespoons snipped fresh chives

sea salt

freshly ground black pepper

To make the omelets, begin by heating a 10-inch skillet over medium-low heat (I use cast-iron for its natural nonstick properties). Crack the eggs into a blender, add the spinach, and purée.

Add the butter to the hot skillet. When the butter has melted, add half of the egg-spinach purée and cook for 60 to 90 seconds on each side. Transfer the omelet to a warm plate, add 2 tablespoons of the smoked salmon, 2 tablespoons of the cheese, and 1 tablespoon of the chives to one side of the omelet then fold it over. Season the omelet with sea salt and freshly ground black pepper. Repeat the process to make the second omelet with the remaining ingredients. Serve immediately.

Yield: 2 omelets

BAKED EGGS WITH GREENS AND BEANS

This nutrient-packed breakfast will keep you going strong all morning long. It is a great way to use up leftover cooked beans. Use any beans you have on hand, such as plain cooked black beans, baked beans, or Mexican spiced pinto beans. If you have leftover sautéed kale, chard, or collard greens, use them in place of the spinach, or use thawed frozen spinach. I like that I can put this meal together in minutes and then let it cook while we are getting ready in the morning.

---

1 tablespoon extra-virgin olive oil or organic butter

1 pound fresh spinach or other greens

2 cups cooked beans

sea salt

freshly ground black pepper

4 large organic eggs

Preheat the oven to 350°F. Lightly grease four 8-ounce ramekins with the olive oil or butter.

Bring a pot of salted water to a boil, add the greens, and blanch for 2 to 4 minutes. Remove with a slotted spoon and transfer to a colander to drain. Transfer the drained greens to a cutting board and chop finely.

Spoon ½ cup of the cooked beans into each ramekin. Evenly distribute the cooked greens among the ramekins. Sprinkle with sea salt and pepper, and crack an egg into each ramekin over the greens and beans. Place the ramekins onto a rimmed baking sheet and bake for about 15 minutes. Serve warm.

Yield: 4 servings

VEGETABLE FRITTATA WITH POTATO CRUST

Serve this nourishing recipe for a Sunday morning breakfast with Lemon–Poppy Seed Muffins (page 176) and a fresh green salad. For a quicker version of this recipe, try eliminating the potato crust. It is just as delicious!

2 teaspoons organic butter or extra-virgin olive oil, plus more for greasing the pie plate

2 cups grated potato (about 1 large baking potato, scrubbed)

½ teaspoon sea salt

1 small onion, diced

2 garlic cloves, finely chopped

1 small red bell pepper, diced

1½ cups finely chopped broccoli

1½ teaspoons dried thyme

½ teaspoon freshly ground black pepper

½ teaspoon sea salt or Herbamare

6 large organic eggs, lightly beaten

½ cup grated raw organic Jack cheese (optional)

Preheat the oven to 375°F. Oil a 9-inch deep-dish pie plate with olive oil or butter.

Place the grated potato into a small bowl with the sea salt. Let rest for about 10 minutes. Squeeze out the excess water, and transfer the grated potato to the prepared pie plate and press evenly into bottom of dish.

In a medium skillet heat the 2 teaspoons olive oil or butter. Add the onion and garlic and sauté over medium heat until soft, about 5 minutes.

Transfer the cooked onion and garlic to a bowl with the bell pepper, broccoli, thyme, black pepper, and sea salt and mix well.

Add the eggs and cheese and mix well. Pour the egg and vegetable mixture over the potato crust. Sprinkle the top with extra grated cheese if desired. Transfer to the oven and bake for 25 to 30 minutes, or until the eggs are cooked through.

Yield: 4 servings

BUTTERNUT SQUASH AND SAGE BREAKFAST HASH

This is one of my favorite autumn breakfasts. I like to serve it with poached eggs and organic sausages. This meal will definitely power you through a busy morning! To make meal preparation faster I will cut up the squash the night before and keep it in my refrigerator in a covered glass container. Just be sure to dice the butternut squash small so it cooks evenly without burning. I like to use ¼-inch cubes.

2 tablespoons extra-virgin olive oil or organic butter

4 cups diced butternut squash

1 small red onion, diced

½ pound cremini mushrooms, diced

2 cups thinly sliced lacinato kale

1 tablespoon finely chopped fresh sage

½ teaspoon sea salt

freshly ground black pepper

Heat the olive oil in an 11- or 12-inch cast-iron skillet over medium heat. Add the squash and onion and sauté for about 5 minutes. Add the mushrooms and sauté for 5 to 7 minutes more, or until the squash is tender. Add the kale, sage, sea salt, and pepper and sauté a minute more, or until the kale is tender. Taste and adjust the salt and seasonings if necessary. Serve.

Yield: 4 to 6 servings

HOME-STYLE POTATOES

These potatoes are great for a hearty Sunday morning breakfast. Serve with scrambled eggs and a fresh green salad for a balanced meal.

6 medium red potatoes, cut into chunks

1 tablespoon extra-virgin olive oil

1 medium red onion, chopped

½ teaspoon sea salt or Herbamare

1 teaspoon garlic powder

1 teaspoon dried oregano

½ teaspoon ground cumin

¼ teaspoon freshly ground black pepper

Place the potatoes in a steamer basket in a medium pot filled with about 2 inches of water. Cover and steam over medium-high heat until tender, but not all the way cooked, about 10 minutes depending on the size of the potato chunks. Remove and set aside to cool.

Heat the olive oil in an 11- or 12-inch cast-iron skillet over medium heat. Add the onion and sauté for 5 to 7 minutes. Add the sea salt, garlic powder, oregano, cumin, and pepper and sauté for 1 minute more.

Add the potatoes to the onion mixture and sauté for 5 to 10 minutes, or until golden brown, being careful not to burn them. If the potatoes begin to stick to skillet, add more olive oil.

Yield: about 4 servings

ZUCCHINI AND POTATO HASH

The combination of the zucchini, potatoes, and kale make a tasty and very nutritious combination to get you going in the morning. If you have a mandoline, you can use it to quickly slice the potatoes and zucchini very thinly—it's a very useful kitchen tool to have on hand! Otherwise, just use a sharp knife to slice the vegetables into thin rounds. Serve this dish with scrambled tofu or eggs and a spoonful of Cultured Vegetables (page 90) for a hearty, balanced breakfast.

1 to 2 tablespoons extra-virgin olive oil or ghee

1 small onion, cut into half-moons

5 to 6 small yellow or red potatoes, sliced into thin rounds

2 medium zucchini, sliced into thin rounds

½ bunch black kale, finely chopped

1 to 2 teaspoons dried thyme

1 garlic clove, crushed

sea salt or Herbamare

Heat the olive oil in an 11- or 12-inch cast-iron skillet over medium heat. Add the onion and sauté for 2 to 3 minutes. Stir in the potatoes, cover the skillet, and cook for 5 to 7 minutes, stirring occasionally, adding water, if necessary, to prevent burning.

Add the zucchini slices, kale, thyme, garlic, and sea salt and gently mix to distribute. Put the cover back onto the skillet and cook for another few minutes, stirring occasionally, until the zucchini and kale are tender. Taste and add more salt or Herbamare if necessary.

Yield: 4 servings

BREAKFAST GREENS

Greens for breakfast? Yes! Greens are great any time of day. Eating fresh organic leafy greens through-out the day will provide you with abundant vitality and health. Greens help to get your digestive juices flowing in the morning, and also are rich in enzymes that assist in the digestion of other parts of your meal. Try fresh greens with your favorite salad dressing, or simply top with the lemon-olive oil dressing below.

4 cups organic salad greens

DRESSING
freshly squeezed juice of 1 large lemon

3 to 4 tablespoons extra-virgin olive oil
1 garlic clove, crushed
¼ teaspoon sea salt

Place the fresh salad greens in a bowl.

To make the dressing, place all the ingredients into a jar with a tight-fitting lid and shake well. Taste and adjust the salt if necessary.

Drizzle the dressing over fresh greens. The dressing will keep in the refrigerator for up to 1 week.

Yield: 2 servings

WARMING MISO SOUP

Miso is a thick paste and is made by fermenting cooked soybeans, koji, sea salt, and different grains for 6 months to 2 years. It is a live food and contains significant amounts of friendly bacteria that promote intestinal health. It is important not to cook the miso for this reason, but rather to add it to already cooked foods. Consuming miso helps to create an alkaline condition in the body, promoting resistance against disease. The salty flavor of miso stimulates digestion, which is why it has been a traditional breakfast food in Japan for centuries. Adding some cooked fish to the soup will help to boost your metabolism even more at your morning meal. For information on gluten-free miso see page 55.

2 teaspoons toasted sesame oil

2 carrots, peeled and cut into matchsticks

3 to 4 shiitake mushrooms, thinly sliced

1 garlic clove, finely chopped

2 to 3 teaspoons finely chopped fresh ginger

4 cups water

1 small strip wakame seaweed, broken into pieces

1 cup thinly sliced baby bok choy leaves

2 to 3 green onions, cut into thin rounds

2 to 3 tablespoons gluten-free miso

1 to 2 tablespoons wheat-free tamari or coconut aminos

1 tablespoon brown rice vinegar or coconut vinegar

2 to 3 teaspoons hot pepper sesame oil

Heat the toasted sesame oil in a 3-quart pot over medium heat. Add the carrots, mushrooms, garlic, and ginger and sauté lightly for about 3 minutes, being very careful not to brown the vegetables.

Add the water and wakame seaweed and bring to a simmer. Cover the pot and cook for 7 to 10 minutes, or until the vegetables are tender.

Turn off the heat and add the bok choy, green onions, and miso that has been mixed with a little water. Then add the tamari, vinegar, and hot pepper sesame oil; stir. Taste and adjust the seasonings if necessary.

Yield: 4 servings

Tip: You can purchase gluten-free, soy-free organic miso from The South River Miso Company (www.South RiverMiso.com).

14

FRESH BREADS AND MUFFINS

What lies behind us and what lies before us are tiny matters compared to what lies within us.
—Ralph Waldo Emerson

Baking is an especially fun activity for children. I have many fond memories of baking bread with my mother when I was a child. All of the recipes in this chapter are gluten-free and some are grain-free as well. I use a variety of flours, including sprouted brown rice, millet, quinoa, buckwheat, almond, and coconut flours. Please see pages 65–67 for a detailed description of these highly nutritious gluten-free flours.

Remember, gluten is a protein found in grains such as wheat, spelt, kamut, rye, barley, and sometimes oats. Gluten-free grain flours all have a chance of being contaminated with gluten because of growing or processing. The least likely to have any cross-contamination issues are brown rice, quinoa, and amaranth flours. Buckwheat and millet grow in similar climates to wheat, and sometimes we've found gluten grains hiding in a bag of whole-grain millet and buckwheat. I prefer to buy certified gluten-free whole raw organic buckwheat groats and grind my own flour. I do the same for millet.

Although I've made my best effort to ensure these baked good recipes use the most nutritious ingredients, eating a diet full of baked goods, no matter how good the ingredients are, won't benefit your overall health. Use these recipes as treats and eat them on occasion. Focus instead on eating mostly fresh fruits, vegetables, meats, legumes, and cooked whole grains.

GLUTEN-FREE SOURDOUGH BREAD

Use the Kombucha Sourdough Bread Starter (page 109) to make bread that rises with natural wild yeasts. You can use any types of organic gluten-free flours in your starter and in this bread recipe—try brown rice, quinoa, millet, sorghum, buckwheat, or amaranth flours. Use this tangy bread for sandwiches or toast in the morning.

WET INGREDIENTS

¼ cup ground chia seeds

½ cup warm water

2 large organic eggs

3 cups sourdough starter (page 109)

¼ cup whole psyllium husks

2 tablespoons extra-virgin olive oil, plus more for greasing the pan

1 tablespoon pure maple syrup

1½ teaspoons sea salt

DRY INGREDIENTS

1 to 1½ cups whole-grain gluten-free flour

½ cup arrowroot powder or tapioca flour

Grease a 9 x 5-inch glass bread pan with olive oil.

Place the ground chia and warm water into a medium mixing bowl or blender, and let it rest for about 5 minutes. Add the eggs and blend on high until smooth, or use an immersion blender in the bowl. If using a blender, pour the mixture into a mixing bowl. Add the sourdough starter, psyllium husks, olive oil, maple syrup, and sea salt; vigorously whisk together.

Add the dry ingredients and stir together well to combine. The dough will be slightly sticky, but should form a loose ball. Place the dough into the bread pan and smooth the top using wet hands. Cover the pan with a plastic bag (I use leftover produce bags) and put in a warm place to rise (I like to place it on top of my refrigerator). Let the bread rise for 3 to 8 hours; the time will depend on the temperature in your house. Rising happens faster in warmer temperatures and slower when your house is cooler. The dough should nearly double in size.

Preheat the oven to 350°F. Once the bread has risen, bake for about 1 hour. Remove from the oven and transfer to a wire rack to cool.

Tip: It is best to use your sourdough starter in its "active and bubbly" stage, which occurs within a few hours after feeding it.

Yield: 1 loaf

SPROUTED BROWN RICE BREAD

This yeast-free bread uses the combination of baking soda, kefir, and eggs to make the bread rise—no yeast required! I use sprouted brown rice flour from Planet Rice, which I buy in 25-pound bags through Azure Standard. It's a lovely flour—light and not as grainy as regular brown rice flour. Plus, since it's sprouted it is much easier to digest.

DRY INGREDIENTS

3 cups sprouted brown rice flour

¾ cup arrowroot powder

1½ teaspoons baking powder

¾ teaspoon baking soda

¾ teaspoon sea salt

WET INGREDIENTS

2 cups plain organic kefir (cow, goat, or coconut)

3 large organic eggs

1 tablespoon pure maple syrup (optional)

Preheat the oven to 350°F. Grease an 8.5 x 4.5-inch glass loaf pan or line with unbleached parchment paper.

In a large bowl, whisk together the dry ingredients. Add the wet ingredients to the dry and vigorously mix together with a wooden spoon until completely incorporated.

Pour the batter into the prepared pan. Bake for approximately 60 minutes. Cool the bread for about 20 minutes, then release the loaf from the pan, transfer to a wire rack, and cool completely before slicing.

Yield: 1 loaf

HEARTY SEED BREAD

Use this hearty, high-protein grain-free bread for small open-faced sandwiches. Try spreading slices with soft goat cheese or the Quick Almond Mayo (page 343), then add a slice of heirloom tomato, fresh basil, and a sprinkling of freshly ground black pepper.

DRY INGREDIENTS

½ cup coconut flour

¼ cup arrowroot powder

½ teaspoon baking soda

¼ teaspoon sea salt

¼ cup pumpkin seeds

¼ cup sunflower seeds

¼ cup hemp seeds

2 tablespoons flaxseeds

WET INGREDIENTS

6 large organic eggs

¼ cup extra-virgin olive oil, plus more for greasing the pan

¼ cup unsweetened applesauce

Preheat the oven to 350°F. Oil an 8.5 x 4.5-inch bread pan.

In a medium mixing bowl, whisk together the dry ingredients.

In a separate smaller mixing bowl, whisk together the wet ingredients. Vigorously whisk the wet ingredients into the dry until combined.

Pour the batter into the prepared pan and bake for 50 to 55 minutes. Remove the bread from the oven and cool completely before slicing.

Yield: 1 loaf

> **Tip:** 1 large egg should measure about ¼ cup. If your eggs are smaller, you will need to use more than 6. You will need a total of 1½ cups of cracked eggs.

BUCKWHEAT SEED BREAD

This is one of the quickest savory breads I make. The baking soda and apple cider vinegar give it its rise without yeast or eggs, while the chia seeds hold in moisture, resulting in a soft, squishy bread. Use it like focaccia bread and cut it in half for sandwiches, or spread some with homemade jam.

DRY INGREDIENTS

1¼ cups freshly ground buckwheat flour

½ cup raw sunflower seeds

½ cup raw pumpkin seeds

½ teaspoon baking soda

½ teaspoon sea salt

WET INGREDIENTS

¼ cup ground chia seeds

1½ cups warm water

2 tablespoons extra-virgin olive oil, plus more for greasing the dish

1 tablespoon pure maple syrup

1 tablespoon apple cider vinegar

Preheat the oven to 350°F. Lightly oil an 8 x 8-inch glass baking dish.

Place all the dry ingredients in a medium mixing bowl and whisk together. Set aside.

Place the ground chia seeds and warm water into a blender and give it a whirl. Let the mixture rest for about a minute. Add the remaining wet ingredients and blend until smooth. Pour the wet ingredients into the dry and stir together with a wooden spoon until combined.

Pour the batter into the prepared dish and bake for approximately 30 minutes.

Yield: about 9 servings

Tip: To grind fresh buckwheat flour, add 2 cups raw buckwheat groats to a high-powered blender and blend until you have a fine flour. You can do this in a coffee grinder as well, ½ cup at a time. I buy raw, organic buckwheat groats from Bob's Red Mill, which is also certified gluten-free.

HERBED FOCACCIA BREAD

This simple grain-free bread recipe contains no yeast and therefore doesn't need to rise. You can whip up a batch of bread while you are making dinner and have it ready to serve with the rest of your meal!

DRY INGREDIENTS
6 tablespoons coconut flour
6 tablespoons arrowroot powder
2 teaspoons dried Italian herbs
¾ teaspoon baking powder
¼ teaspoon sea salt

WET INGREDIENTS
4 large organic eggs
3 tablespoons water
2 tablespoons extra-virgin olive oil, plus more for greasing the dish
1 to 2 garlic cloves, chopped (optional)

Preheat the oven to 350°F. Grease an 8 x 8-inch glass baking dish with olive oil.

In a medium mixing bowl, whisk together the dry ingredients.

In another mixing bowl, whisk together the wet ingredients. Pour the wet ingredients into the dry and vigorously whisk together.

Pour the batter into the prepared dish and bake for about 25 minutes. Cool the bread before serving.

Yield: 6 to 8 servings

GLUTEN-FREE HAMBURGER BUNS

I like to use sprouted brown rice flour in this recipe, but any combination of gluten-free flours will work. If desired, sprinkle the tops of the buns with sesame seeds before rising.

WET INGREDIENTS

2 cups warm water (105° to 110°F)

1 tablespoon active dry yeast

1 teaspoon pure maple syrup or organic cane sugar

2 tablespoons extra-virgin olive oil

1 tablespoon pure maple syrup or honey

½ cup ground golden flaxseeds

¼ cup whole psyllium husks

DRY INGREDIENTS

2¼ cups brown rice flour, plus more flour for kneading

¾ cup arrowroot powder or tapioca flour

1½ teaspoons sea salt

Place the warm water in a bowl or 4-cup liquid glass measuring cup, add the yeast and the teaspoon of maple syrup or sugar, and whisk together. Let proof for 5 to 10 minutes to activate the yeast. The mixture should get foamy or bubbly. If not, dump it out and start over. While the yeast is activating, mix together the dry ingredients in a large bowl.

After the yeast is activated, whisk the olive oil, the 1 tablespoon of maple syrup or honey, the ground flaxseeds, and the psyllium husks into the water-yeast mixture. Let stand for 1 to 2 minutes to let the flaxseeds and psyllium release their gelatinous substances, then whisk again.

Pour the wet ingredients into the dry and mix together with a large wooden spoon until thick.

Turn the dough out onto a floured wooden board. Knead in more flour, a little at a time, until the dough holds together and isn't too sticky.

Divide the dough into six to eight equal-size balls. On the floured board, roll each piece of dough into a nice round ball. Place each ball onto a baking sheet lined with unbleached parchment paper and set in a warm spot to rise. I like to place it on top of a large pan filled partially with water that is set on the stovetop on low heat. Let rise for 60 minutes.

Preheat the oven to 375°F. Bake the buns for about 35 minutes, or until done. Cool completely, then slice in half.

Yield: 6 hamburger buns

VEGAN CINNAMON ROLLS

I like to make these for my family as a special treat once or twice a year. If you can tolerate dairy products, then frost the cooled cinnamon rolls with the Honey–Cream Cheese Frosting (page 412), or for a dairy-free option, frost with the Cashew-Honey Icing (page 411).

WET INGREDIENTS

2 cups warm water (105° to 110°F)

2¼ teaspoons dry active yeast

1 teaspoon organic sugar or pure maple syrup

¼ cup pure maple syrup

2 tablespoons melted virgin coconut oil

½ cup ground golden flaxseeds

¼ cup whole psyllium husks

DRY INGREDIENTS

2 cups sorghum flour

1 cup millet flour or brown rice flour

1 cup blanched almond flour

¾ cup tapioca flour or arrowroot powder

1¼ teaspoons sea salt

FILLING

¼ cup virgin coconut oil, softened, plus more for greasing the pans

½ cup coconut sugar

1 tablespoon ground cinnamon

Place the warm water, yeast, and the organic sugar into a 4-cup liquid glass measuring cup and whisk together. Let the mixture rest for a few minutes to activate the yeast. You should see a bit of bubbling and/or foaming. Add the maple syrup, coconut oil, ground flaxseed, and psyllium husks and whisk together and let rest for about 2 to 3 minutes to thicken.

In a large bowl, whisk together the dry ingredients. Use only 1 cup of sorghum flour to start.

Pour the wet ingredients into the dry and whisk together. Then gradually add the remaining cup of sorghum flour, kneading it in until the dough forms a ball and isn't sticky. You may only need ½ cup of the remaining flour. Every batch is a little different.

Grease two 9-inch cake pans with coconut oil.

Place the dough onto a piece of unbleached parchment paper that is lightly floured with tapioca flour. Roll out into a large rectangle about 12 to 14 inches x 18 to 20 inches. Spread the ¼ cup coconut oil evenly onto the dough. Then sprinkle with coconut sugar and cinnamon. Roll the dough toward you into a long log. Using a serrated knife, cut 10 to 12 rolls. Place the rolls into two cake pans. Cover and let rise in a warm spot for about 1 hour.

Preheat the oven to 350°F. Place the cinnamon rolls into the oven and bake for 30 to 35 minutes.

Yield: about 1 dozen rolls

ALMOND-COCONUT PIZZA CRUST

Create your own grain-free pizzas with this crust! Make sure to use a pizza stone—it's what makes the crust crispy on the bottom.

DRY INGREDIENTS

2 cups blanched almond flour

¼ cup ground golden flaxseeds

¼ cup coconut flour

1 tablespoon Italian seasoning

½ teaspoon sea salt

WET INGREDIENTS

½ cup warm water

2 large organic eggs

2 teaspoons extra-virgin olive oil, plus more for the pizza stone

Preheat the oven to 375°F. Lightly oil a 12-inch round pizza stone and set aside.

In a medium bowl, whisk together the dry ingredients. Add the wet ingredients and whisk to incorporate.

Place the dough onto the oiled pizza stone and pat into a large circle. Sometimes it helps to oil your hands so they don't stick to the dough while doing this. Bake the pizza crust for 20 to 25 minutes, then add any desired toppings and return to the oven until the toppings are cooked and heated through, 5 to 10 minutes more.

Yield: 1 pizza crust

BUCKWHEAT PIZZA CRUST

Use this simple vegan, gluten-free crust to create your favorite pizza. Sometimes we spread the cooked crust with fresh pesto, sliced tomatoes, and fresh basil leaves.

WET INGREDIENTS

1 cup warm water (105° to 110°F)

2¼ teaspoons active dry yeast (1 package)

2 teaspoons pure maple syrup

1 tablespoon ground chia seeds

2 tablespoons extra-virgin olive oil, plus more for the pizza stone

DRY INGREDIENTS

2 cups freshly ground buckwheat flour

1 cup arrowroot powder

¾ teaspoon sea salt

In a small bowl, whisk together the warm water, yeast, and maple syrup. Let it proof until foamy and bubbly, about 5 minutes. Whisk in the ground chia seeds and olive oil.

In a medium mixing bowl, whisk together the dry ingredients. Pour the wet ingredients into the dry and stir with a wooden spoon to incorporate. The dough will be very sticky; don't be tempted to add more flour. Cover the bowl and let it rise in a warm spot for about 45 minutes.

Preheat the oven to 400°F. Oil a pizza stone with olive oil. Place the dough onto the pizza stone and pat into a large circle using oiled hands. Bake for about 20 minutes. Add the toppings and bake for 5 to 10 minutes more.

> **Tip:** To grind fresh buckwheat flour, add 2 cups raw buckwheat groats to a high-powered blender and blend until you have a fine flour. You can do this in a coffee grinder as well, ½ cup at a time. I buy raw, organic buckwheat groats from Bob's Red Mill, which are also certified gluten-free.

Yield: 1 pizza crust

INJERA

Injera is a traditional Ethiopian flat bread made from fermented teff flour. Its lightness comes from trapped gas bubbles from the fermentation process. You can use any gluten-free whole-grain flour, or a combination of a few, in your sourdough starter (page 109) to make this bread. Make sure you use your starter when it is active and bubbly or within a few hours of feeding it. Serve injera with meat, bean, or vegetable soups and stews.

4 tablespoons virgin coconut oil or ghee
sea salt

2 cups sourdough starter (page 109)

Heat a 10-inch cast-iron skillet over medium heat. Make sure your skillet is hot before adding the oil. Then add 1 tablespoon of the coconut oil and a generous sprinkling of sea salt. Add ½ cup of starter to the hot pan and let it cook for 60 to 90 seconds, then flip using a wide spatula and cook for 60 to 90 seconds more.

Repeat with the remaining 3 tablespoons oil and the starter. Serve the bread hot.

Yield: 4 flatbreads

QUINOA TORTILLAS

Use these tortillas to make the Smashed Yam and Black Bean Quesadillas (page 299) or the Fish Tacos (page 320). They are soft and pliable when warm, but straight out of the fridge, like most gluten-free tortillas, they will crack. All you need to do to make them pliable again is to place one on a wire rack over a pot of simmering water and steam for 30 seconds on each side. I use an 8-inch cast-iron tortilla press to get them superthin and then cook them in a cast-iron skillet.

1½ cups quinoa flour
½ cup arrowroot powder
½ teaspoon sea salt

¾ cup water
virgin coconut oil, for cooking

In a small mixing bowl, whisk together the quinoa flour, arrowroot, and sea salt. Add the water and mix with a wooden spoon. Add more water, 1 tablespoon at a time, if the dough feels dry. Knead the dough a little in the bowl, then let it rest for a few minutes while the skillet heats up.

Preheat a 10-inch cast-iron skillet over medium heat. Divide the dough into four equal-size balls. Place a piece of unbleached parchment paper on the bottom of a tortilla press then place one of the balls in the center, cover with a second sheet of parchment paper, and press to form a thin, round tortilla.

Add about 1 teaspoon of coconut oil to the hot skillet. Gently remove the top sheet of parchment, place the tortilla into skillet, then remove the second sheet of parchment. Cook for 1 to 2 minutes on each side. Repeat making tortillas with the remaining dough. Transfer the cooked tortillas to a plate and flip another plate over the top to keep the tortillas warm and soft. Let them sit for about 20 minutes inside the plates; this way they will be nice and pliable for serving.

Yield: four 8-inch tortillas

Variation: You can experiment with this recipe using different gluten-free whole-grain flours in place of the quinoa flour, but keep in mind that each flour will require a different amount of water. For example, brown rice flour requires about 1 cup of water per batch! I prefer quinoa flour because the end result is quite pliable.

SPROUTED FLOUR BISCUITS

I like using sprouted flours in my cooking and baking. These types of flours are lighter, have a better flavor, and are more easily digested compared to their nonsprouted counterparts. Use this biscuit dough to dollop over chicken pot pie filling or my Home-Style Chicken and Vegetable Stew (page 326) and then bake it for about 25 minutes—it makes a hearty supper casserole for a cold winter's evening!

1½ cups sprouted brown rice flour

¾ cup sprouted chickpea (garbanzo bean) flour

¾ cup arrowroot powder

1 tablespoon baking powder

¾ teaspoon sea salt

10 tablespoons organic palm shortening

1 cup milk (dairy or nondairy)

2 tablespoons ground chia seeds

Preheat the oven to 425°F. Line a baking sheet with unbleached parchment paper.

In a mixing bowl, whisk together the flours, arrowroot powder, baking powder, and sea salt. Cut in the shortening using your fingers or a pastry cutter until pea-size crumbs form.

Pour the milk into a small bowl and whisk in the chia seeds; let rest for about 5 minutes. Then pour the milk-chia mixture into the flour mixture, and using a fork, mix it together. Knead the dough slightly to form a ball.

Pat the dough ball out on a floured surface into a 1-inch-thick round. Cut the dough into rounds with a biscuit cutter. Alternatively, you can drop the dough by the large spoonful onto the baking sheet; you should have 8 biscuits. Bake for about 15 minutes. Serve warm or at room temperature.

Yield: 8 biscuits

SPICED BANANA BREAD

Spread a slice of this grain-free banana bread with Orange-Honey-Fig Jam (page 360), and serve with afternoon tea. It also makes a nutritious treat packed in your child's lunch box.

DRY INGREDIENTS

¾ cup coconut flour

¼ cup arrowroot powder

¼ cup ground golden flaxseeds

2 teaspoons baking powder

½ teaspoon baking soda

½ teaspoon sea salt

½ teaspoon ground nutmeg

½ teaspoon ground cardamom

WET INGREDIENTS

5 large organic eggs

1¼ cups mashed ripe banana (about 3 medium)

¼ cup melted virgin coconut oil, plus more for greasing the pan

¼ cup pure maple syrup

Preheat the oven to 350°F. Coat an 8.5 x 4.5-inch bread loaf pan with coconut oil.

In a medium mixing bowl, whisk together the dry ingredients. In another mixing bowl, beat together the wet ingredients with an electric mixer. Pour the wet ingredients into the dry and beat together.

Pour batter into the prepared pan and bake for approximately 50 minutes. Cool for about 20 minutes in the pan, then loosen the sides with a knife, and turn over onto a wire rack, allowing to cool completely.

Yield: 1 loaf

APPLE-CRANBERRY OATMEAL MUFFINS

I love making these muffins as a special treat for my children in the fall. Full of warming spices and hearty oats, they are packed with goodness.

DRY INGREDIENTS

1 cup brown rice flour

½ cup gluten-free rolled oats

1½ teaspoons baking powder

½ teaspoon baking soda

¼ teaspoon sea salt

1½ teaspoons ground cinnamon

1 teaspoon ground ginger

¼ teaspoon ground cloves

WET INGREDIENTS

1 cup grated apple

½ cup unsweetened applesauce

¼ cup melted virgin coconut oil or organic butter, plus more for greasing the pan

¼ cup coconut sugar

2 large organic eggs

OTHER INGREDIENTS

½ cup fresh or frozen cranberries

½ cup chopped walnuts or pecans (optional)

½ cup raisins or dried currants (optional)

Preheat the oven to 350°F. Coat a 12-cup muffin pan with coconut oil or line with unbleached paper liners.

In a medium mixing bowl, whisk together the dry ingredients. In a separate mixing bowl, whisk together the grated apple, applesauce, melted oil, coconut sugar, and eggs. Pour the wet ingredients into the dry and vigorously whisk together. Fold in the cranberries and walnuts, pecans, raisins, or currants if using.

Spoon the batter into the prepared muffin cups, filling them about halfway. Bake for about 25 minutes. Cool on a wire rack before serving.

Yield: 1 dozen muffins

Variations: Replace the grated apple with grated zucchini or carrots. Replace the cranberries with fresh or frozen blackberries, blueberries, or raspberries.

> **Tip:** Always use organic rolled oats as the nonorganic varieties are sprayed with gut-damaging herbicides. I buy certified gluten-free, organic oats online; see the Resources section (page 429) for more information.

BANANA-WALNUT MUFFINS

Serve these egg-free, gluten-free muffins in lieu of cupcakes for a young child's birthday party. I use sprouted brown rice flour in my recipes because I find it easier to digest and more nutritious, but regular brown rice flour works as well.

DRY INGREDIENTS

2 cups brown rice flour

½ cup arrowroot powder

2 teaspoons baking powder

½ teaspoon baking soda

¼ teaspoon sea salt

1 teaspoon ground cinnamon

WET INGREDIENTS

2 tablespoons ground chia seeds

¾ cup warm water

1¼ cups mashed ripe bananas (about 3 medium)

⅓ cup coconut sugar

⅓ cup melted virgin coconut oil, plus more for greasing the pan

1 to 2 teaspoons vanilla extract

OTHER INGREDIENTS

½ cup chopped walnuts

½ cup dark chocolate chips

Preheat the oven to 350°F. Coat a 12-cup muffin pan with coconut oil or line with paper muffin cups.

In a medium mixing bowl, whisk together the dry ingredients.

In another mixing bowl, vigorously whisk together the ground chia seeds and warm water. Let rest for about 5 minutes. Add the mashed bananas, coconut sugar, melted coconut oil, and vanilla and beat together. Add the wet ingredients to the dry and mix together well. Fold in the walnuts and chocolate chips.

Spoon the batter into the prepared muffin cups. Bake for about 25 minutes. Cool on a wire rack before serving.

Yield: 1 dozen muffins

BLUEBERRY-ALMOND MUFFINS

Serve these nourishing muffins with sautéed kale and sausages for breakfast, or pack one in your lunch. You can also make them into mini muffins and serve them for a child's tea party!

DRY INGREDIENTS

2 cups blanched almond flour

¼ cup coconut flour

2 teaspoons baking powder

½ teaspoon baking soda

½ teaspoon sea salt

WET INGREDIENTS

4 large organic eggs

⅓ cup melted virgin coconut oil, plus more for greasing the pan

⅓ cup pure maple syrup

¼ cup coconut milk or cashew milk

2 teaspoons vanilla extract

OTHER INGREDIENTS

1 heaping cup fresh blueberries

Preheat the oven to 350°F. Line a 12-cup muffin pan with unbleached paper liners.

Whisk together the dry ingredients.

In a separate bowl, whisk together the wet ingredients. Add the wet ingredients to the dry and vigorously whisk together until combined. Fold in blueberries.

Spoon the batter into the lined muffin cups. Bake 25 to 30 minutes. Cool on a wire rack before serving.

Yield: 1 dozen muffins

> **Tip:** You can purchase organic blanched almond flour online from www.Nuts .com!

CARROT-RAISIN BUCKWHEAT MUFFINS

If you are a buckwheat lover then you will to enjoy these gluten-free muffins. Be sure to use freshly ground buckwheat flour from the raw groats. This type of flour tastes and behaves much differently than regular roasted buckwheat flour you buy in the store. Serve these with a green smoothie for a quick breakfast.

DRY INGREDIENTS

2½ cups buckwheat flour

½ cup arrowroot powder or tapioca flour

2 teaspoons baking powder

½ cup coconut sugar

1 teaspoon baking soda

½ teaspoon sea salt

2 teaspoons ground cinnamon

1 teaspoon ground ginger

WET INGREDIENTS

2 cups unsweetened applesauce

¼ cup melted virgin coconut oil, plus more for greasing the pans

2 teaspoons vanilla extract

1 cup grated carrots

½ to 1 cup raisins (soaked for 10 minutes in ¼ cup water)

Preheat the oven to 375°F. Coat a 12-cup muffin pan with coconut oil or line with unbleached paper muffin cups.

In a large bowl, combine the buckwheat flour, arrowroot, sugar, baking soda, baking powder, sea salt, and spices and mix well.

Put the applesauce in a separate bowl and add the melted coconut oil, vanilla, carrots, and raisins and whisk to combine. Pour the wet ingredients into the dry and mix to incorporate. The batter will seem thick; don't be tempted to add more liquid.

Spoon the batter into the prepared muffin pans and bake at 375°F for 25 to 30 minutes. Loosen the sides of the muffins with a knife and gently remove them from the pans. Transfer to a wire rack to cool.

Yield: 1 to 1½ dozen muffins

> **Tip:** To grind fresh buckwheat flour, add 2 cups raw buckwheat groats to a high-powered blender and blend until you have a fine flour. You can do this in a coffee grinder as well, ½ cup at a time. I buy raw, organic buckwheat groats from Bob's Red Mill, which are also certified gluten-free.

LEMON–POPPY SEED MUFFINS

These muffins are lemony and not too sweet, perfect to serve for breakfast with scrambled eggs and steamed kale.

DRY INGREDIENTS

½ cup coconut flour

½ cup arrowroot powder

2 tablespoons poppy seeds

1 teaspoon baking soda

¼ teaspoon sea salt

WET INGREDIENTS

6 large organic eggs, at room temperature

¼ cup melted virgin coconut oil, plus more for greasing the pan

¼ cup unsweetened applesauce

¼ cup pure maple syrup

freshly squeezed juice of 1 large lemon

1 to 2 teaspoons finely grated lemon zest

Preheat the oven to 350°F. Coat a 12-cup muffin pan with coconut oil or line with paper muffin cups.

In a medium mixing bowl, whisk together the dry ingredients.

In a smaller mixing bowl, whisk together the wet ingredients. Pour the wet ingredients into the dry and immediately whisk together until combined.

> **Tip:** If you would like a sweeter muffin, add ¼ to ½ teaspoon liquid stevia or an additional tablespoon of maple syrup to the wet ingredients.

Spoon the batter into the prepared muffin cups, filling each cup halfway. Bake for 25 to 30 minutes. Cool on a wire rack before serving.

Yield: 1 dozen muffins

PUMPKIN–GOJI BERRY MUFFINS

Serve these nutritious muffins on a chilly holiday morning along with scrambled eggs and sautéed kale. My children also like to pack them in their lunch boxes. If you don't have goji berries—an antioxidant-rich superfood—then use dried cranberries or chopped pecans, or omit them altogether.

DRY INGREDIENTS

½ cup coconut flour

¼ cup arrowroot powder

1 teaspoon baking powder

½ teaspoon baking soda

⅛ teaspoon sea salt

1½ teaspoons pumpkin pie spice

½ cup goji berries

WET INGREDIENTS

½ cup pumpkin purée

⅓ cup pure maple syrup

¼ cup melted virgin coconut oil

4 large organic eggs

1 teaspoon vanilla extract

Preheat the oven to 350°F. Line a 12-cup muffin pan with unbleached paper liners or coat with coconut oil.

In a large mixing bowl, whisk together the dry ingredients. In a separate mixing bowl, whisk together the wet ingredients. Pour the wet into the dry and vigorously mix together until combined. Spoon the batter equally into the prepared muffin cups.

Bake for about 25 minutes. Cool on a wire rack before serving. Store leftover muffins in an airtight glass container for up to 4 days.

Yield: 1 dozen muffins

CORN-FREE BAKING POWDER

Here is a recipe for an allergen-free baking powder. In addition to being sensitive to gluten, dairy, and eggs, many people also have allergies or sensitivities to corn. Cornstarch is one of the main ingredients in baking powder. You can store your homemade baking powder in a tightly covered glass jar almost indefinitely. Just be sure to label it!

¼ cup baking soda

½ cup cream of tartar

½ cup arrowroot powder

Place all the ingredients into a glass jar and shake well. Store your baking powder in a cool, dry place.

Yield: ¾ cup

15

SOUPS

Of soup and love, the first is best.
—Old Spanish Proverb

Soup is probably as old as the history of cooking as food historians say. The act of combining different ingredients in a large pot to create a nutritious, filling, and easily digested food was inevitable. Soups, stews, and porridges evolved according to local ingredients and tastes.

Soup is a wonderful way to enjoy a variety of vegetables, herbs, beans, and meats in a savory form. The ingredients in the simmering soup slowly release their vital nutrients into the liquid; which includes many minerals and trace minerals, vitamins, and phytochemicals. Serve soup with a fresh green salad or cultured vegetables to maximize digestion of vital nutrients. Soup, which is very economical, is easy to make and can be made in large batches and then frozen for later use.

Before embarking on the recipes, please review this important information on how to cook beans, which will be necessary in order to make many of the soup and vegetarian main dish recipes in this book.

HOW TO COOK BEANS

It is important to buy dried beans from a store that has a rapid turnover. Buy organic beans that are in the bulk bins from your local co-op or health food store. It is best to use dried beans within a few months of purchasing them.

Store

Store dried beans in glass jars or another type of airtight container in the coolest and driest place in your kitchen. This will preserve their freshness and make them last longer. Beans stored in this way can be kept for 6 to 9 months. Mark the date of purchase on your bean containers so you will know to discard them if they are older than 6 months. Older beans become very dry and hard and will take much longer to cook until tender.

Sort

Sort through your beans and pick out any stones, foreign matter, or discolored; shriveled beans. Then rinse them to remove any dirt or debris. You can do this by placing the dried beans into a bowl and adding cool water, then take your hand and swirl the beans around. Pour off the water through a strainer and give them one final rinse with cool water.

Soak

Soaking your beans decreases cooking times dramatically and allows the gas-producing sugars in beans to be released into the soaking water.

Smaller beans do not require any soaking; these include green or brown lentils, red lentils, green or yellow split peas, black-eyed peas, mung beans, and adzuki beans.

Larger beans need be soaked for at least 8 hours, preferably 24. These include chickpeas, pinto beans, pink beans, black beans, lima beans, navy beans, kidney beans, Great Northern beans, Christmas limas, and cannellini beans.

Place the rinsed beans in a large bowl with twice as much water as beans. So for 1 cup of dry beans use 2 cups of water. Soak for 8 to 24 hours or overnight. Drain and rinse the beans.

Sprout

For increased digestibility you can easily sprout your beans after soaking. Drain the soaking water from the beans and leave them in the bowl. Rinse twice daily, then once you see a small sprout forming (this usually takes about 2 days), cook them according to the directions below.

```
Bean Conversions

One 15-ounce can of beans = 1½ cups cooked,
    drained beans
One pound dry beans = 6 cups cooked,
    drained beans
One pound dry beans = 2 cups dry beans
One cup dry beans = 2 to 3 cups cooked,
    drained beans
```

Stovetop Cooking

For Small Beans or Legumes (green or brown lentils, red lentils, green or yellow split peas, black-eyed peas, mung beans, and adzuki beans):

1. Place the rinsed beans into a heavy-bottomed, stainless steel pot. Use 2 to 2½ cups of water per cup of dry beans.
2. Add herbs or spices if desired, and one 2-inch piece of kombu seaweed. Herbs that aid in digestion of beans include cumin, fennel, ginger, and winter savory.
3. Bring the beans, water, and kombu to a boil. Reduce the heat, cover, and simmer. See the bean cooking chart on pages 182–183 for cooking times. Salt the beans at the end of the cooking time.

For Large Beans (chickpeas, pinto beans, pink beans, black beans, lima beans, navy beans, kidney beans, Great Northern beans, Christmas limas, and cannellini beans):

1. Place the soaked, rinsed beans in a heavy-bottomed stainless steel pot. Use 3 cups of fresh water per 1 cup of dry beans that have been soaked.
2. Add herbs or spices if desired, and one 3-inch piece of kombu seaweed.
3. Bring the beans, water, and kombu to a boil. Reduce the heat, cover, and simmer. Add water as needed during cooking to make sure beans are always covered with liquid. A well-cooked bean can easily be mashed on the roof of your mouth with your tongue. See the bean cooking chart on pages 182–183 for cooking times.

```
Tip: Remember, never add salt or acids, such
as tomatoes, vinegars, and citrus, to your pot
of cooking beans. These will toughen the outer
layer of the beans and may prevent them from
cooking thoroughly. Always add salt and any
acid at the end of the cooking time. Salt and
acids help to bring out the flavor of beans and
are important in creating a delicious bean dish.
```

Pressure-Cooking Beans

Directions below are for both small unsoaked beans and large soaked beans.

1. Place the rinsed beans into the pressure cooker. Use about 3 cups of water per cup of dry beans. The beans need to be completely covered with water to cook evenly.
2. Add herbs or spices if desired, and one 2- or 3-inch piece of kombu seaweed.

3. Lock the lid into place, place on the stovetop over medium-high, and bring cooker to high pressure.
4. Cook for the time indicated on the Bean Cooking Times chart. The timing begins when full pressure is reached.
5. Let the pressure come down naturally. Then remove the lid and test for doneness.
6. If the beans are almost done, but need a little more time, then simmer on the stovetop until done. If they need considerably more time, then place the lid back on and bring to high pressure. Cook for only a few minutes more.
7. Now add salt and flavorings if desired.

The chart below gives approximate cooking times for large soaked beans and small unsoaked beans. Always check beans for doneness at least 5 to 10 minutes before the minimum time indicated (stovetop method) for small beans, and 20 to 30 minutes before the minimum time indicated for large beans.

> **Ingredient Tip:** Kombu is a sea vegetable that contains glutamic acid, which helps to tenderize and break down the indigestible, gas-producing sugars, raffinose and stacchiose, in beans. Kombu is also a rich source of many important trace minerals. These minerals are released into the cooking water of the beans. Kombu can be purchased in the dried form in either the bulk or macrobiotic section from your local co-op or health food store.

Bean Cooking Times

Beans (1 cup dry)	Approximate Stovetop Cooking Times	Approximate Pressure Cooking Times	Yield Cooked Beans in Cups
Adzuki	1 hour	10–15 minutes	2 cups
Black (turtle)	1½–2 hours	5–10 minutes	2 cups
Black-eyed pea	30 minutes	8–11 minutes	2¼ cups
Cannellini	1–1½ hours	8–12 minutes	2 cups
Christmas lima	1–1½ hours	8–10 minutes	1¼ cups
Cranberry	1½–2 hours	8–11 minutes	2¼ cups
Garbanzo	1–1½ hours	12–16 minutes	2½ cups
Great Northern	1–1½ hours	8–11 minutes	2¼ cups
Kidney	1½–2 hours	10–14 minutes	2 cups
Lentils (brown or green)	40–50 minutes	6–8 minutes	2 cups
Lima (large)*	45 minutes–1 hour	4–6 minutes	2 cups
Lima (baby)	45 minutes–1 hour	5–6 minutes	2 cups
Navy	1–1½ hours	6–8 minutes	2 cups
Pink	1–1½ hours	4–6 minutes	2 cups

(Continued)

Pinto	1–1½ hours	4–6 minutes	2¼ cups
Red lentil	20–25 minutes	—	2 cups
Scarlet runner	1½–2 hours	12–14 minutes	1¼ cups
Soybeans (beige)	2–3 hours	8–12 minutes	2¼ cups
Soybeans (black)*	1½ hours	20–22 minutes	2½ cups
Split peas	45 minutes	8–10 minutes	2 cups

Note: Large lima beans and black soybeans have delicate skins and need salt added to the cooking water to keep them intact during stovetop cooking. When pressure-cooking large lima beans and soybeans, add 2 tablespoons oil per cup of beans.

Pressure-cooking times are for minutes under high pressure only. Timing begins when full pressure has been reached.

HOMEMADE BEEF STOCK

Homemade beef stock contains many healing nutrients—gelatin for good digestion as well as strong nails and bones, and marrow for vitamins B12 and A. Beef stock can be used to make bean and vegetable soups, such as minestrone, or beef stew. It can also be sipped on when you are ill or having digestive complaints. I freeze beef stock in quart jars to have on hand for cooking. When purchasing beef bones, look for knuckle and marrow bones from organic pastured animals. Sometimes you can buy these bones from a local farmer, or you can find them in the frozen section of your health food store.

2 to 3 pounds beef bones	2 bay leaves
1 large onion, chopped	1 tablespoon whole black peppercorns
1 head garlic, cut in half crosswise	1 tablespoon sea salt
2 to 3 carrots, chopped	2 to 3 sprigs fresh rosemary
3 celery stalks, chopped	16 cups water
½ cup sun-dried tomatoes	¼ cup dry red wine

Place all the ingredients into an 8-quart stockpot and bring to a boil. Reduce the heat to low, cover, and simmer for 6 to 12 hours. Let cool to room temperature, then strain into clean, widemouthed, 1-quart jars. Refrigerate for up to a week or freeze for up to a year.

Yield: 4 quarts

> **Tip:** To safely freeze stock in glass jars without the danger of cracking, be sure to leave at least an inch of space from the top of the jar. Let the filled jars cool completely, then freeze with the lids off. Once frozen, screw on the lids.

HOMEMADE CHICKEN STOCK

Chicken stock is rich in nutrients that support healthy digestion. Use it in place of water in soups and stews, or sip on it when you are feeling under the weather. Always use organic or pastured chicken for the healthiest stock. Once the stock is done, you can pull the meat from the bones and use it to make enchiladas, chicken salad, or chicken noodle soup.

2 pounds organic chicken wings

2 pounds organic chicken thighs, bone in, skin on

1 large onion, chopped

1 head garlic, cut in half crosswise

3 celery stalks, chopped

2 carrots, chopped

3 to 4 sprigs fresh thyme

2 to 3 sprigs fresh rosemary

1 handful fresh parsley

2 bay leaves

1 tablespoon whole black peppercorns

1 tablespoon sea salt

1 tablespoon apple cider vinegar

16 cups water (4 quarts)

Place all the ingredients into an 8-quart stockpot, cover, and bring to a boil. Reduce the heat to low and simmer for 3 to 4 hours. Strain the stock through a colander into another pot or large bowl. Pull the meat from the bones and place it in a container in your refrigerator for future use. You can use the bones and skin again for another round of stock if desired.

Pour the stock into clean, widemouthed, 1-quart jars, cover, and place into your refrigerator to chill. Once cooled you can freeze the stock (see Tip on page 184).

Yield: 4 quarts

Tip: To add more gut-healing nutrients, such as gelatin, to the stock, add 1 to 2 chicken feet. You can usually find these in the frozen section of your local health food store or from a local organic chicken farmer.

HOMEMADE VEGETABLE STOCK

Making your own vegetable stock is very easy. I like to save vegetable scraps from a few days' worth of cooking and make a large pot of stock on the weekends. You can create many different flavors of stock by varying the herbs and vegetables you use. Freeze your stock in widemouthed, 1-quart jars for later use.

12 cups water

1 large onion, coarsely chopped

1 leek, chopped and well rinsed

2 to 3 carrots, chopped

4 celery stalks, chopped

4 garlic cloves, chopped

1 strip kombu seaweed

½ bunch fresh parsley

3 bay leaves

1 teaspoon whole black peppercorns

1 handful fresh herbs (thyme, rosemary, savory, marjoram)

vegetable scraps (carrot peels, celery tops, onion skins)

1 to 2 teaspoons sea salt or Herbamare

Place all the ingredients into an 8-quart stockpot and bring to a boil. Cover, reduce the heat to low, and simmer for 2 to 3 hours.

Strain the stock into another pot, discard the vegetables, and pour into clean, widemouthed, 1-quart jars. Store the stock in the refrigerator or freezer (see Tip on page 184).

Yield: 3 quarts

ASIAN SOUP STOCK

This delicious and medicinal soup stock can be used as a base for a soup or stew, or simply sipped when you have a cold or flu. I like to freeze at least half of this when I make it because you never know when you will need it!

12 cups water	3 to 4 cups chopped shiitake mushrooms
1 large onion, chopped	1 strip kombu seaweed
1 head garlic, cut in half crosswise	1 lemongrass stalk, chopped (optional)
one 2-inch piece fresh ginger, sliced	½ to 1 teaspoon crushed red chili flakes
3 celery stalks, chopped	1 to 2 teaspoons sea salt
2 carrots, chopped	

Place all the ingredients into an 8-quart stockpot and bring to a boil. Cover, reduce the heat to low, and simmer for 2 to 3 hours.

Place a strainer over a large bowl or pot and pour the stock through it. You can discard the vegetables, though the shiitake mushrooms are especially good to nibble on!

The stock may be frozen for later use or stored in widemouthed, 1-quart jars in the refrigerator for 5 to 7 days (see Tip on page 184).

Yield: 3 quarts

Variation: Add 2 pounds bone-in, skin-on organic chicken for a more nourishing stock.

BONE BROTH SOUP

Use this soup to help treat an upset tummy. It's the perfect meal to eat when the gut is so out of balance that no other foods will digest properly. The gelatin and amino acids in bone broth help to heal a leaky gut, and the cooked vegetables are easily digested. Use either the beef or chicken stock recipe on the previous pages. Add small amounts of slow-cooked organic chicken or beef if desired.

---

2 quarts Homemade Beef Stock (page 184) or Homemade Chicken Stock (page 185)

1 medium onion, finely diced

3 to 4 carrots, diced

3 to 4 celery stalks, diced

1 garlic clove, crushed

1 teaspoon dried thyme

1 to 2 medium zucchini, diced

2 to 3 cups chopped bok choy

½ cup finely chopped fresh parsley

sea salt or Herbamare

Place the stock, onion, carrots, celery, garlic, and thyme into a 3-quart pot, cover, and simmer for 10 to 15 minutes. Add the zucchini and bok choy and simmer 5 to 7 minutes more, or until the zucchini is tender. Add the parsley, and season to taste with sea salt or Herbamare.

Yield: 4 to 6 servings

Variation: In the wintertime, use diced butternut squash, celery root, rutabagas, or sweet potatoes.

BUTTERNUT SQUASH, KALE, AND WHITE BEAN SOUP

I like to make this soup when the winter squash are coming into season, which happens just as my children are going back to school in the fall. They like to pack this soup in small stainless steel Thermoses for their school lunch. Serve with the Hearty Seed Bread (page 161).

---

2 tablespoons extra-virgin olive oil

1 large onion, chopped

3 celery stalks, chopped

1 small butternut squash, peeled, seeded, and cubed

8 cups Homemade Chicken Stock (page 185) or Homemade Vegetable Stock (page 186)

2 to 3 tablespoons chopped fresh rosemary

3 to 4 cups cooked cannellini beans

2 to 3 cups chopped kale

freshly ground black pepper

sea salt

Heat the olive oil in a 6-quart pot over medium heat. Add the onion and sauté for 5 to 10 minutes. Add the celery, butternut squash, stock, and rosemary, cover, and simmer for about 15 minutes, or until the squash is tender.

Add the cooked beans, kale, pepper, and sea salt and simmer for 4 to 5 minutes more. Taste and adjust the salt and seasonings if necessary.

Yield: 6 to 8 servings

FALL PINTO BEAN AND YAM SOUP

This soup is a celebration of the flavors of autumn and the abundant harvest that this season has to offer. Serve this soup with the Autumn Harvest Salad (page 221) and cooked quinoa. If you do not want to cook your own beans then use three cans of organic beans. Just add them to the soup where you would add the freshly cooked beans.

BEANS

2 cups dry pinto beans (soaked overnight)

6 to 8 cups water

4 garlic cloves, peeled

1 strip kombu seaweed

SOUP

2 tablespoons extra-virgin olive oil

1 large onion, chopped

5 garlic cloves, crushed

1 to 2 jalapeño peppers, chopped

2 small yams, peeled and diced

3 carrots, cut into rounds

1 tablespoon ground cumin

1 teaspoon paprika

½ teaspoon chipotle chile powder

8 cups bean cooking liquid or water

4 cups chopped fresh tomatoes

2 to 3 ears organic fresh corn, kernels cut off cobs

1 small bunch black kale, finely chopped

1 cup chopped fresh cilantro

freshly squeezed juice of ½ lime

2 to 3 teaspoons sea salt or Herbamare

To cook the beans, rinse and drain the soaked beans and place them into a 6-quart pot with the water, garlic, and kombu and bring to a boil. Reduce the heat to a gentle simmer and cook for approximately 1 hour, or until the beans are soft and mash easily. Remove the pot from the heat. Drain the beans and reserve the cooking liquid.

To make the soup, heat the olive oil in an 8-quart pot over medium heat. Add onion and sauté for about 5 minutes.

Add the garlic, jalapeño peppers, yams, carrots, cumin, paprika, and chipotle chile powder and sauté, stirring, for 5 minutes more. Add the reserved bean cooking liquid or water and mix well to remove any spices that have stuck to the bottom of the pot.

Add the cooked beans, tomatoes, and corn kernels and mix well. If the soup needs more liquid, add more water.

Cover the pot and simmer the soup until the vegetables are tender, 20 to 25 minutes. Add the kale, cilantro, lime juice, and sea salt or Herbamare and simmer for about 5 minutes more. Taste and adjust the salt and lime juice if needed.

Yield: 8 servings

FRAGRANT LENTIL SOUP

Garam masala is an Indian spice blend that can be found in the bulk spice section of your local co-op or health food store. It is the secret ingredient in this great-tasting soup! Serve this easy-to-make soup with the Winter Quinoa Salad (page 287) for a festive winter meal.

---

1 tablespoon extra-virgin olive oil

1 large onion, chopped

4 garlic cloves, crushed

3 large carrots, diced

1 tablespoon dried thyme

1 teaspoon garam masala

2 cups green lentils, rinsed and drained

8 cups water, Homemade Vegetable Stock (page 186), or Homemade Beef Stock (page 184)

2 cups chopped tomatoes (see Tip on page 204)

4 cups baby spinach leaves

1 to 2 teaspoons sea salt or Herbamare

2 tablespoons red wine vinegar

Heat the olive oil in a 6-quart pot over medium heat. Add the onion and sauté for about 5 minutes, or until soft.

Add the garlic, carrots, thyme, and garam masala and sauté for 5 to 7 minutes more.

Add the lentils and water, cover the pot, and simmer for 35 to 40 minutes.

Add the tomatoes, spinach, sea salt, and red wine vinegar and simmer for 10 minutes more.

Yield: 6 servings

> **Tip:** If you are gluten-sensitive be sure to sort through your lentils and pick out any gluten grains, then rinse the lentils very well. Lentils can be cross contaminated with gluten grains during growing and processing.

FRENCH LENTIL SOUP

French lentils, also called *lentilles de Puy*, are named after Le Puy in Auvergne, a volcanic area in the center of France with the ideal soil and climate for the growth of the lentils. French lentils have a delicate taste and a fine green skin with steel blue speckles. They usually can be found in the bulk section of your local co-op or health food store.

1 tablespoon extra-virgin olive oil
1 medium onion, chopped
3 garlic cloves, crushed
2 celery stalks, diced
2 large carrots, diced
3 small red potatoes, diced
1 teaspoon dried thyme
2 teaspoons paprika

1 teaspoon Italian seasoning
2 cups French lentils, rinsed and drained
8 cups water
2 cups chopped tomatoes (see Tip on page 204)
1 tablespoon red wine vinegar
2 to 3 teaspoons sea salt or Herbamare
½ cup chopped fresh basil
½ cup chopped fresh parsley

Heat the olive oil in an 8-quart pot over medium heat. Add the onion and sauté for about 5 minutes, or until soft. Add the garlic and sauté 2 minutes more. Add the celery, carrots, potatoes, thyme, paprika, and Italian seasoning and sauté for another 5 minutes, stirring frequently.

Add the French lentils and water, cover, and simmer over low heat for 25 minutes.

After the lentils are cooked and the vegetables are tender, add the tomatoes, vinegar, sea salt, and fresh herbs and mix well. Simmer, uncovered, for another 5 minutes.

Yield: 6 servings

LEMON AND LENTIL SOUP

This soup is a great dish to prepare when you don't have a lot of time; we use a food processor for all of the chopping, which cuts the preparation time in half. Serve this soup over cooked brown jasmine or basmati rice (see page 265). This soup also freezes well for later use.

1 small onion, roughly chopped

5 garlic cloves, peeled

2 tablespoons extra-virgin olive oil

2 cups red lentils, rinsed and drained

8 cups Homemade Vegetable Stock (page 186) or water

4 to 5 cups baby spinach

1 small handful fresh parsley

½ cup freshly squeezed lemon juice

1 to 2 teaspoons sea salt or Herbamare

Put the onion and garlic into a food processor fitted with the "s" blade and pulse until finely chopped.

Heat the olive oil in a 6-quart pot. Add the finely chopped onions and garlic and sauté for about 5 minutes, or until soft.

Add the red lentils and the stock or water, cover the pot, and simmer for about 25 minutes, or until the lentils are very soft and cooked through.

While the lentils are cooking, put the spinach and parsley into the food processor and pulse until minced.

Add the minced parsley and spinach to the cooked lentils along with the lemon juice and sea salt. Simmer the soup on low for another 3 to 5 minutes. Taste and add more salt or lemon juice if desired. Serve over cooked brown jasmine or brown basmati rice.

Yield: 4 to 6 servings

LILY'S LEMONGRASS SOUP

Our daughter, Lily, created this recipe when she was 4½ years old. She has been cooking in the kitchen with me ever since she was a baby and now creates her own recipes. She did all of the cutting and preparation for this soup, adding all ingredients of her choice, with no input from me. Our younger daughter, Grace, was standing next to Lily on a stool while she was cooking this and decided to add some cooked rice to the soup. After refining the recipe, I added the soup stock, garlic, and kaffir lime leaves. This soup has now become a regular part of our family's meal plans!

---

6 cups Asian Soup Stock (page 187)

2 fresh lemongrass stalks, cut into 3-inch pieces

3 to 4 kaffir lime leaves

3 carrots, chopped

3 to 4 celery stalks, chopped

3 to 4 garlic cloves, crushed

1 teaspoon freshly grated ginger

sea salt or Herbamare

1 to 2 cups cooked brown jasmine rice (optional)

4 to 5 green onions, sliced

½ cup chopped fresh cilantro

crushed red chili flakes

Place the stock, lemongrass, and kaffir lime leaves into a 6-quart pot. Cover and simmer for about 35 minutes. Remove the lemongrass and lime leaves from the pot.

Add the carrots, celery, garlic, ginger, and sea salt to taste and simmer for another 7 to 10 minutes, or until the vegetables are crisp-tender.

Add the cooked rice, if using, green onions, and cilantro. Taste and adjust the salt and seasonings if necessary.

Garnish each bowl with a pinch or two of red chili flakes.

Yield: 4 to 6 servings

Variation: Add cooked chicken to the soup for more protein, B vitamins, and selenium.

MINESTRONE SOUP

This is a simple, classic soup that everyone will enjoy. The soup can be made in large batches and then frozen into serving-size containers. The addition of the large amount of fresh herbs really makes this recipe stand out from others. Use Homemade Beef Stock (page 184) for a more flavorful and nutritious soup.

---

1 tablespoon extra-virgin olive oil

1 medium onion, finely chopped

8 garlic cloves, crushed

3 celery stalks, chopped

2 large carrots, peeled and diced

½ teaspoon dried crushed rosemary

½ teaspoon freshly ground pepper

8 cups Homemade Vegetable Stock (page 186) or Homemade Beef Stock (page 184)

4 cups chopped tomatoes

¼ cup tomato paste

½ pound green beans, ends trimmed and cut into pieces

2 medium zucchini, diced

2 cups cooked kidney beans

2 cups cooked chickpeas

2 tablespoons chopped fresh thyme

½ cup chopped fresh basil

¼ cup chopped fresh oregano

1 cup chopped fresh parsley

1 to 2 teaspoons sea salt or Herbamare

Heat the olive oil in an 8-quart pot over medium heat. Add the onion and sauté for about 5 minutes, or until soft.

Add the garlic, celery, carrots, crushed rosemary, and pepper and sauté for another 5 minutes, stirring frequently.

Add the beef or vegetable stock, tomatoes, and tomato paste and stir well. Cover, and cook for 7 to 10 minutes, or until the carrots are slightly tender but not cooked all the way through.

Add the green beans, zucchini, kidney beans, chickpeas, fresh herbs, and sea salt, cover, and simmer until all of the vegetables are tender, about 7 minutes more. Taste and adjust the salt and seasonings if desired.

Yield: 6 to 8 servings

MOROCCAN CHICKPEA AND POTATO SOUP

This soup is a favorite among children and adults alike, making it a very family friendly meal. It is flavorful yet simple to please many tastes. This soup is delicious served with freshly cooked quinoa, olives, and steamed chard. Remember to plan ahead for this recipe and soak the beans before you go to bed the night before.

2 tablespoons extra-virgin olive oil

1 large onion, chopped

6 garlic cloves, crushed

1 teaspoon curry powder

1 teaspoon ground cardamom

½ teaspoon ground turmeric

½ teaspoon freshly ground black pepper

1½ cups dried chickpeas (soaked overnight)

10 to 12 cups water

4 large carrots, diced

4 to 5 red or yellow potatoes, diced

¼ cup tomato paste

¼ cup freshly squeezed lemon juice

1 to 2 teaspoons sea salt

½ cup chopped fresh parsley

Heat the olive oil in an 8-quart pot over medium heat. Add the onion and sauté for 4 to 5 minutes. Add the garlic and spices and sauté for 1 minute more.

Drain the soaked chickpeas and rinse well. Add the chickpeas and 10 to 12 cups of fresh water to the pot and bring to a boil. Reduce the heat to low and simmer, partially covered, for about 45 minutes.

Add the carrots and potatoes to the pot and simmer for 15 to 20 minutes more, or until the vegetables are tender and the chickpeas are completely cooked. Then add the tomato paste, lemon juice, sea salt, and parsley, stir well, and simmer for a few minutes more. Taste and adjust the salt and seasonings if desired.

Yield: 6 to 8 servings

QUINOA CORN CHOWDER

We like to make this hearty chowder in late summer when the sweet corn and peppers are in abundance, plus it's a great way to use up leftover roasted chicken and cooked quinoa! Use the Homemade Chicken Stock (page 185) or the Homemade Vegetable Stock (page 186) for best results. The raw cashew butter gives the chowder a creaminess without using dairy.

1 tablespoon extra-virgin olive oil or virgin coconut oil

1 large onion, chopped

1 leek, chopped and well rinsed

2 to 3 garlic cloves, crushed

3 celery stalks, chopped

3 to 4 carrots, diced

1 large poblano pepper, diced

4 to 5 ears organic sweet corn, kernels cut from the cobs

8 cups Homemade Chicken Stock (page 185) or Homemade Vegetable Stock (page 186)

2 to 3 tablespoons raw cashew butter

3 cups cooked quinoa

2 cups cooked chopped chicken (optional)

2 to 3 cups chopped kale

2 teaspoons sea salt or Herbamare

freshly ground black pepper

GARNISH

chopped fresh cilantro or parsley

chopped serrano chiles

Heat the oil in an 8-quart pot over medium heat. Add the onion and leek and sauté about 5 minutes. Add the garlic, celery, carrots, poblano pepper, and corn kernels and sauté a few minutes more. Add the stock and cashew butter; cover, and simmer for 20 to 25 minutes, stirring occasionally.

Add the cooked quinoa, chopped chicken if using, kale, Herbamare, and plenty of freshly ground black pepper, cover, and simmer 5 to 10 minutes more. Taste and adjust the salt and seasonings if necessary. Serve garnished with cilantro or parsley. If you like your chowder spicy, sprinkle your bowl with chopped fresh serrano chiles!

Yield: about 8 servings

Variation: Replace the cooked quinoa with cooked wild rice.

> **Tip:** To cut kernels from the cob, stand the cob up over a plate or a wide, shallow bowl and cut downward along the kernels, using a serrated knife. Keep rotating the cob until you have cut off all the kernels.

RED LENTIL DAL

Dal is an Indian stew made with lentils and spices, which is usually served over rice. It is very easy to make and portions can be frozen for later use. Serve this hearty dal with Indian Fried Rice (page 273) and the Cabbage Salad with Cilantro Vinaigrette (page 226).

2 tablespoons virgin coconut oil

1½ teaspoons whole cumin seeds

1½ teaspoons black mustard seeds

1 large onion, diced

3 garlic cloves, crushed

2 teaspoons ground turmeric

2 teaspoons ground cumin

⅛ to ¼ teaspoon cayenne pepper

2 large carrots, peeled and diced

3 medium red potatoes, cubed

2½ cups red lentils, rinsed and drained

6 cups water

one 14-ounce can coconut milk

2 cups chopped tomatoes

2 teaspoons sea salt or Herbamare

Heat the coconut oil in an 8-quart pot over medium heat. Add the cumin seeds and black mustard seeds and sauté until they begin to pop. Quickly add the onion and garlic and sauté until soft, about 5 minutes.

Add the turmeric, ground cumin, cayenne, carrots, and potatoes and sauté a few minutes more.

Add the red lentils, water, coconut milk, and chopped tomatoes and stir well to combine. Bring to a boil, cover, and simmer for about 45 minutes. Season with the sea salt and serve.

Yield: 6 to 8 Servings

SPICY BLACK BEAN SOUP

Not only are black beans high in molybdenum, folate, fiber, protein, and manganese, they are also high in antioxidant compounds called anthocyanins. These compounds work synergistically with other compounds found in whole foods to protect against cancer and other diseases. This soup can be made with less spice if you leave out the jalapeño pepper. Serve bowls of soup dolloped with Coconut Milk Yogurt (page 104).

1 tablespoon extra-virgin olive oil	¼ teaspoon chipotle chile powder
1 medium onion, chopped	pinch cayenne pepper
1 medium red bell pepper, diced	2 to 3 cups water
1 large carrot, diced	6 cups cooked black beans
1 small jalapeño pepper, finely diced	2 cups chopped tomatoes
1 teaspoon ground cumin	1 cup fresh or frozen organic corn kernels
1 teaspoon paprika	½ cup chopped fresh cilantro
½ teaspoon dried oregano	2 teaspoons sea salt or Herbamare
½ teaspoon chili powder	1 tablespoon apple cider vinegar

Heat the olive oil in a 6-quart pot over medium heat. Add the onion and a pinch of sea salt and sauté until slightly golden. Add the bell pepper, carrot, and jalapeño pepper and sauté, stirring occasionally, for a few minutes more. Add the spices and stir to coat.

Add the water, black beans, tomatoes, and corn kernels and more water if necessary. Reduce the heat to medium-low and simmer until the vegetables are fork-tender, 20 to 25 minutes.

Remove the pot from the heat and add the cilantro. Season with sea salt or Herbamare. Stir in the vinegar. Taste and adjust the salt and seasonings if necessary.

Yield: 6 servings

SPLIT PEA SOUP WITH FRESH VEGETABLES AND HERBS

Split peas are an excellent source of molybdenum, soluble fiber, protein, and B vitamins. The fiber in peas helps to stabilize blood sugar levels and reduce cholesterol. Serve this soup with a green salad and a cooked whole grain for a balanced meal.

---

2 cups split peas, rinsed and drained

5 cups water

3 bay leaves

1 tablespoon extra-virgin olive oil

1 medium onion, diced

4 garlic cloves, crushed

2 medium carrots, diced

2 celery stalks, diced

1 medium red bell pepper, diced

1 tablespoon dried thyme

1 teaspoon ground dried rosemary

1 teaspoon sea salt

3 cups Homemade Vegetable Stock (page 186) or Homemade Chicken Stock (page 185)

¼ cup fresh basil, chopped

½ cup fresh parsley, chopped

1 tablespoon white wine vinegar

½ teaspoon freshly ground black pepper

Place the split peas into a 6-quart pot with the water and bay leaves. Cover, and simmer on medium-low heat for 45 minutes, stirring occasionally. Add more water if needed.

Heat the olive oil in a large skillet over medium heat. Add the onion and garlic and cook until they begin to soften, 3 to 5 minutes. Add the carrots, celery, and bell pepper and sauté for a minute. Add the thyme, rosemary, and sea salt and sauté 3 to 5 minutes more.

Add the cooked vegetables to the pot with the cooked split peas, then add the stock, and stir well. Simmer over medium-low heat until the vegetables are tender. Add the fresh basil, parsley, white wine vinegar, and black pepper. Adjust the salt and seasonings if necessary.

Yield: 6 servings

SUMMER VEGETABLE SOUP

This colorful soup celebrates the bounty of the summer harvest. You can really get creative here and use whatever vegetables you have growing in your garden. Try adding fresh corn kernels, different dark leafy greens, or even a combination of different types of tomatoes.

1 tablespoon extra-virgin olive oil

1 medium onion, diced

3 to 4 garlic cloves, crushed

2 to 3 large carrots, diced

½ pound green or yellow wax beans, cut into 1-inch pieces

2 to 3 cups diced fresh tomatoes

6 to 8 cups Homemade Vegetable, Chicken, or Beef Stock (pages 186, 185, 184)

2 zucchini, diced

4 cups thinly sliced greens (kale, chard, collards, cabbage)

¼ cup finely chopped fresh herbs (basil, oregano, chives, marjoram)

2 cups cooked beans (cranberry, baby lima, or chickpeas)

1 to 2 teaspoons sea salt or Herbamare

freshly ground black pepper

Heat the olive oil in a 6-quart pot over medium heat. Add the onion and sauté for about 5 minutes, or until soft. Add the garlic and carrots and sauté a few minutes more.

Add the green beans, tomatoes, and stock and simmer, covered, for 10 to 15 minutes, or until the vegetables are tender but not all the way cooked.

Add the zucchini, greens, fresh herbs and cooked beans and simmer for 5 to 7 minutes more, or until the zucchini is cooked. Season with sea salt and pepper to taste.

Yield: 6 to 8 servings

THREE-BEAN CHILI

Serve this warming soup with Easy Polenta (page 290) and Apple-Spiced Collard Greens (page 246). Freeze portions in serving-size containers for later use.

---

1 cup dried pinto beans (soaked overnight)
1 cup dried kidney beans (soaked overnight)
1 cup dried black beans (soaked overnight)
8 to 10 cups water
1 tablespoon extra-virgin olive oil
1 large onion, chopped
4 to 5 garlic cloves, crushed
4 large carrots, peeled and sliced
1 large green bell pepper, chopped

1 tablespoon ground cumin
1 tablespoon chili powder
2 teaspoons dried oregano
4 cups diced tomatoes
2 cups tomato purée
4 to 5 cups reserved bean cooking liquid or water
2 teaspoons sea salt or Herbamare

Rinse the beans and place them in a large bowl. Add at least twice as much water as there are beans and soak overnight or for 8 to 24 hours.

Drain off all of the soaking water from the beans, rinse well, and place into an 8- quart pot with the fresh water. Simmer for 1 to 1½ hours, or until the beans are tender and cooked. Drain the beans in a colander over a bowl, reserving the cooking liquid.

Rinse out the pot and place it back on the stovetop. Add the olive oil and heat over medium heat. Add the onion and sauté for about 5 minutes, or until soft. Then add the garlic, carrots, bell pepper, cumin, chili powder, and oregano and sauté for another 3 minutes or so.

Add the diced tomatoes, tomato purée, reserved bean cooking liquid, and cooked beans and simmer for 20 to 25 minutes, or until the vegetables are tender. Season to taste with sea salt or Herbamare.

Yield: 6 to 8 servings

VEGETARIAN CHIPOTLE CHILI

This recipe is very fast and easy to prepare and makes a great weeknight meal. Serve with Basic Sticky Brown Rice (page 266) and the Arugula Salad with Lime Vinaigrette (page 218) for a complete meal.

1 tablespoon extra-virgin olive oil	2 teaspoons ground cumin
1 large onion, chopped	6 to 8 cups cooked kidney beans
3 garlic cloves, crushed	6 cups diced plum tomatoes
2 large carrots, diced	2 teaspoons chili powder
2 medium zucchini, diced	¾ teaspoon chipotle chile powder
1 medium red bell pepper, diced	2 to 3 cups water
2 teaspoons sea salt or Herbamare	1 cup chopped fresh cilantro

Heat the olive oil in an 8-quart pot over medium heat. Add the onion and sauté until softened. Add the garlic and carrots, stir to coat with olive oil, and sauté for a few minutes more.

Add the zucchini, bell pepper, sea salt, and cumin and sauté, stirring, for about 1 minute.

Add the kidney beans, tomatoes, chili powder, and chipotle chile powder to the pot. Add the water, a little at a time, until you reach the desired consistency. Simmer the chili, covered, for 15 to 20 minutes, or until the vegetables are tender. Stir in the cilantro. Taste and adjust salt and spices if necessary.

Yield: 6 to 8 servings

Variation: Place the tomatoes onto two large baking sheets and broil in the oven for 8 to 10 minutes; then add to the soup. This will give the soup more flavor.

WINTER VEGETABLE AND WHITE BEAN SOUP

Navy beans or Great Northern beans work very well in this soup. If you are pinched for time use two cans of organic beans instead of cooking your own. Serve this warming soup in the winter with the Herbed Focaccia Bread (page 163) and the Braised Kale with Garlic and Ginger (page 247).

¼ cup extra-virgin olive oil

1 large onion, diced

2 teaspoons sea salt

2 celery stalks, diced

2 large carrots, diced

6 to 8 garlic cloves, crushed

2 shallots, minced

1 tablespoon chopped fresh rosemary

1 teaspoon dried thyme

8 cups Homemade Vegetable Stock (page 186) or Homemade Chicken Stock (page 185)

4 cups diced tomatoes

2 medium yellow potatoes, diced

1 small rutabaga, peeled and diced

1 small yam, peeled and diced

1 small delicata squash, diced

4 cups cooked white beans

2 cups Savoy cabbage, chopped

Heat the olive oil in an 8-quart pot over medium heat. Add the onion and sea salt and sauté until softened, about 5 minutes.

Add the celery, carrots, garlic, shallots, rosemary, and thyme and sauté for about 5 minutes.

Add the vegetable or chicken stock, diced tomatoes, potatoes, rutabaga, yam, squash, and cooked white beans. Cover, reduce the heat to low, and simmer for 20 to 25 minutes, or until the vegetables are tender.

Stir in the Savoy cabbage and simmer for 5 minutes more. Taste and adjust the salt and herbs if necessary.

Yield: 8 servings

Tip: I like to freeze whole plum tomatoes in late summer to use in winter soups like this one. When ready to use, take them out of the freezer and run them under hot water to remove the skins, then chop while they are still frozen.

CELERY ROOT, PEAR, AND PARSNIP SOUP

Starchy root vegetables such as celery root and parsnips provide a source of clean-burning, low-glycemic carbohydrates. Serve this soup in lieu of bread with a meal. It's hearty, warming, and very satisfying on a chilly autumn evening.

2 tablespoons extra-virgin olive oil or organic butter

1 medium onion, chopped

2 medium celery roots, peeled and chopped

1 large parsnip, peeled and chopped

2 ripe pears, cored and chopped

3 garlic cloves, chopped

1 teaspoon dried thyme

6 cups Homemade Chicken Stock (page 185) or Homemade Vegetable Stock (page 186)

½ cup dry white wine

1 to 2 teaspoons sea salt or Herbamare

freshly ground black pepper

Heat the olive oil or butter in a 6-quart pot over medium heat. Add the onion and sauté for 5 to 7 minutes, or until softened and beginning to change color. Add the celery roots, parsnip, pears, garlic, thyme, stock, and wine, cover, and simmer for about 30 minutes. Season with the sea salt and pepper.

Using an immersion blender, purée the soup, or let it cool slightly and transfer the soup to a blender and purée. Reheat if necessary and serve.

Yield: 6 servings

CREAMY BUTTERNUT SQUASH SOUP

This is a wonderful warming fall soup. If you like a little less spice, then add half the amount of red chili flakes. This soup freezes very well, so stock your freezer while squash is in season!

2 tablespoons virgin coconut oil

1 large onion, chopped

6 garlic cloves, crushed

1 teaspoon crushed red chili flakes

one 4- to 5-pound butternut squash, peeled and cubed

3 to 4 cups chopped tomatoes

two 14-ounce cans coconut milk

4 cups Homemade Vegetable Stock (page 186) or water

½ cup chopped fresh cilantro

2 teaspoons sea salt or Herbamare

Heat the coconut oil in an 8-quart pot heat over medium heat. Add the onion and sauté for about 5 minutes. Add the garlic and red chili flakes and sauté for 1 to 2 minutes more, stirring frequently so the garlic doesn't burn.

Add the squash, tomatoes, coconut milk, and vegetable stock, cover, and simmer over low heat for about 30 minutes, or until the squash is very tender.

When the squash is cooked, stir in the cilantro. Using a stainless steel immersion blender, purée the soup in the pot. If you like your soup a little chunky, then purée only half of it. Season to taste with sea salt or Herbamare.

Yield: 6 to 8 servings

CREAMY CAULIFLOWER SOUP

When purchasing cauliflower, make sure the tops are white. If the florets have begun to spot brown or purple, it is past its nutritional peak. Cauliflower is an excellent source of the disease-fighting nutrients indole-3-carbinol and sulforaphane. These two nutrients act together in the body to destroy and sweep out cancerous cells.

2 tablespoons extra-virgin olive oil	2 teaspoons dried thyme
1 leek, chopped and well rinsed	1 large cauliflower head, cut into chunks
2 garlic cloves, crushed	6 cups water
2 celery stalks, chopped	¼ cup fresh tarragon, chopped
2 teaspoons sea salt or Herbamare	½ cup chopped fresh parsley
¼ teaspoon ground white pepper	½ cup raw cashews

Heat the olive oil in a 6-quart pot over medium heat. Add the sliced leeks and sauté for about 2 minutes. Then add the garlic and celery and sauté, stirring, for another 3 minutes, or until the celery begins to soften. Add the sea salt, white pepper, and thyme. Add the cauliflower and stir to coat with oil and spices.

Add the water; if the water is insufficient to cover the cauliflower then add more water, a little at a time until it is about ½ inch above the vegetables. Cook, covered, over medium-low heat for 20 to 25 minutes, or until the cauliflower is soft. When the cauliflower is soft, stir in the tarragon and parsley.

Remove 1 cup of the broth from the pot with the cauliflower and add it to a blender with the raw cashews. Blend on high until the mixture resembles a smooth cream. Add a few cups of soup to the cashew mixture and purée until smooth. Pour the puréed mixture into a clean pot.

Continue to purée the soup, working in batches, until it is all blended. Stir to combine the cashew cream–soup mixture with the rest of the soup. For a thinner soup, add more water. Taste and adjust the salt and spices if needed.

Gently reheat the soup over low heat and serve.

Yield: 6 servings

GINGERED CARROT SOUP

Ginger lovers will enjoy this light and creamy soup. Serve it with the Spiced Citrus Salmon (page 316) and a mixed green salad for a colorful, nutrient-rich meal.

---

1 tablespoon virgin coconut oil

1 medium onion, chopped

3 garlic cloves, crushed

2 tablespoons grated fresh ginger

½ to 1 teaspoon ground cumin

½ teaspoon ground cinnamon

¼ teaspoon ground allspice

2 pounds carrots, peeled and chopped

6 cups water or Homemade Chicken Stock (page 185)

2 to 3 tablespoons freshly squeezed lemon juice

1 to 2 teaspoons sea salt or Herbamare

coconut milk, for garnish (optional)

Heat the coconut oil in a 6-quart pot over medium heat. Add the onion and sauté until soft, about 5 minutes. Add the garlic, ginger, and spices; and continue to sauté for 1 minute more.

Add the carrots, stir to coat with oil and spices, and cook 3 to 4 minutes. Add the water or broth, cover, and simmer until the carrots are soft, about 30 minutes. Stir in the lemon juice.

Using a stainless steel immersion blender, purée the soup in the pot, or cool the soup briefly and transfer the soup to a blender and blend on high until puréed, working in batches until all of the soup is puréed. Season with sea salt to taste.

For added taste and appearance, serve in individual bowls with a swirl of coconut milk if desired.

Yield: 6 servings

ROASTED RED PEPPER SOUP

This soup has a medium rating for spiciness; if you like it mild add ½ teaspoon less of the crushed red chili flakes, or add ½ teaspoon more for a hotter soup. Serve this soup with baked fish or chicken and a green salad.

1 tablespoon virgin coconut oil

1 large onion, diced

2 tablespoons chopped garlic

½ to 1 teaspoon crushed red chili flakes

1 teaspoon sea salt or Herbamare

two 14-ounce cans coconut milk

4 cups Homemade Vegetable Stock (page 186) or Homemade Chicken Stock (page 185)

4 to 5 red bell peppers, roasted

4 cups chopped tomatoes

¼ cup minced fresh parsley

¼ cup minced fresh basil

Heat the coconut oil in a 6-quart pot over medium heat. Add the onion, garlic, red chili flakes, and sea salt and sauté until tender.

Add the coconut milk, stock, bell peppers, and tomatoes to the pot and simmer for 20 minutes, covered, stirring occasionally.

Purée the soup in blender in batches then return to pot, or use an immersion blender to purée the soup in the pot. Cook on low heat for about 5 minutes, then add the parsley and basil, and cook for 5 minutes more, stirring often. Taste and adjust the salt and spices if necessary.

Yield: 6 servings

Tip: To roast the red bell peppers, place them in a baking dish under the broiler until the skin is charred, turning frequently, 8 to 10 minutes. Remove the peppers from the dish and place them into a paper bag or a covered glass bowl. Let steam for about 10 minutes. Remove the peppers and peel off charred skin. Cut the peppers and remove and discard the stem and seeds.

ROASTED TOMATO-FENNEL SOUP

I like to make this soup in late summer when the plum tomatoes and fresh fennel are plentiful. I freeze it in quart jars to enjoy when the weather cools. Serve with the Herbed Focaccia Bread (page 163) and a green salad.

---

12 to 14 plum tomatoes (about 3 pounds)
2 medium fennel bulbs
1 large leek
¼ cup extra-virgin olive oil
1 teaspoon sea salt

4 cups Homemade Chicken Stock (page 185) or Homemade Vegetable Stock (page 186)
1 handful fresh basil leaves
freshly ground black pepper

Preheat the oven to 400°F. Set out two large, rimmed baking sheets or glass baking pans.

Cut the tomatoes in half lengthwise and distribute them evenly between the two baking sheets. Cut the green stems off the fennel bulbs. Chop the fennel bulb into large pieces and transfer them to the baking sheets. Trim the ends off the leek, cut in half lengthwise, and rinse well under cool running water to remove dirt, then chop into large pieces and distribute equally between the two baking sheets.

Add 2 tablespoons of olive oil and ½ teaspoon sea salt to the vegetables on each baking sheet and toss together. Roast in the oven for about 45 minutes. Transfer the roasted vegetables along with any pan juices to a 6-quart pot. Discard any pieces of vegetable that are very browned (sometimes a few leek pieces can get too browned when I make this). Add the stock and purée using an immersion blender (or add ingredients to a blender), then add the basil leaves and barely blend them so they are just in little pieces, not completely puréed. Place the pot on the stovetop and heat the soup on low. Season with sea salt and pepper to taste. Serve.

Yield: 6 servings

THAI COCONUT VEGETABLE SOUP

I love the flavors of Thai food. This recipe embodies those flavors without being too difficult to prepare. The Asian Soup Stock (page 187) is especially delicious in this soup, though a basic vegetable or chicken stock will do. Fish, chicken, shrimp, or tofu can easily be added to this soup if you desire. Unlike most soups, which improve with age, this soup tastes best immediately after it is made.

2 cups Homemade Vegetable Stock (page 186) or Homemade Chicken Stock (page 185)

one 14-ounce can coconut milk

1 teaspoon crushed red chili flakes

6 to 8 garlic cloves, crushed

1 small onion, cut into half-moons

2 to 3 carrots, peeled and cut into matchsticks

1 red bell pepper, cut into strips

1 medium zucchini, sliced into half moons

2 cups thinly sliced bok choy or cabbage leaves

½ cup chopped fresh cilantro

sea salt or Herbamare

Pour the stock into a 4-quart pot. Add the coconut milk, red chili flakes, garlic, onion, carrots, and bell pepper and simmer for 15 minutes, covered, or until the vegetables are just tender.

Add the zucchini and simmer for 5 minutes more. Remove the pot from the heat and add the sliced bok choy leaves and cilantro. Season to taste with sea salt or Herbamare. Garnish with extra red chili flakes if desired.

Yield: 4 servings

CHICKEN NOODLE AND VEGETABLE SOUP

Soup is a great way to make use of the whole chicken. By simmering the chicken with vegetables, water, and herbs, vital nutrients from the bone marrow are released into the broth. Don't skip the fresh rosemary! It is the secret ingredient to this great-tasting soup.

BROTH

1 whole organic chicken (about 4 pounds)
1 large onion, cut into quarters with skin on
1 head garlic, cut in half crosswise
3 celery stalks, chopped
1 large carrot, chopped
2 bay leaves
1 strip kombu seaweed
2 teaspoons whole black peppercorns
½ bunch fresh parsley, chopped
4 sprigs fresh rosemary
3 sprigs fresh marjoram
3 sprigs fresh thyme
1 tablespoon sea salt or Herbamare
12 cups water

SOUP

1 large onion, diced
3 large carrots, peeled and sliced into rounds
3 celery stalks, chopped
3 to 4 red potatoes, cubed
½ bunch fresh parsley, chopped
1 to 2 tablespoons finely chopped fresh rosemary
1 teaspoon dried thyme
½ package quinoa spaghetti noodles
4 cups chopped kale
sea salt or Herbamare
freshly ground black pepper

To make the broth, rinse the chicken and put it in an 8-quart pot; add the remaining ingredients for the broth. Place the pot over medium-high heat, and bring to a gentle boil. Reduce the heat to a low simmer and cover with a lid. Simmer for 1½ to 2 hours, or until the chicken falls easily off the bone.

Place a large strainer over a clean large pot and pour the contents of the broth through the strainer to separate the broth from the vegetables and chicken. Remove the chicken and transfer to a plate to cool. Discard the vegetables and herbs.

To make the soup, place the pot of broth back on the stovetop over medium heat; add the chopped onion, sliced carrots, celery, cubed potatoes, and herbs; simmer for 15 to 20 minutes.

Remove the chicken meat from the bones, cut into pieces if necessary, and add to the soup. Then add a half package of quinoa noodles into the simmering soup. Cook until tender; just a few minutes. Stir in the kale and cook for another 5 minutes. Season with sea salt or Herbamare and freshly ground black pepper to taste.

Yield: 8 servings

Variation: Instead of noodles, add a few cups of cooked brown rice or quinoa, or add more vegetables!

TURKEY AND WILD RICE SOUP

This soup makes a wonderful fall or winter soup. Serve with the Spinach Salad with Pecans and Dried Cherries (page 237). Soup freezes well for later use.

BROTH

2 to 3 pounds organic turkey breast, bone in, skin on

1 large onion, chopped

1 large carrot, chopped

3 celery stalks, chopped

½ bunch fresh parsley, chopped

2 sprigs fresh rosemary

3 sprigs fresh thyme

1 teaspoon whole black peppercorns

1 tablespoon sea salt or Herbamare

8 cups water

RICE

1 cup wild rice

2 cups water

SOUP

2 tablespoons extra-virgin olive oil

1 large leek, sliced and well rinsed

2 large carrots, diced

4 celery stalks, diced

2 teaspoons dried thyme

1 teaspoon dried sage

4 cups fresh baby spinach leaves

½ bunch fresh parsley, chopped

To make the broth, place all the ingredients for the broth into an 8-quart pot and bring to a boil. Cover, reduce the heat to a low simmer, and cook for about 2 hours, or until the meat easily falls off the bone.

To make the rice, rinse and drain the wild rice. Place into a medium saucepan with the water and bring to a boil. Reduce the heat to a simmer and cook for about 45 minutes. Set aside.

When the turkey is cooked, place a colander over a large clean pot and strain the broth into it. Transfer the turkey breast to a plate to cool. Discard the vegetables and herb sprigs.

To make the soup, heat the olive oil in a clean 6- or 8-quart pot over medium heat. Add the sliced leek and sauté a few minutes until tender. Stir in the carrots, celery, thyme, and sage. Add the broth to the vegetable mixture and simmer over medium-low heat for 20 minutes, or until vegetables are tender.

While the vegetables are simmering, remove the skin from the turkey and pull the meat from the bones. Cut the meat into pieces and then add it to the pot of simmering vegetables and herbs.

Add the cooked wild rice, baby spinach, and parsley and stir well. Remove the soup from the heat and season to taste with sea salt or Herbamare.

Yield: 6 servings

16

FRESH SALADS AND VEGETABLES

The ultimate value of life depends upon awareness and the power of contemplation rather than upon mere survival.

—*Aristotle*

Vegetables offer us a wide variety of potent antioxidants, anticancer agents, phytochemicals, vitamins, minerals, and more. Let your eyes guide you when choosing vegetables from the store or the market. The beautiful array of colors offered by vegetables give us the good chemicals we need to maintain optimal health. Chances are that the colors that you are most attracted to are the chemicals that your body needs most at that moment. Not only do these plants give us all of the potent nutrients we need, they also offer our taste buds a wide variety of wonderful flavors.

A diet high in fresh organic vegetables has been associated with a decrease in almost every disease. At the same time, a diet low in fresh vegetables has been associated with a higher risk for almost every disease. Try to make vegetables and greens a regular part of every meal.

Tips for adding more vegetables to your diet:

✓ Prepare a raw vegetable platter each day or as often as you like. Choose vegetables like celery, carrots, bell peppers, cucumbers, summer squash, sugar snap peas, cauliflower, or romaine lettuce. It is fun to create a beautiful design on a plate or platter that you will be attracted to. Leave it on the countertop at home so everyone can munch throughout the day. Set a bowl of bean dip beside the vegetables and your beautiful platter will disappear in no time.
✓ Add spinach, bell peppers, onions, and zucchini to your eggs in the morning. You can even add some fresh herbs for added flavor and nutrients.

✓ Top a plate of mixed greens with chopped raw vegetables and drizzle them with your favorite salad dressing.
✓ Use puréed vegetables to add to muffins and breads. You can also make many exciting soups using puréed vegetables, spices, and broths.
Make a variety of soups and stews to which you can add almost an endless amount of chopped vegetables.
✓ Make vegetable juices with a variety of vegetables and fruits. Experiment and find a combination that you like best. One of my favorite combinations is pear, pineapple, beet, fennel, carrot, and parsley.
✓ Create tantalizing smoothies with different greens, vegetables, and fruits. Try a combination of 50 to 60% fruit and 40 to 50% greens. You can use kale, lettuce, dandelion greens, carrot tops, radish greens, spinach, cabbage, and more. See "Smoothies," chapter 12 for green smoothie recipes.

HOW TO SELECT AND STORE FRESH PRODUCE

Whenever possible, we prefer to purchase organic vegetables and fruits from our local farmers' market. Buying locally supports the local economy and benefits small farmers. It is also wonderful to connect with the farmers who grow your food. Chances are, if you have a health food store or food co-op in town, their produce is grown locally. Purchase fresh, organic produce frequently from a store that has a rapid turnover. If possible, make more frequent trips to the store and buy smaller amounts of produce.

Choose vibrant, brightly colored vegetables and fruits.

Dull-looking or wilted vegetables have been sitting on the shelf too long. Choose crisp, colorful produce that is free of any discolored areas and slime.

Buy only the produce that you plan on using within the next few days.

Longer storage time cannot only cause the produce to spoil, but also significantly reduce nutrient levels and flavor. Delicate produce such as leafy greens, fresh herbs, broccoli, summer squash, and soft, ripe fruits is best used within a few days. Other produce, such as winter squash, onions, garlic, and root vegetables can be stored for longer periods of time without leading to spoilage or significantly reducing nutrient levels.

Choose local, seasonal fruits and vegetables.

When you purchase in-season produce, it is much fresher, the nutritional value is significantly higher, and the flavors are far superior to food that has traveled thousands of miles. Imagine the difference in flavor and texture from a just-picked local organic strawberry compared to a strawberry that has traveled across the country to get to your grocery store. Buying local, organic produce also reduces carbon emissions from transport, thus reducing the impact on global warming.

Don't wash vegetables before storing.

Wash your vegetables before you use them, not before you store them. They need to be stored dry. If you are purchasing your vegetables at a grocery store, they are usually sprayed with cold water throughout the day. This keeps them fresh and crisp in the store, but at home in a plastic bag they may mold rather quickly. Make sure you dry them well. Wrap leafy greens with a cloth or paper towel and then place them in a plastic bag in the crisper drawer in your refrigerator. Berries can quickly degrade if they are wet; be sure to eat them, freeze them, or cook with them very soon after purchasing. Other vegetables that are damp can simply be dried off before storing.

Store fresh produce according to its type.

Place root vegetables, such as potatoes and yams, in a cool, dark place. Exposure to light can cause potatoes to turn green. The green pigment contains the toxic alkaloid, solanine. Green sections of potatoes should be removed before cooking. Pumpkins and other winter squashes can be stored in a dry place for 2 to 3 months. Onions and garlic should be stored in a separate basket that allows for plenty of airflow.

Root vegetables such as carrots, parsnips, and beets can be stored in the refrigerator for several weeks. Cut the leaves from root vegetables before storing as the flow of sap continues to the leaves at the expense of the root.

Cabbage can be kept in the refrigerator for several weeks also. Store other vegetables in the refrigerator crisper drawer for up to a week. Apples, berries, and cherries are best kept in the refrigerator, while other fruits can be kept on the countertop in a well-ventilated container until ripe.

Ripe fruits can be stored in the refrigerator in an open plastic bag until ready to use. Tropical and citrus fruits, as well as avocados and tomatoes, are best kept at room temperature.

ARUGULA SALAD WITH LIME VINAIGRETTE

This is a light and zesty salad that pairs well with a spicy black bean dish or any dish with Mexican flair. Fresh organic sweet corn kernels freshly cut off the cob are another delicious addition to this salad.

SALAD

6 cups arugula leaves

2 cups mixed organic salad greens

½ cup raw pumpkin seeds, toasted

1 small red bell pepper, sliced into rings

1 avocado, cubed

3 to 4 green onions, sliced

DRESSING

¼ cup extra-virgin olive oil

1 to 2 teaspoons finely grated lime zest

¼ cup freshly squeezed lime juice

1 tablespoon brown rice vinegar or coconut vinegar

1 garlic clove, crushed

¼ teaspoon sea salt

¼ teaspoon ground cumin

pinch ground cardamom

To prepare the salad, rinse the arugula and salad greens to remove any dirt or sand. Bunched arugula can sometimes have quite a bit of dirt on it. Spin dry with a salad spinner and transfer to a large salad bowl.

In a skillet over medium-low heat, toast the pumpkin seeds until you hear a "pop." Transfer the seeds to a small bowl to cool.

Add the pumpkin seeds, red pepper rings, avocado cubes, and green onion slices to the salad bowl with the greens.

To make the dressing, whisk together all the ingredients in a small bowl. Pour the dressing over the salad and toss to coat. Serve immediately.

Yield: 4 to 6 servings

ARUGULA SALAD WITH WHITE NECTARINE VINAIGRETTE

Adding fruit to olive oil and vinegar creates a luscious, fruity salad dressing. If you don't have a white nectarine, use a white or yellow peach instead. This dressing pairs well with any type of spicy salad green. Try mustard greens or a spicy salad mix in place of the arugula.

SALAD

1 large bunch arugula

1 cup raw walnuts, roasted and chopped

1 nectarine, sliced

DRESSING

½ ripe white nectarine

6 tablespoons extra-virgin olive oil

¼ cup white wine vinegar

1 small garlic clove

¼ to ½ teaspoon sea salt

1 to 2 tablespoons finely chopped fresh parsley

To prepare the salad, rinse and drain the arugula. Tear the larger leaves into pieces if necessary. Place into a large salad bowl. Sprinkle with roasted walnuts and add the sliced nectarine.

To make the dressing, place all the ingredients except for the parsley into a blender and blend on high until puréed. Add the parsley and blend on low speed until incorporated; if you blend the parsley too long it will turn the dressing green.

Pour the dressing over the salad and toss to coat. Serve immediately. Store any extra dressing in a glass jar in the refrigerator for up to 1 week.

Yield: 4 to 6 servings

ASIAN CABBAGE SLAW

Serve this colorful slaw recipe with grilled chicken, baked fish, or stir-fried tofu and brown rice. If you want to prepare this ahead of serving, simply make the salad and store it in the refrigerator. Keep the dressing in a glass jar and pour it over the salad when ready to serve.

SALAD

3 cups thinly sliced red cabbage

3 cups thinly sliced green cabbage

2 carrots, grated

3 to 4 green onions, thinly sliced

½ cup chopped fresh cilantro

½ cup sesame seeds, toasted

DRESSING

¼ cup toasted sesame oil

3 tablespoons brown rice vinegar or coconut vinegar

1 tablespoon wheat-free tamari or coconut aminos

1 tablespoon pure maple syrup

1 garlic clove

one 1-inch piece fresh ginger

To prepare the salad, place all the ingredients into a large bowl and toss to combine.

To make the dressing, place all the ingredients into a blender and blend until combined. Alternatively, you can add all the ingredients to a widemouthed pint jar and use an immersion blender to combine. Pour the dressing over the salad and toss to coat. Serve immediately.

Yield: 6 servings

AUTUMN HARVEST SALAD WITH BALSAMIC VINAIGRETTE

This is an excellent salad to serve in early autumn when the fall harvest of greens is available and the green apples and fresh figs are in season. Make a double batch of the dressing to have on hand for a quick salad of mixed greens. Dried figs can easily replace the fresh figs in this recipe.

SALAD

8 cups mixed organic salad greens

1 to 2 cups finely sliced red cabbage

1 green apple, diced

3 to 4 fresh black mission figs, cut into wedges

½ cup dried currants

2 to 3 green onions, sliced

½ cup raw walnuts, lightly roasted

½ cup raw pumpkin seeds, toasted

DRESSING

4 tablespoons extra-virgin olive oil

3 tablespoons balsamic vinegar

1 tablespoon pure maple syrup

2 teaspoons Dijon mustard

¼ teaspoon sea salt

Preheat the oven to 350°F.

To prepare the salad, rinse and dry the salad greens. Place in a large bowl along with the cabbage, apple, figs, currants, and green onions and toss gently to combine.

Spread the walnuts out in a small glass baking dish and lightly roast for 12 to 14 minutes. Remove the nuts from the oven and cool slightly, then chop. Add them to the salad.

Heat a skillet over medium heat. Add the pumpkin seeds and toast, keeping them moving in the skillet, until they begin to "pop." Remove from the heat, and let cool slightly. Sprinkle on top of salad.

To make the dressing, place all the ingredients in a jar with a tight-fitting lid and shake well. Pour the dressing over the salad and gently toss to coat. Serve immediately.

Yield: 4 to 6 servings

BASIL-FETA–CRANBERRY BEAN SALAD

Fresh cranberry beans can be found at your local farmers' market in the summertime. The beans are white with dark pink speckles and are easy to shell. Have your children shell them in the backyard on a sunny afternoon. It's a great activity to keep them busy and feeling like part of the family team! Serve this salad over cooked quinoa or fresh lettuce leaves.

4 cups fresh cranberry beans
6 cups cold water
1 small red onion, finely diced
1 cup packed fresh basil leaves
¼ cup extra-virgin olive oil

freshly squeezed juice of 1 lemon
¾ to 1 teaspoon sea salt or Herbamare
freshly ground black pepper
crumbled organic feta cheese (optional)

Put the beans in a 4-quart pot and cover with about 6 cups of water. Bring to a boil, then reduce the heat to a high simmer and cook for 25 to 30 minutes. Drain the beans in a colander and set aside to cool.

Place the cooled beans into a medium bowl, add the remaining ingredients, and gently toss together. Serve the salad at room temperature, or refrigerate for up to 4 days.

Yield: 4 to 6 servings

BEET AND FENNEL SALAD WITH ORANGE VINAIGRETTE

Fresh fennel is an excellent source of fiber, vitamin C, folate, potassium, and the phytonutrient anethole. Anethole helps to reduce inflammation and works to prevent the occurrence of cancer. Serve this salad with cooked quinoa and baked wild salmon for a balanced meal.

SALAD

1 cup raw walnuts, lightly roasted

3 small beets, peeled and cubed

8 cups mixed organic salad greens

1 small fennel bulb, sliced

1 avocado, cubed

4 green onions, sliced

½ cup chopped fresh basil

DRESSING

1 teaspoon finely grated orange zest

¼ cup freshly squeezed orange juice

¼ cup extra-virgin olive oil

1 tablespoon balsamic vinegar

1 tablespoon chopped fresh fennel fronds

¼ teaspoon sea salt

¼ teaspoon ground cinnamon

Preheat the oven to 350°F.

To prepare the salad, spread out the walnuts in a glass baking dish and roast in the oven for 12 to 14 minutes, or until the walnuts give off a nutty aroma. Set aside to cool.

Place the cubed beets in a steamer basket over about 2 inches of water in a 2-quart pot. Place a lid on the pot and cook over medium heat for 10 to 15 minutes or until tender. Transfer to a dish to cool completely.

To make the dressing, whisk together all the ingredients in a small bowl.

To assemble the salad, in a large salad bowl, combine the mixed greens, beets, walnuts, fennel, avocado, green onions, and basil. Pour over the dressing and toss to coat. Serve immediately.

Yield: 4 to 6 servings

BEET, KALE, AND WALNUT SALAD

Beets are a nutrient-dense food, particularly rich in folic acid, which protects us from heart disease, birth defects, and certain cancers. Kale is a powerful anticancer food rich in organosulfur compounds. Walnuts are very high in omega-3 fatty acids, which reduce inflammation, protect against cardiovascular disease, and improve cognitive function. Serve this dish with the Wild Salmon with Lemon, Garlic, and Thyme (page 318).

SALAD

3 to 4 beets, peeled and cubed

1 bunch kale, rinsed and chopped

1 cup raw walnuts, lightly roasted

½ cup organic feta cheese (optional)

freshly ground black pepper (optional)

DRESSING

3 tablespoons extra-virgin olive oil

2 tablespoons balsamic vinegar

1 tablespoon pure maple syrup

2 tablespoons finely chopped fresh basil

¼ teaspoon sea salt

Preheat the oven to 350°F.

To prepare the salad, place the cubed beets in a steamer basket over about 2 inches of water in a 2- or 3-quart pot. Place a lid on the pot and cook over medium heat for 10 to 15 minutes or until tender. Transfer to a bowl to cool completely.

Place the chopped kale into the steamer basket and steam for 5 to 10 minutes, or until tender but still bright green. Transfer to the bowl with the beets.

Spread the walnuts out in a small glass baking dish and roast in the oven for 12 to 14 minutes. Let cool completely. Transfer to the bowl with the beets and kale.

To make the dressing, whisk together all the ingredients in a small bowl.

To assemble the salad, pour the dressing over the beets, kale, and walnuts, and toss to coat. Top with the feta cheese and freshly ground black pepper if desired.

Yield: 4 to 6 servings

BERRY-HAZELNUT SALAD WITH HONEY–POPPY SEED VINAIGRETTE

This Northwest-inspired salad utilizes fresh greens, hazelnuts, and whatever combination of berries you desire—try strawberries, blueberries, blackberries, salmonberries, thimbleberries, or raspberries.

SALAD

8 cups mixed organic salad greens

2 cups mixed fresh berries

½ cup raw hazelnuts, roasted

3 to 4 green onions, sliced into rounds

DRESSING

¼ cup extra-virgin olive oil

3 tablespoons red wine vinegar

1 tablespoon raw honey

1 tablespoon poppy seeds

¼ teaspoon sea salt

To prepare the salad, rinse and dry the greens and place them into a large salad bowl. Rinse and drain the berries and add them to the bowl with the greens. Chop the hazelnuts and add them to the salad along with the green onions.

To make the dressing, place all the ingredients into a glass jar and shake well. Pour the dressing over the salad just before serving and toss to coat. Serve immediately.

Yield: 4 to 6 servings

> **Tip:** To roast hazelnuts, preheat the oven to 350°F. Spread the nuts out in a shallow baking dish. Roast in the oven for 15 to 18 minutes. Transfer to a plate and let cool before chopping.

CABBAGE SALAD WITH CILANTRO VINAIGRETTE

Cabbage is a rich source of powerful phytochemicals that help fight against cancer. Raw cabbage is also very detoxifying to the body, improving digestion and elimination, while killing harmful bacteria and viruses in the gut. This salad is delicious served with the Lemon Millet Patties (page 288) and the Navy Beans in a Homemade Barbecue Sauce (page 307).

SALAD

4 to 6 cups chopped Napa or Savoy cabbage

4 green onions, sliced into rounds

1 large carrot, grated

½ cup sunflower seeds, toasted

DRESSING

¼ cup chopped fresh cilantro

¼ cup extra-virgin olive oil

3 tablespoons brown rice vinegar or coconut vinegar

¼ teaspoon sea salt

pinch cayenne pepper

To prepare the salad, place the cabbage, green onions, carrot, and toasted sunflower seeds into a large salad bowl.

To make the dressing, place all the ingredients into a blender and blend until smooth. Pour the dressing over the salad and toss to coat well. Serve immediately.

Yield: 4 servings

> **Tip:** To toast the sunflower seeds, heat a 10-inch skillet over medium-low heat and add the seeds. Toast the seeds by keeping the pan moving over the stovetop for about 5 minutes, or until the seeds are lightly browned.

CARROT-HIJIKI SALAD WITH SWEET MISO DRESSING

Serve this mineral-rich salad at your next potluck or holiday gathering. It also pairs well with baked wild salmon and cooked brown rice. We buy gluten-free, soy-free miso from the South River Miso Company. Miso is a live food rich in beneficial bacteria!

SALAD

¼ cup hijiki

1 pound carrots, grated (about 4 cups)

4 green onions, sliced into thin rounds

½ cup chopped fresh cilantro

¼ cup sesame seeds, toasted

DRESSING

3 tablespoons toasted sesame oil

3 tablespoons brown rice syrup

2 tablespoons gluten-free miso

2 tablespoons brown rice vinegar

1 tablespoon wheat-free tamari or coconut aminos

1 to 2 teaspoons hot pepper sesame oil

1 teaspoon grated fresh ginger

1 garlic clove, crushed

To prepare the salad, place the hijiki into a small saucepan and cover with about 2 cups water. Let soak for about 5 minutes, then place the pot on the stovetop and simmer for about 25 minutes, or until the hijiki is tender. Drain off the water.

Transfer the hijiki to a large bowl with the carrots, green onions, cilantro, and toasted sesame seeds.

To make the dressing, whisk together all the ingredients in a small bowl. Pour the dressing over the carrot mixture and toss well to coat. Serve immediately, or store in the refrigerator for up to 3 days. The salad is best served the day it is made.

> **Tip:** To toast the sesame seeds, heat a 10-inch skillet over medium-low heat and add the seeds. Toast the seeds by keeping the pan moving over the stovetop for about 5 minutes, or until the seeds are lightly browned and smell quite fragrant.

Yield: 4 to 6 servings

CHICKEN FAJITA SALAD WITH SPICY AVOCADO DRESSING

When we make meals like this we like to place everything out on the countertop and let the children make their own plates with the ingredients they prefer most. If you want the dressing less spicy, then remove the seeds from the pepper before blending. If you want it really spicy, leave the seeds intact and just cut the stem off before blending.

CHICKEN

4 organic boneless chicken breasts, cut into strips

freshly squeezed juice of 1 lime

2 teaspoons ground cumin

1 teaspoon paprika

¼ to ½ teaspoon chipotle chile powder

½ teaspoon sea salt

virgin coconut oil, for cooking

SALAD

1 head romaine lettuce, thinly sliced

1 small head Napa cabbage, thinly sliced

2 heirloom tomatoes, cut into wedges

1 to 2 sweet bell peppers, cut into strips

½ cup chopped fresh cilantro

DRESSING

2 small avocados

¾ cup water

¼ cup freshly squeezed lime juice

1 jalapeño pepper, stemmed, seeded if desired

1 garlic clove, peeled

1 small handful fresh cilantro

½ teaspoon sea salt

To prepare the chicken, place all the ingredients except for the oil into a medium bowl or glass pan and stir gently. Cover and marinate on the countertop for 20 to 30 minutes, or refrigerate and marinate for up to 3 hours.

Heat a large stainless steel or cast-iron skillet over medium-high heat. Add about 1 tablespoon of the coconut oil. Add some of the chicken, making sure not to crowd the skillet (if you crowd the skillet, the temperature drops and the chicken loses its natural juices and becomes dry). Sauté each batch of chicken for 3 to 4 minutes, or until cooked through. Transfer to a serving plate.

For the salad, place the romaine and cabbage into a large salad bowl and toss together. Arrange the tomatoes and bell peppers on a plate. Put the chopped cilantro into a small bowl.

To make the dressing, place all the ingredients into a blender and blend until smooth and creamy. Pour the dressing into a jar or serving pitcher. Place everything on the table or countertop and invite your diners to assemble their own salads.

Yield: about 6 servings

CUCUMBER-DILL SALAD

Serve this refreshing salad as a summer afternoon snack or as part of a balanced dinner. It pairs well with grilled chicken, baked salmon, or quinoa and beans.

SALAD

2 English cucumbers, sliced

2 tablespoons minced red onion

2 tablespoons finely chopped fresh dill

DRESSING

2 tablespoons coconut vinegar

1 tablespoon extra-virgin olive oil

1 teaspoon raw honey

¼ to ½ teaspoon sea salt

To prepare the salad, combine the cucumbers, minced onion, and dill in a large salad bowl.

To make the dressing, whisk together all of the ingredients in a small bowl. Pour the dressing over the salad and gently toss together. Serve immediately.

Yield: 6 servings

CUCUMBER, TOMATO, BASIL SALAD

The skin of cucumbers contains the minerals silica, magnesium, and potassium. Silica is an essential component to healthy connective tissue. The flesh of cucumbers contains good amounts of vitamin C. Eating cucumbers regularly can improve the look and feel of your skin and hair. Cucumbers, tomatoes, and basil are abundant during the summer months. This salad is easy and quick to prepare. Serve it as part of a summer picnic or as a simple late-afternoon snack.

2 medium cucumbers, sliced

3 to 4 firm tomatoes, quartered and sliced

½ cup thinly sliced fresh basil

1 to 2 garlic cloves, finely chopped

2 tablespoons extra-virgin olive oil

2 tablespoons red wine vinegar

sea salt

freshly ground black pepper

Place the sliced cucumbers and tomatoes into a shallow serving dish. Add the basil, garlic, olive oil, and vinegar.

Toss gently to combine. Season to taste with sea salt and pepper. Toss again and serve.

Yield: 2 to 4 servings

FRESH GARDEN SALAD WITH HERBAL VINAIGRETTE

This salad is rich in fiber. Many plant fibers are used as foods to feed beneficial bacteria in the intestinal tract that make a short-chained fatty acid called butyrate. This fatty acid is used by the body to regulate appetite and fat storage leading to a leaner body. This salad is perfect to include as part of an evening summer meal when the tomatoes, cucumbers, lettuce, and fresh herbs are sweet and bountiful.

SALAD

1 head green leaf lettuce
1 large ripe tomato, chopped
1 small cucumber, sliced
1 large carrot, shredded
2 green onions, sliced
½ cup raw sunflower seeds, toasted
fresh sprouts

DRESSING

freshly squeezed juice of 1 small lemon
⅓ cup extra-virgin olive oil
2 tablespoons balsamic vinegar
2 teaspoons Dijon mustard
1 tablespoon pure maple syrup
3 tablespoons chopped fresh basil
2 tablespoons chopped fresh chives
1 tablespoon chopped fresh oregano
1 garlic clove, crushed
½ teaspoon sea salt

To prepare the salad, tear the lettuce leaves into pieces, rinse, and spin dry in a salad spinner. Transfer the lettuce to a large salad bowl. Add the remaining salad ingredients.

To make the dressing, in a separate small bowl, whisk together the all the ingredients. Toss the salad with the dressing when ready to serve.

Yield: 4 to 6 servings

LEMON–OLIVE OIL CHICKPEA SALAD

This nutrient-dense salad makes a perfect light lunch when served over salad greens! Pack a small container in your child's lunch box along with a slice of Hearty Seed Bread (page 161) and a container of organic green grapes for a balanced meal.

6 cups cooked chickpeas

1 medium cucumber, diced

3 carrots, diced

½ cup diced red onion

½ cup chopped fresh parsley

1 to 2 tablespoons chopped fresh oregano

¼ cup extra-virgin olive oil

1 teaspoon finely grated lemon zest

3 to 4 tablespoons freshly squeezed lemon juice

1 teaspoon sea salt

freshly ground black pepper

Place all the ingredients for the salad into a medium bowl and toss to combine. Taste and add more sea salt and pepper if necessary. Serve immediately, or store in the refrigerator for up to 4 days. Bring to room temperature before serving.

Yield: about 6 servings

LETTUCE AND CABBAGE SALAD WITH CREAMY GINGER DRESSING

Ginger contains a compound called gingerol. This compound acts as a powerful anti-inflammatory, reducing pain in people with arthritis. This delicious salad dressing will keep you coming back for more. It can also be drizzled over steamed vegetables or cooked whole grains. Store the dressing in a glass jar in the refrigerator for up to 10 days. When ready to use, place the jar under warm running water to thin out the olive oil.

SALAD

1 head red leaf lettuce

½ head red cabbage, chopped

2 large carrots, shredded

4 green onions, sliced

1 cup chopped fresh cilantro

DRESSING

⅓ cup sesame seeds

½ cup chopped celery

3 to 4 tablespoons chopped fresh ginger

½ cup extra-virgin olive oil

3 tablespoons brown rice vinegar or coconut vinegar

3 tablespoons wheat-free tamari or coconut aminos

2 tablespoons water

1 tablespoon pure maple syrup

⅛ teaspoon ground white pepper

To prepare the salad, tear the lettuce leaves into pieces, rinse, and spin dry in a salad spinner. Transfer the lettuce to a large salad bowl. Add the remaining salad ingredients.

To make the dressing, heat a skillet over medium-low heat. Add the sesame seeds and dry toast for about 2 minutes. Be sure to keep the seeds moving in the skillet to prevent burning. Remove from the heat and place the seeds into a blender with the remaining dressing ingredients. Blend on high until very smooth and creamy. When ready to serve, pour the dressing over the salad and serve immediately.

Yield: 4 to 6 servings

ITALIAN GREENS SALAD WITH RED WINE VINAIGRETTE

This crisp, refreshing salad pairs well with any dish that has Italian flavors. Try serving it with some cooked brown rice pasta and Fresh Marinara Sauce (page 356), or with a chicken or fish dish.

SALAD

1 small head romaine lettuce

1 small red onion, sliced into thin rounds

½ small red bell pepper, cut into rings

½ cup Kalamata olives, pitted

¼ cup fresh parsley, chopped

3 plum tomatoes, sliced

5 pepperoncini peppers, chopped

½ cup grated organic Parmesean cheese (optional)

DRESSING

¼ cup extra-virgin olive oil

¼ cup red wine vinegar

1 teaspoon Dijon mustard

1 teaspoon pure maple syrup or raw honey

½ teaspoon sea salt

1 teaspoon dried Italian seasoning

1 teaspoon paprika

1 garlic clove, crushed

To prepare the salad, tear the lettuce leaves into pieces, rinse, and spin dry in a salad spinner. Transfer the lettuce to a large salad bowl.

Gently toss in the onion, bell pepper, olives, parsley, tomatoes, and pepperoncini. Sprinkle with the grated cheese if using.

To make the dressing, place all the ingredients in a jar with a tight-fitting lid and shake. Pour the dressing over the salad and serve immediately. Leftover dressing will keep in the refrigerator for up to 10 days.

Yield: 4 to 6 servings

PEAR AND HAZELNUT SALAD WITH CREAMY CRANBERRY DRESSING

Serve this salad when cranberries, pears, and hazelnuts are in season in autumn. It is also delicious served at a festive holiday meal.

SALAD

1 head red leaf lettuce

1 firm ripe pear, cored and thinly sliced

½ small red onion, sliced into thin rounds

1 cup raw hazelnuts, roasted

½ cup crumbled organic feta cheese (optional)

DRESSING

2 teaspoons plus ¼ cup extra-virgin olive oil

2 shallots, peeled and thinly sliced

1 cup fresh cranberries

1 teaspoon finely grated orange zest

¼ cup freshly squeezed orange juice

3 tablespoons balsamic vinegar

1 to 2 tablespoons pure maple syrup

½ teaspoon sea salt or Herbamare

To prepare the salad, tear the lettuce leaves into pieces, rinse, and spin dry in a salad spinner. Transfer the lettuce to a large salad bowl. Add the remaining salad ingredients.

Heat a small skillet over medium heat. Add the 2 teaspoons of olive oil and shallots and sauté for 3 to 5 minutes, or until soft. Add the cranberries and continue to sauté until the cranberries are soft and have "popped."

Transfer the mixture to a blender along with orange zest, orange juice, vinegar, maple syrup, the remaining ¼ cup olive oil, and the sea salt and blend on high until smooth. For a thinner consistency, add a few tablespoons of water and blend again.

Drizzle the dressing over the salad and serve immediately. Extra dressing can be stored in a glass jar in the refrigerator for up to 10 days.

Yield: 4 to 6 servings

> **Tip:** To roast hazelnuts, preheat the oven to 350°F. Spread the nuts out in a shallow baking dish. Roast in the oven for 15 to 18 minutes. Transfer to a plate and let cool before chopping.

STEAMED SALMON, SPINACH, AND FENNEL SALAD

Steaming is a great way to prepare salmon. It is fast, easy, and helps the body retain much of the essential fatty acids. Serve this salad as part of a weekend brunch in the springtime or as a light evening meal. This delicious salad recipe is an adaptation of a salad from Bastyr University instructor, Mary Shaw.

SALAD

1 large fennel bulb

½ to 1 pound wild Alaskan salmon fillet

1 bunch spinach, rinsed and torn into pieces

½ red onion, cut into thin rounds

½ cup finely chopped fresh basil

DRESSING

¼ cup extra-virgin olive oil

2 to 3 tablespoons raw apple cider vinegar

1 teaspoon finely grated orange zest

2 to 3 tablespoons freshly squeezed orange juice

½ teaspoon ground cinnamon

¼ teaspoon sea salt

To make the salad, cut the green stalks from the fennel bulb and place them into a 10-inch skillet. Fill the skillet with water until it reaches the tops of the fennel, about ½ to 1 inch of water. Place the salmon fillet over the top of the fennel, cover the skillet, and steam the fish over medium heat for 10 to 15 minutes, or until the salmon is cooked through.

While the salmon is cooking, trim the ends off the fennel bulb and thinly slice it into small strips. Place the sliced fennel, spinach, onion, and basil into a large bowl and gently toss to combine.

To make the dressing, combine all the ingredients for the dressing in a small bowl and mix well.

To assemble the salad, when the salmon is cooked, remove the skin and discard along with the fennel tops. Break the salmon flesh into small pieces and place into the bowl with the spinach. Drizzle the dressing over the salad and toss gently to coat. Serve immediately.

Yield: 4 to 6 servings

SPINACH SALAD WITH PECANS AND DRIED CHERRIES

Spinach can protect you against osteoporosis, heart disease, colon cancer, arthritis, and other diseases all at the same time. Spinach is a rich source of vitamin K1 and is very high in different flavonoid compounds, which function as antioxidants and as anticancer agents in the body. In addition, spinach contains a special carotenoid, called neoxanthin, which has shown to be helpful in the treatment of prostate cancer.

PECANS

1 cup raw pecans

1 tablespoon extra-virgin olive oil

2 tablespoons pure maple syrup

1 teaspoon Dijon mustard

pinch sea salt

SALAD

8 ounces spinach leaves, rinsed and spun dry

½ cup dried organic cherries

½ small red onion, sliced into thin rounds

DRESSING

3 tablespoons extra-virgin olive oil

2 tablespoons balsamic vinegar

1 tablespoon pure maple syrup

1 teaspoon Dijon mustard

¼ teaspoon sea salt

¼ teaspoon fresh ground black pepper

Preheat the oven to 375°F.

To prepare the pecans, place the pecans, olive oil, maple syrup, Dijon mustard, and the pinch of sea salt into a pie plate and mix together. Bake in the oven for 12 to 15 minutes. Let cool slightly, then transfer to a plate to cool.

To assemble the salad, place the spinach into a salad bowl. Add the pecans, cherries, and onion.

To make the dressing, place all of the ingredients into a small jar with a tight-fitting lid and shake well. Dress the salad just before serving.

Yield: 4 to 6 servings

RAW KALE SALAD WITH LEMON AND PUMPKIN SEEDS

Dark green leafy vegetables, such as kale, are very alkalizing to the body, especially with the addition of fresh lemon juice. When we eat a diet rich in alkalizing foods, we decrease our risk for many diseases. Serve this nourishing salad with cooked beans and rice, or baked chicken and yams.

SALAD

2 bunches kale (about 8 cups chopped)

1 cup raw pumpkin seeds, toasted

½ cup finely diced red onion

¼ cup dried currants

DRESSING

¼ cup extra-virgin olive oil

1 teaspoon finely grated lemon zest

3 tablespoons freshly squeezed lemon juice

1 tablespoon raw honey or coconut nectar

1 garlic clove, crushed

½ to 1 teaspoon sea salt or Herbamare

To prepare the salad, rinse the kale and remove the tough ribs that run along the middle of each leaf, then finely chop the leaves. Transfer the kale to a large salad bowl and set aside.

To make the dressing, whisk together all the ingredients in a small bowl. Pour the dressing over the chopped kale in the salad bowl. Using clean hands, massage the dressing into the kale for about 2 minutes. Set aside and let it rest for about 10 minutes; this will help to soften the kale leaves.

Add the toasted pumpkin seeds, onion, and currants and toss together. Serve immediately.

Yield: 6 servings

ROASTED BEET SALAD WITH BASIL-BALSAMIC VINAIGRETTE

Roasting beets may sound a bit complicated, but once you do it you will realize how easy it is, especially using my method below. Sometimes I will roast as many as I can fit into my pan and then store them in my refrigerator for quick salads or breakfasts. Just make sure to leave the skins on the roasted beets until you are ready to use them.

SALAD

1 bunch beets

1 head red leaf lettuce, rinsed and spun dry

1 small red onion, sliced into thin rounds

½ cup raw pumpkin seeds, toasted

DRESSING

6 tablespoons balsamic vinegar

½ cup packed fresh basil leaves

1 garlic clove, peeled

1 teaspoon Dijon mustard

½ teaspoon sea salt

½ cup extra-virgin olive oil

To roast the beets, preheat the oven to 350°F. Cut the greens off the beets and rinse them well to remove any dirt. Place the beets into a casserole dish, cover with a lid, and roast for 45 to 90 minutes depending on the size of the beets. Smaller beets take less time while larger ones take more. Once they are fork-tender, remove the dish from the oven and let the beets cool completely. Once cooled, peel the skins from the beets using your fingers (they should slip right off). Cut the beets into halves or quarters.

To assemble the salad, tear the lettuce leaves into pieces and place into a large salad bowl. Add the beets, onion, and toasted pumpkin seeds.

To make the dressing, place the vinegar, basil, garlic, mustard, and sea salt into a blender and blend until smooth. With the blender on low, slowly add the olive oil. Pour the dressing over the salad. Extra dressing can be stored in a small glass jar in the refrigerator for up to 10 days.

Yield: 4 to 6 servings

SMOKED SALMON AND YAM SALAD WITH CREAMY CHIPOTLE-LIME DRESSING

This is one of our favorite salads to have on hand for meals on-the-go! Take out a portion and place it into a small glass container with fresh salad greens for a healthy lunch. Serve the salad with sliced avocado and lime wedges.

SALAD

3½ to 4 pounds yams, peeled and cubed

½ pound smoked salmon

1 red bell pepper, diced

4 to 5 green onions, sliced into rounds

½ cup chopped fresh cilantro

DRESSING

½ cup raw cashews

6 to 8 tablespoons water

¼ cup freshly squeezed lime juice

¼ cup extra-virgin olive oil

1 small garlic clove

¾ to 1 teaspoon sea salt or Herbamare

¼ to ½ teaspoon chipotle chile powder

To make the salad, cook the cubed yams in a steamer basket over about 2 inches of water in a 2- or 3-quart pot. Place a lid on the pot and cook over medium-high heat. Steam for 15 to 20 minutes, or until fork-tender. Transfer to a plate or platter to cool completely.

In a large bowl, combine the cooled yams and remaining salad ingredients and gently toss together.

To make the dressing, add all ingredients to a high-powered blender and blend on high until smooth and creamy. For a thinner dressing, add more water. Taste and adjust the salt and seasonings if necessary. Pour the dressing over the salad and gently toss to coat. Serve. The salad keeps in the refrigerator for up to 4 days.

Yield: 6 servings

Variation: If you are vegan or allergic to fish, replace the smoked salmon with 2 to 3 cups of cooked black beans.

STRAWBERRY SALAD WITH CANDIED PUMPKIN SEEDS

You can find raw pumpkin seeds (also called *pepitas*) in the bulk section of your local food co-op or health food store. We use coconut nectar, a slightly sweet liquid sweetener mainly composed of fructooligosaccharides—sugars that feed beneficial bacteria in your gut.

CANDIED PUMPKIN SEEDS

1 cup raw pumpkin seeds

2 tablespoons coconut nectar

SALAD

1 head red leaf lettuce, rinsed and spun dry

2 to 3 green onions, sliced into thin rounds

1 pint fresh strawberries, hulled and quartered

DRESSING

½ cup extra-virgin olive oil

6 tablespoons organic red wine vinegar

2 tablespoons honey or coconut nectar

2 tablespoons poppy seeds

½ teaspoon sea salt

To make the candied pumpkin seeds, first line a plate with unbleached parchment paper and set aside; otherwise the seeds will stick mercilessly. Heat a 10-inch skillet over medium heat, add the seeds, and toast them, keeping them moving in the skillet. They should puff up and "pop" and turn slightly golden. If they brown, it means your heat was too high. It should take about 5 minutes depending on your stove. Turn off the heat and immediately add the coconut nectar. Stir it into the seeds using a wooden spoon. The nectar should get stringy, and when this happens, remove them from the skillet and transfer to the parchment-lined plate. Let them cool completely to crisp up.

To assemble the salad, tear the lettuce into pieces and place into a salad bowl. Add the green onions and strawberries. Break up the cooled candied pumpkin seeds and sprinkle over the salad.

To make the dressing, place all the ingredients into a small jar with a tight-fitting lid and shake well. Pour the desired amount of dressing over salad and toss to coat. Store leftover dressing in the refrigerator for up to 10 days.

Yield: 4 to 6 servings

WHOLE MEAL SALAD WITH LEMON-TAHINI DRESSING

This nutrient-dense salad creates an energizing lunch. The diverse array of flavors and textures is a delight to the taste buds! I often like to add some steamed cubed beets, which add even another dimension of color and flavor. Any dressing will work here, but the Lemon-Tahini Dressing below is especially luscious.

SALAD

4 to 6 cups torn lettuce (green, red, or butter leaf lettuce)

4 to 6 pieces sautéed organic tofu

1 handful raw almonds, soaked or sprouted

1 small avocado, cubed

1 carrot, chopped

2 green onions, sliced

LEMON-TAHINI DRESSING

¼ cup sesame tahini

2 to 3 teaspoons finely grated lemon zest

¼ cup freshly squeezed lemon juice

2 tablespoons water

2 tablespoons extra-virgin olive oil

1 garlic clove, crushed

¼ teaspoon sea salt

OPTIONAL ADDITIONS

alfalfa sprouts

steamed cubed beets

cherry tomatoes

chopped celery

To assemble the salad, evenly distribute the lettuce between two bowls or plates. Place the tofu pieces on top of the lettuce. Top with the soaked almonds, avocado, chopped carrot, green onions, and any other optional additions you might want to add.

To make the dressing, whisk all the ingredients in a small bowl. Taste and add more salt or garlic if desired. Pour the desired amount of dressing over each salad. Store extra dressing in a glass jar in the refrigerator for up to 10 days.

Yield: 2 servings

Variation: Replace the tofu with one organic grilled chicken breast, cut into strips.

GREEN BEANS WITH GARLIC DRESSING

Serve these scrumptious green beans as a side dish to the Sunny Sunflower Seed Burgers, (page 293), or as a side dish to any baked fish or chicken dish. Green beans are an excellent source of beta-carotene and vitamin C.

SALAD

2 pounds green beans, ends trimmed
½ cup sliced or chopped almonds
1 tablespoon chopped fresh thyme

DRESSING

2 tablespoons extra-virgin olive oil
1 tablespoon freshly squeezed lemon juice
1 teaspoon Dijon mustard
2 garlic cloves, crushed
½ teaspoon finely grated lemon zest
½ teaspoon sea salt
¼ teaspoon freshly ground black pepper

To prepare the beans for the salad, blanch the beans in a large pot of boiling water for 4 minutes or until crisp-tender. Plunge them into ice water to stop the cooking and set the color; drain well.

To make the dressing, whisk all the ingredients in a small bowl.

To assemble the salad, place the beans, almonds, and thyme in a large serving bowl, add the dressing, and toss well to coat.

Yield: 4 to 6 servings

PICNIC POTATO SALAD

Olives are an excellent source of vitamin E and monounsaturated fats. The anti-inflammatory actions of the monounsaturated fats and vitamin E in olives may help to reduce the severity of asthma, osteo-arthritis, and rheumatoid arthritis—three conditions where much of the damage is caused by high levels of free radicals. This recipe was inspired by something I tasted at the Bellingham Community Food Co-op's deli. Serve this dish as part of a summer meal, or try it with the Lemon Millet Patties (page 288) and the Navy Beans in a Homemade Barbecue Sauce (page 307).

---

5 medium red potatoes, cut into chunks

1 pint cherry tomatoes

1 cup Kalamata olives

1 small leek, sliced in half lengthwise then chopped

1 cup chopped fresh parsley

½ teaspoon sea salt

½ teaspoon freshly ground black pepper

3 tablespoons red wine vinegar

3 tablespoons extra-virgin olive oil

Place the potato chunks in a steamer basket over about 2 inches of water in a 2- or 3-quart pot. Place a lid on the pot and cook over medium-high heat. Steam until tender but not mushy, 10 to 12 minutes. Remove from heat and let cool.

To assemble the salad, transfer the cooled potatoes to a large bowl with the cherry tomatoes, olives, leek, parsley, sea salt, and pepper and toss gently to combine.

Drizzle the vinegar and olive oil over the potato mixture and toss gently to coat.

Yield: 4 to 6 servings

SUMMER SQUASH AND CANNELLINI BEAN SALAD

This vegetable dish makes a great addition to any summer picnic. Summer squash include pattypan, crookneck, and zucchini. Cannellini beans are a traditional white Italian bean, sometimes known as white kidney beans. They have a very smooth texture with an elusive nutty flavor. Please refer to pages 180–183 for how to cook beans.

SALAD

6 small summer squash, diced

1 small red onion, finely chopped

3 cups cooked cannellini beans

¾ cup chopped olive oil–packed, sun-dried tomatoes

1 cup chopped fresh parsley

DRESSING

⅓ cup extra-virgin olive oil

¼ cup red wine vinegar

2 teaspoons Dijon mustard

1 tablespoon chopped fresh rosemary

1 tablespoon minced shallots

½ teaspoon sea salt or Herbamare

freshly ground black pepper

To assemble the salad, combine the squash, onion, cooked beans, sun-dried tomatoes, and parsley in a large salad bowl.

To make the dressing, whisk the olive oil, vinegar, mustard, rosemary, shallots, sea salt, and pepper in a small bowl. Alternatively, you could place all the dressing ingredients in a blender and blend until smooth and creamy.

When ready to serve, pour the dressing over the salad and toss to coat.

Yield: 2 to 4 servings

Tip: If you can't find olive oil–packed sun-dried tomatoes, then use regular sun-dried tomatoes (often found in the bulk or raw food section of your local health food store). Just rehydrate them for about 10 minutes in a bowl of warm water first.

APPLE-SPICED COLLARD GREENS

Cooked greens are a warming way to eat your greens in the fall and winter when the weather can be a bit chilly for a cold fresh salad. These greens are great served with the Spicy Black-Eyed Pea Stew (page 308) or with the Three-Bean Chili (page 202).

1 tablespoon extra-virgin olive oil

4 to 6 garlic cloves, crushed

¼ to 1 teaspoon crushed red chili flakes

2 to 3 bunches collard greens, rinsed and chopped

¼ to ½ cup organic apple cider or apple juice

1 to 2 tablespoons raw apple cider vinegar

½ teaspoon sea salt

Heat the olive oil in a large pot over medium heat. Add the garlic and sauté 30 seconds. Add the red chili flakes, greens, and apple cider or juice and continue to cook, stirring, until tender.

After 4 to 6 minutes, or when the greens are tender, remove the pot from the heat. Add the raw apple cider vinegar and season with sea salt to taste. Toss gently and serve.

Yield: 2 to 4 servings

BRAISED KALE WITH GARLIC AND GINGER

Kale is powerful anticancer food. It is rich in glucosinolates, which are a group of phytonutrients that lessen the occurrence of a wide variety of cancers. A study published in the September 2004 issue of the *Journal of Nutrition* shows sulforaphane helps to stop the proliferation of breast cancer cells, even in the later stages of their growth. Serve these scrumptious greens as part of a fall or winter meal.

1 tablespoon extra-virgin olive oil or virgin coconut oil

4 to 6 garlic cloves, crushed

1 teaspoon grated fresh ginger

2 to 3 bunches kale, rinsed and chopped

¼ to ½ cup water or Asian Soup Stock (page 187)

OPTIONAL SEASONINGS

brown rice vinegar

coconut vinegar

ume plum vinegar

freshly squeezed lemon juice

coconut aminos

wheat-free tamari

sea salt

toasted sesame seeds

Heat the oil in a 6- or 8-quart pot over medium heat. Add the garlic and ginger and sauté for 15 to 30 seconds. Quickly add the chopped greens and water or stock and continue to cook, stirring occasionally, until tender.

After 4 to 6 minutes, or when the greens are tender, remove the pot from the heat and add your favorite seasonings. Our favorite is a combination of coconut aminos and coconut vinegar. Toss gently and serve.

Yield: 2 to 4 servings

GARLIC AND SESAME SPINACH

The combination of spinach, garlic, and sesame is truly delightful. This recipe is very easy to prepare and cooks in a snap! Serve it with a cooked whole grain and the Coconut-Lime Chicken (page 325).

1 tablespoon toasted sesame oil

¼ cup raw sesame seeds

4 to 5 garlic cloves, crushed

8 cups baby spinach leaves

2 to 3 teaspoons brown rice vinegar or coconut vinegar

2 to 3 teaspoons wheat-free tamari or coconut aminos

Heat an 11- or 12-inch skillet over medium heat and add the sesame oil. Then add the sesame seeds and stir for 1 to 2 minutes.

Add the garlic and sauté for 30 seconds, then add the baby spinach leaves and sauté until wilted but still bright green, adding water if needed, 2 to 3 minutes.

Remove from the heat and add the brown rice vinegar and tamari to taste.

Yield: 2 to 4 servings

MEDITERRANEAN CHARD

This quick-and-easy-greens dish is wonderful served with the White Bean and Vegetable Stew (page 309), and cooked brown basmati rice. Or serve it with baked halibut or salmon.

1 tablespoon extra-virgin olive oil

½ cup raw pine nuts

4 to 5 garlic cloves, crushed

2 bunches chard, rinsed and chopped

freshly squeezed juice of 1 lemon

¼ to ½ cup Kalamata olives, pitted and chopped

¼ teaspoon sea salt

Heat the olive oil in a large pot or skillet over medium heat. Add the pine nuts and sauté until slightly golden, 3 to 5 minutes. Add the garlic and sauté for 30 seconds more.

Add the wet chard greens and sauté until wilted and bright green, making sure all the greens reach the heat of the skillet, 3 to 4 minutes.

Remove from the heat and add the lemon juice, olives, and sea salt. Taste and season with more salt if needed. Serve immediately.

> **Tip:** When sautéing dark leafy greens, it helps to have them wet before adding to the pan. This prevents burning and helps them cook properly.

Yield: 4 servings

STEAMED GREENS WITH A SPICY PEANUT CURRY SAUCE

I love the flavor of curry spices and peanut butter. This is a special treat because we rarely eat peanut butter. In fact, you can easily substitute the peanut butter for cashew butter or sunflower seed butter, which is equally delicious. Try using a single green or a combination of a few. Kale, collards, rapini, mustard, chard, or spinach all work well; though our favorite always seems to be black kale.

6 to 8 cups finely chopped greens

SAUCE
1 tablespoon virgin coconut oil
1 to 2 small shallots, minced
4 to 5 garlic cloves, minced
1 teaspoon freshly grated ginger
½ teaspoon ground cumin
½ teaspoon ground coriander

1½ teaspoons curry powder
¼ teaspoon cayenne pepper, or as desired
½ cup organic unsalted peanut butter
¾ to 1 cup water or coconut milk
1 to 2 tablespoons wheat-free tamari or coconut aminos
1 tablespoon brown rice vinegar or coconut vinegar

To prepare the greens, place the greens in a steamer basket over about 2 inches of water in a 2- or 3-quart pot. Place a lid on the pot and cook over medium-high heat. Steam for 7 to 10 minutes, or until the greens are very tender.

While the greens are steaming, make the sauce. Heat the coconut oil in a small saucepan over medium heat. Add the shallots, garlic, and ginger and sauté for about 5 minutes, being careful not to burn. Add the spices and mix well. Add the peanut butter, water, tamari, and brown rice vinegar and whisk to combine. Simmer over low heat for a few minutes until thickened. For a thinner sauce, add more water or coconut milk. For a smoother sauce, try blending it in a blender before serving.

Place the cooked greens into a serving bowl and pour the sauce over them. Serve immediately.

Yield: 4 to 6 servings

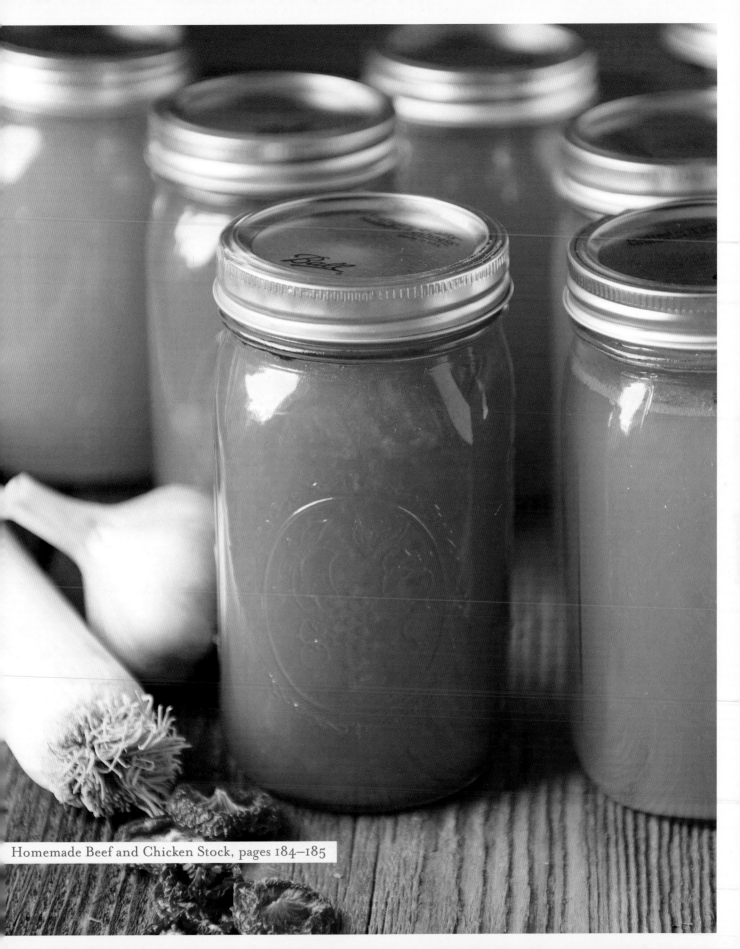

Homemade Beef and Chicken Stock, pages 184–185

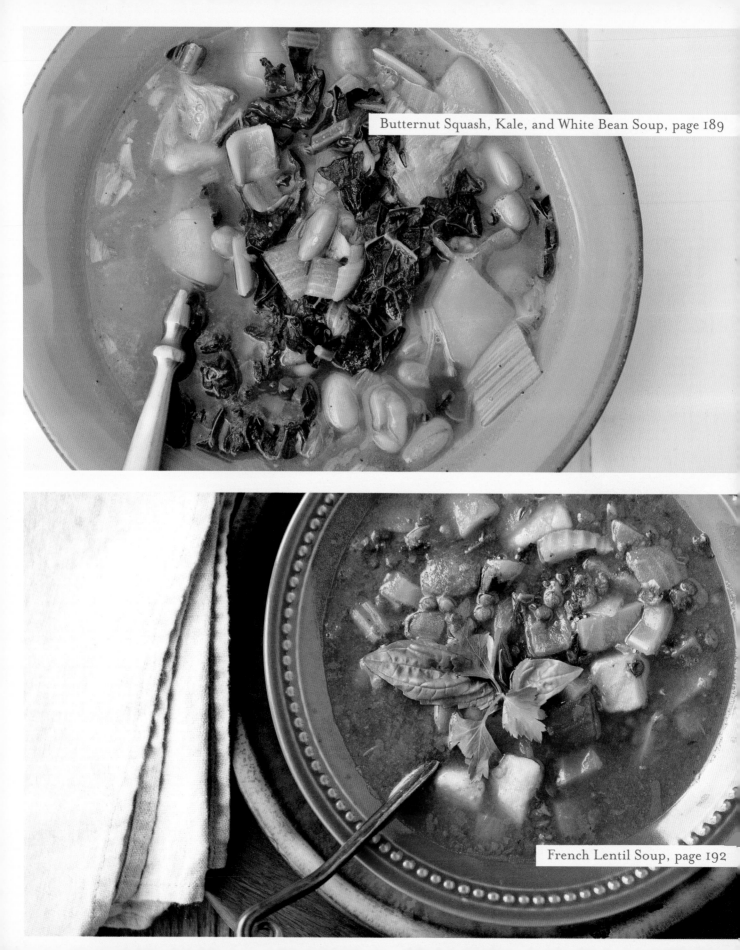

Butternut Squash, Kale, and White Bean Soup, page 189

French Lentil Soup, page 192

Quinoa Corn Chowder, page 197

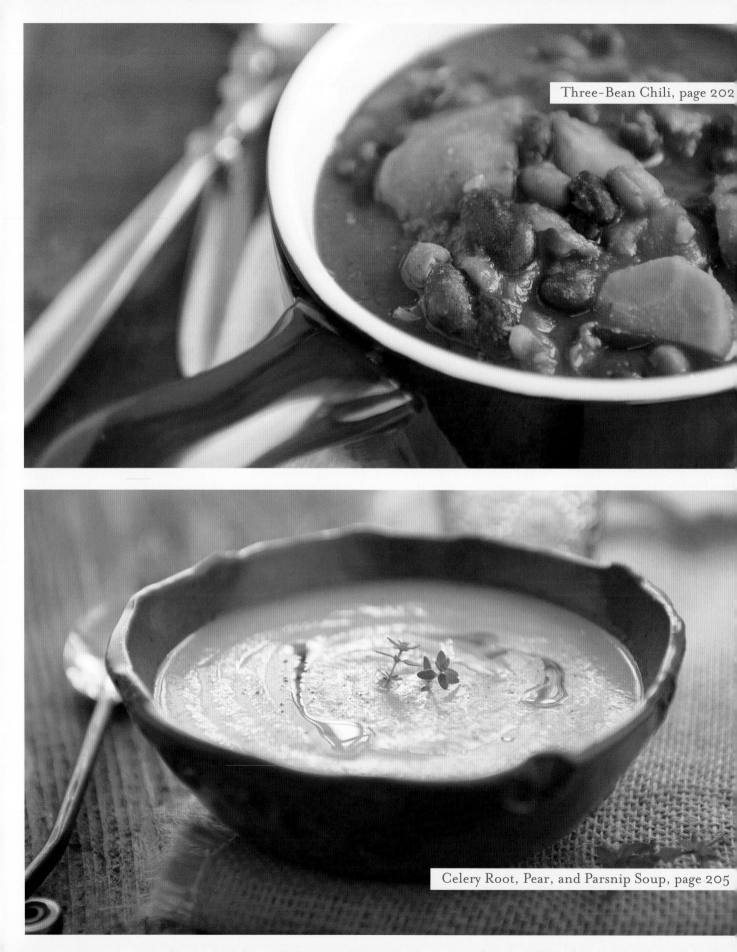

Three-Bean Chili, page 202

Celery Root, Pear, and Parsnip Soup, page 205

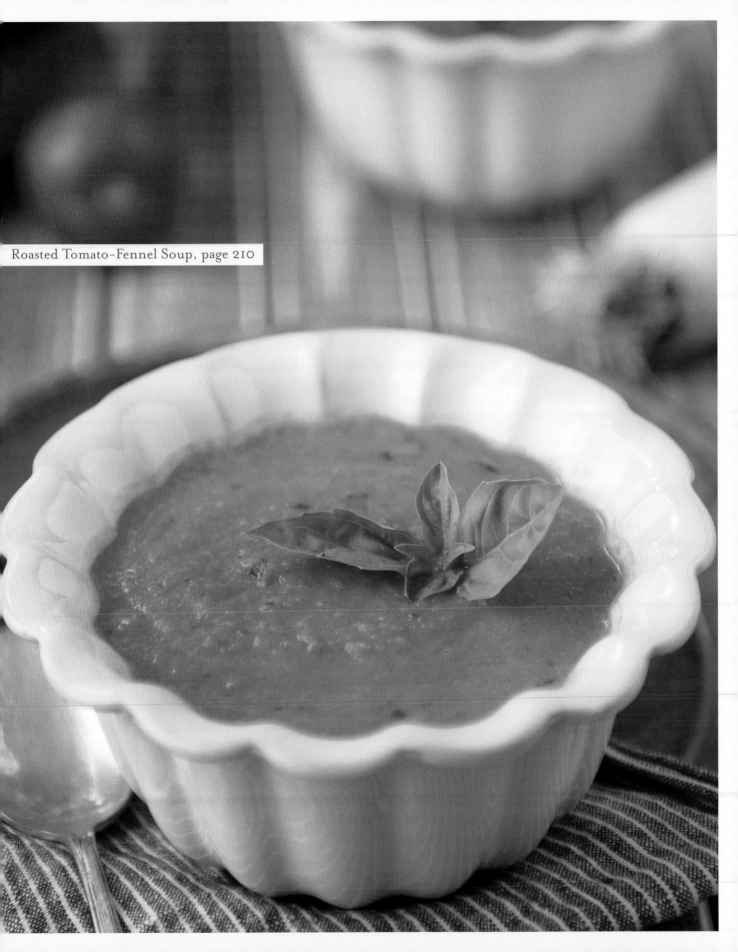

Roasted Tomato-Fennel Soup, page 210

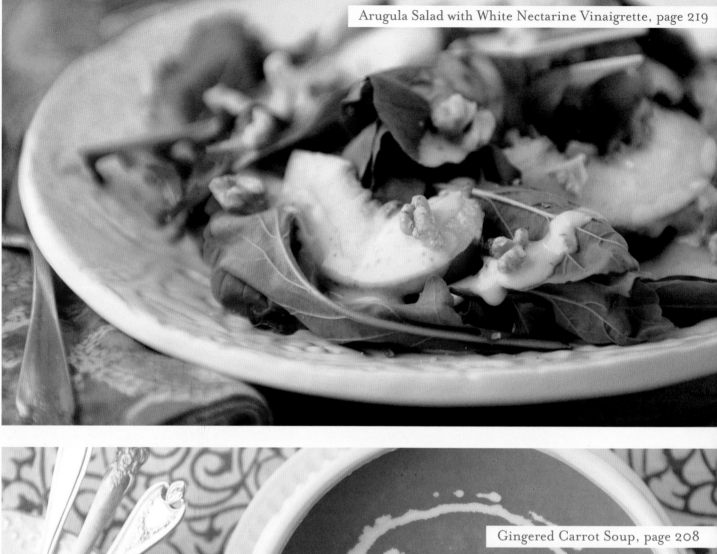

Arugula Salad with White Nectarine Vinaigrette, page 219

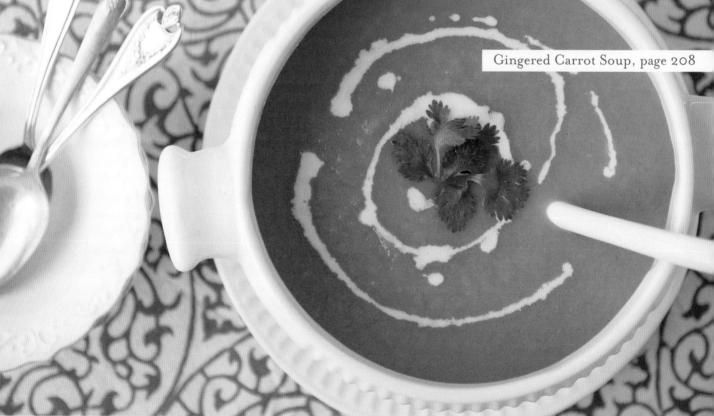

Gingered Carrot Soup, page 208

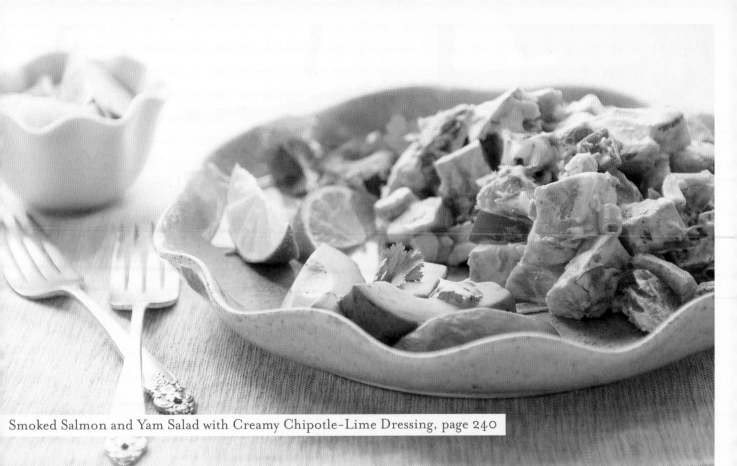

Smoked Salmon and Yam Salad with Creamy Chipotle-Lime Dressing, page 240

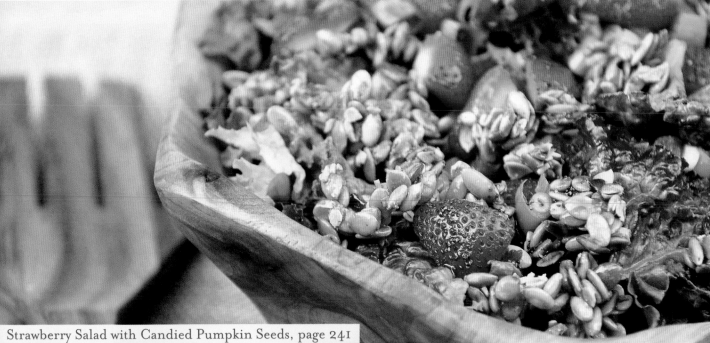

Strawberry Salad with Candied Pumpkin Seeds, page 241

Steamed Vegetables with Lemon-Garlic Dressing, page 255

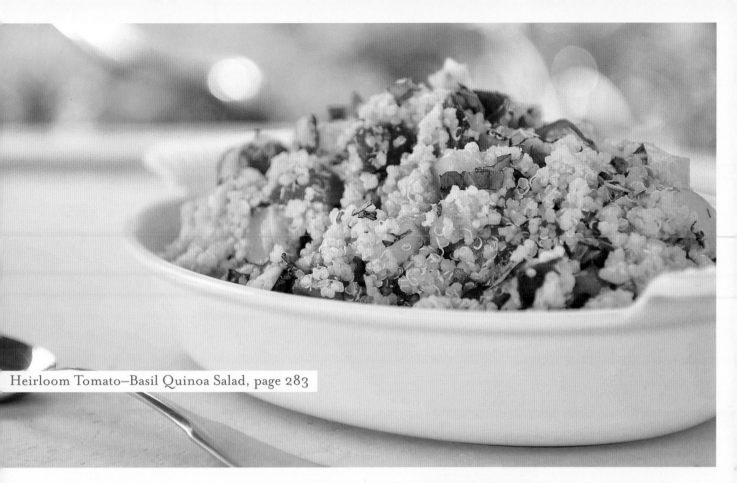

Heirloom Tomato–Basil Quinoa Salad, page 283

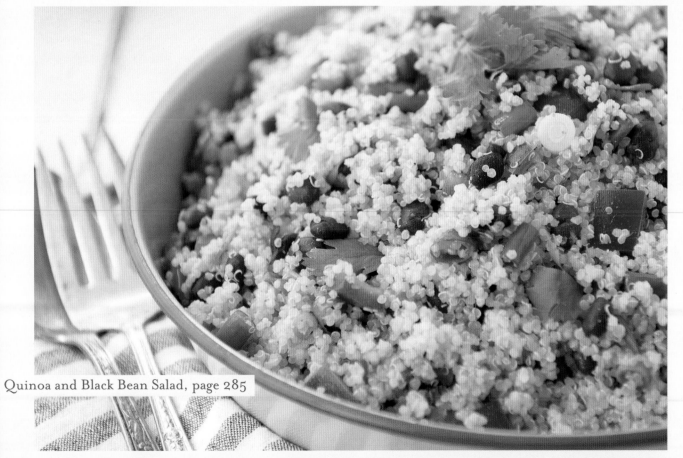

Quinoa and Black Bean Salad, page 285

Lemon Millet Patties, page 288

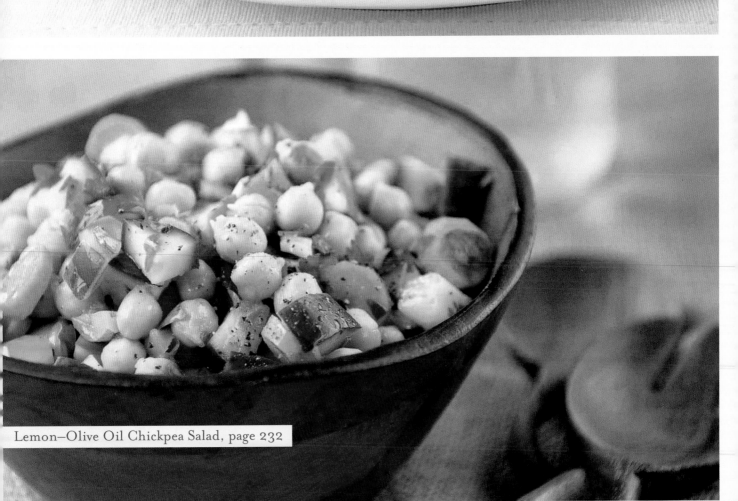

Raw Thai Wraps with Cilantro-Pumpkin Seed Pâte, page 298

Lemon–Olive Oil Chickpea Salad, page 232

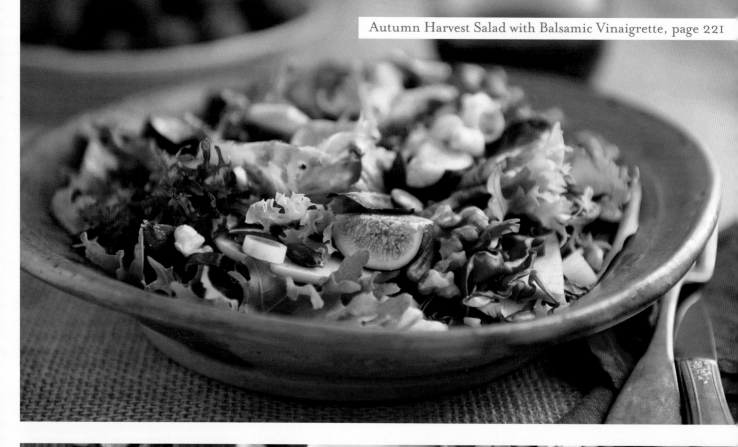

Autumn Harvest Salad with Balsamic Vinaigrette, page 221

Basil–Feta–Cranberry Bean Salad, page 222

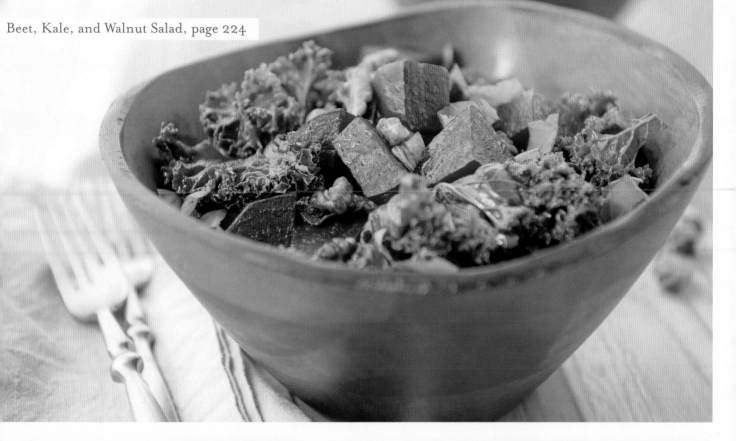

Beet, Kale, and Walnut Salad, page 224

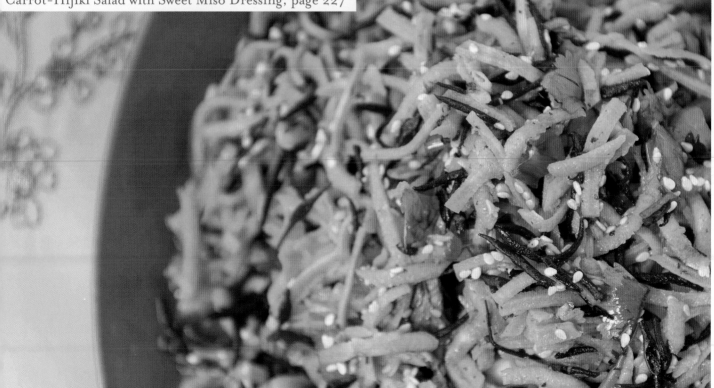

Carrot-Hijiki Salad with Sweet Miso Dressing, page 227

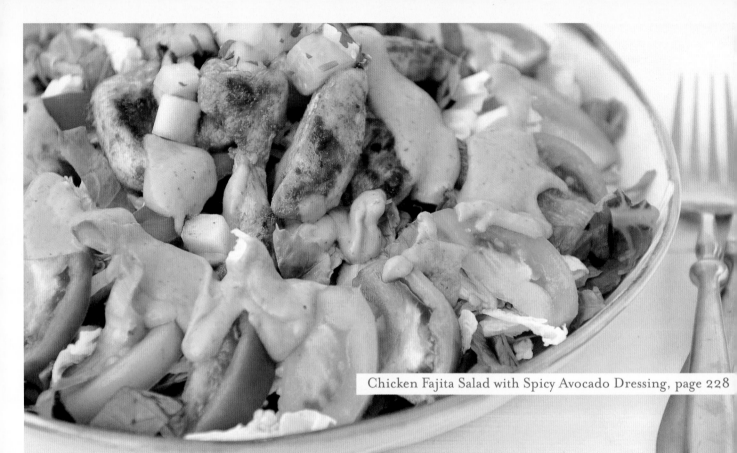

Chicken Fajita Salad with Spicy Avocado Dressing, page 228

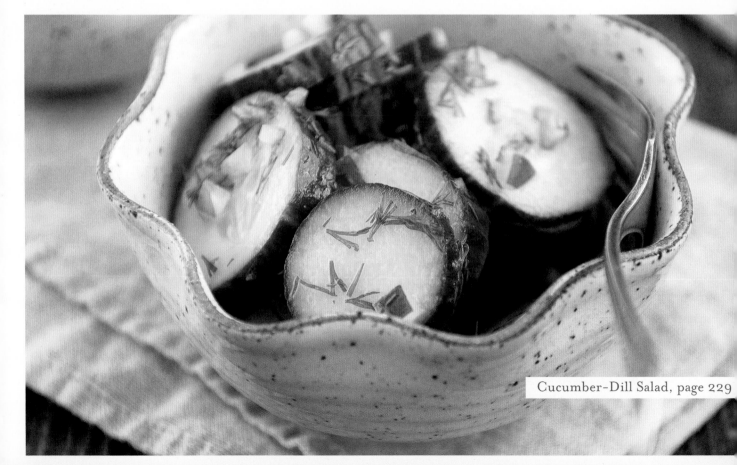

Cucumber-Dill Salad, page 229

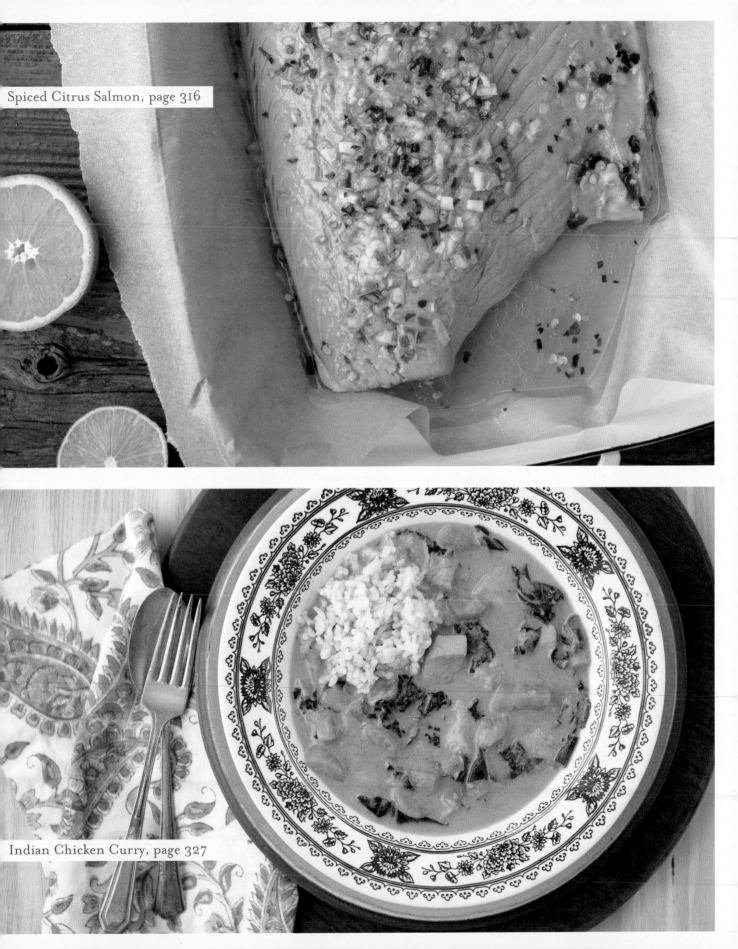

Spiced Citrus Salmon, page 316

Indian Chicken Curry, page 327

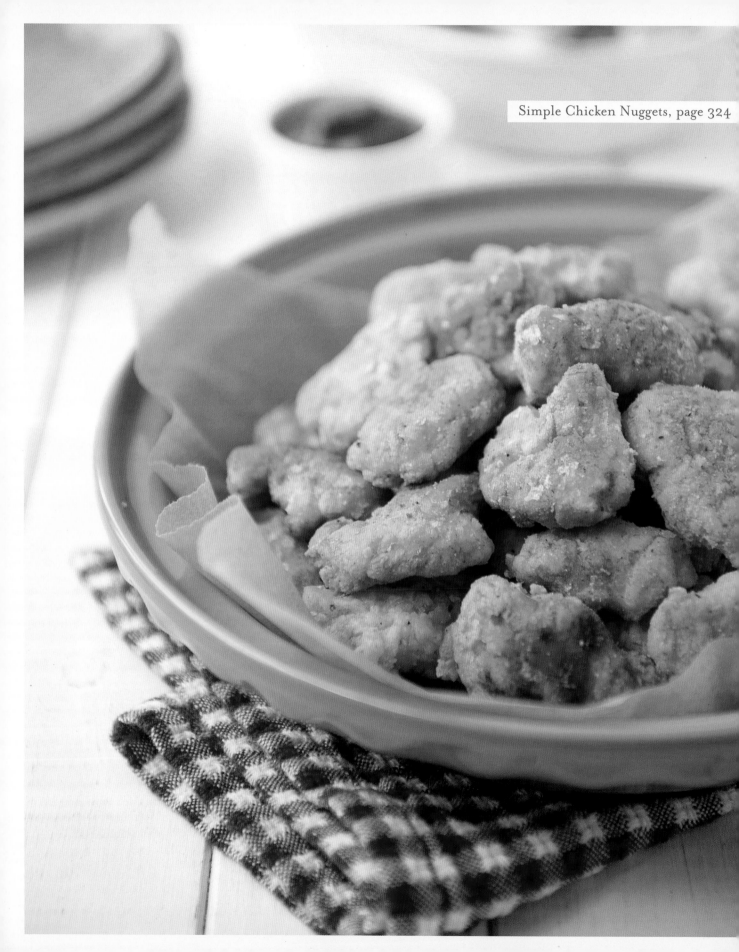

Simple Chicken Nuggets, page 324

QUICK CRUCIFEROUS STIR-FRY

This stir-fry, rich in cruciferous vegetables, offers significant cancer protection. The anticancer effects of these vegetables come from the phytochemicals like sulforaphane and indoles. These chemicals suppress not only tumor growth, but also cancer cell metastasis. You can add cubed marinated organic chicken or tofu to this stir-fry if desired. Serve with brown basmati rice (see page 265).

1 tablespoon virgin coconut oil

1 medium onion, chopped

2 carrots, peeled and sliced ¼ inch thick on the diagonal

2 to 3 garlic cloves, crushed

2 teaspoons minced fresh ginger

1 head broccoli, cut into florets

2 cups chopped baby bok choy

3 to 4 cups chopped Napa or Savoy cabbage

¼ to ½ cup water

½ tablespoon kudzu, mixed with a few tablespoons water

1 to 2 tablespoons wheat-free tamari or coconut aminos

1 tablespoon brown rice vinegar or coconut vinegar

Heat the coconut oil in a large stainless steel skillet or wok over medium-high heat. Add the onion and sauté for about 3 minutes, being careful not to brown.

Add the carrots and sauté 2 to 3 minutes more. Add the garlic, ginger, and broccoli and sauté for a few minutes more. Keep the vegetables moving in the skillet. Add the bok choy, cabbage, and ¼ cup of water, mix well, cover, and cook for just a couple of minutes more, or until the vegetables are crisp-tender and still brightly colored.

Reduce the heat to the lowest possible setting and add the kudzu-water mixture, tamari, and vinegar and stir gently for about 30 seconds, or until the liquid is clear. Add additional water if necessary.

Yield: 4 to 6 servings

Variation: If you don't have kudzu, use 1 tablespoon of arrowroot powder mixed with a few tablespoons of water instead.

SAUTÉED ASPARAGUS WITH GARLIC AND LEMON

Asparagus is a great source of vitamin K1, folate, vitamin C, beta-carotene, and potassium. Asparagus also contains a large amount of inulin, which is a carbohydrate that our bodies cannot digest. The health-promoting friendly bacteria in our large intestine, such as *Bifidobacteria* and *Lactobacilli*, do digest it though. When we feed the friendly bacteria in our gut, their growth increases, which keeps out the more harmful bacteria that can have negative effects on our health. Serve this wonderful springtime dish with fish or poached eggs.

1 to 1½ pounds asparagus	1 tablespoon freshly squeezed lemon juice
1 tablespoon extra-virgin olive oil	¼ teaspoon sea salt
3 garlic cloves, crushed	

Trim the bottom ends off the asparagus. The ends are usually too tough and woody for consumption. Cut the asparagus spears into 3-inch pieces.

Heat the olive oil in a large skillet over medium heat. Add the crushed garlic and sauté 30 seconds. Add the asparagus and sauté for 5 to 6 minutes or until crisp-tender.

Remove the skillet from the heat and add the lemon juice and sea salt and stir well. Serve immediately.

Yield: 2 to 4 servings

SAUTÉED CABBAGE WITH CUMIN SEEDS

Serve this simple vegetable dish alongside a bean or chicken curry. Sometimes we serve it with roasted organic chicken and baked yams on a chilly winter evening.

1 tablespoon whole cumin seeds	4 cups sliced green cabbage
1 tablespoon virgin coconut oil	sea salt

Heat an 11- or 12-inch skillet over medium-high heat. Add the cumin seeds and toast them for about 30 seconds. Then add the coconut oil and cabbage and sauté for 4 to 5 minutes. Season to taste with sea salt.

Yield: 4 servings

SAUTÉED PATTYPAN SQUASH WITH LEMON AND CAPERS

Summer squash is an excellent source for manganese and vitamin C. This dish is best made in the summer when pattypan squash is in season. Serve with cooked fresh cranberry beans or grilled fish, and cooked quinoa for a simple summer meal.

1 tablespoon extra-virgin olive oil

2 garlic cloves, crushed

4 to 5 medium pattypan squash, chopped

¼ cup chopped fresh parsley

2 tablespoons freshly squeezed lemon juice

3 tablespoons capers

sea salt or Herbamare

In a large skillet, heat the olive oil over medium heat. Add the garlic and chopped squash and sauté for about 1 minute. Cover and cook until tender, stirring occasionally, 3 to 4 minutes.

Transfer to a bowl and add the parsley, lemon juice, capers, and sea salt to taste. Toss to coat. Serve immediately.

Yield: 4 servings

CURRIED VEGETABLES

Turmeric, one of the ingredients in this dish, acts as an excellent anti-inflammatory. Turmeric is especially effective in arthritis sufferers where it acts not only as an anti-inflammatory but also as an antioxidant to neutralize some of the free radicals that are causing the joint pain. Serve this dish with a lentil dal and brown jasmine rice for a colorful, flavorful meal.

1 tablespoon virgin coconut oil
1 large onion, chopped
1 teaspoon ground coriander
1 teaspoon ground cumin
1½ teaspoons curry powder
½ teaspoon ground turmeric
¼ teaspoon ground cinnamon
pinch cayenne pepper
4 to 5 garlic cloves, crushed
3 large carrots, sliced diagonally

2 small yams, peeled and sliced diagonally
2 cups diced tomatoes
½ cup water
1 large red bell pepper, cut into large pieces
2 medium zucchini, sliced diagonally
1 tablespoon arrowroot powder, mixed with
    ½ cup cold water
1 teaspoon sea salt
1 cup chopped fresh cilantro

Heat the coconut oil in a large skillet or pot over medium heat. Add the onion and sauté until soft, about 5 minutes. Add the coriander, cumin, curry powder, turmeric, cinnamon, and cayenne and sauté for 1 minute more.

Add the garlic, carrots, and yams and gently mix to coat with oil and spices. Add diced tomatoes and water and cook for 5 to 10 minutes, covered, stirring frequently, adding additional water to prevent sticking or burning.

When the vegetables are beginning to get tender, add the bell pepper and zucchini and gently mix. Cover and cook until the zucchini and other vegetables are tender but not mushy.

Add the arrowroot mixture and simmer for 1 minute more. Remove from heat and season with the sea salt and cilantro and mix gently.

Yield: 4 servings

STEAMED VEGETABLES WITH LEMON-GARLIC DRESSING

Lightly steaming your vegetables is a great way to lock in nutrients while increasing digestibility. You can vary the vegetables to what is in season.

VEGETABLES

2 carrots, cut into thin strips

1 medium zucchini, cut into thin strips

1 yellow squash, cut into thin strips

1 small red bell pepper, cut into thin strips

¼ cup finely chopped fresh parsley, for garnish

DRESSING

freshly squeezed juice of ½ lemon

2 tablespoons extra-virgin olive oil

1 garlic clove, crushed

½ teaspoon finely grated lemon zest

¼ teaspoon sea salt or Herbamare

To prepare the vegetables, place the cut vegetables in a steamer basket over about 2 inches of water in a 2- or 3-quart pot. Place a lid on the pot and cook over medium heat. Steam for 5 to 7 minutes or until crisp-tender. Transfer to a bowl.

To make the dressing, whisk together all the ingredients in a small bowl. Pour the dressing over the steamed vegetables, add the parsley, and toss. Taste and add more sea salt or Herbamare if desired.

Yield: 4 servings

OVEN FRIES

This recipe is a favorite of children. Serve with the Sunny Sunflower Seed Burgers (page 293), organic ketchup, and steamed broccoli for a healthy, kid-friendly meal. These fries are delicious on their own or with the optional spices below.

---

4 medium organic russet potatoes or sweet
   potatoes
¼ cup extra-virgin olive oil or melted coconut oil
½ teaspoon sea salt or Herbamare
freshly ground black pepper

OPTIONAL SPICES
½ teaspoon ground turmeric
1 to 2 teaspoons garlic powder
1 tablespoon paprika

Preheat the oven to 425°F.

Scrub the potatoes well and remove any eyes or discolored areas. Leave the peels on. Cut into wedges and place into a large bowl. Add the oil, sea salt or Herbamare, and pepper; toss to coat. Add optional spices if desired.

Arrange the potatoes in a single layer in a 9 x 13-inch glass baking dish. Bake until golden and fork-tender, 30 to 40 minutes.

Yield: 4 servings

BALSAMIC ROASTED BEETS

Serve these delicate and flavorful beets as an appetizer dipped in plain organic yogurt, or as a side dish to your evening meal. They are also wonderful on salads, drizzled with a balsamic vinaigrette.

---

1 bunch beets, trimmed and peeled
2 to 3 tablespoons balsamic vinegar

2 tablespoons extra-virgin olive oil
¼ teaspoon sea salt

Preheat the oven to 400°F.

Cut beets into quarters and then cut into slices about ¼ inch thick. Place the beet slices into a 9 x 13-inch pan and toss with the vinegar, olive oil, and sea salt.

Roast for 35 to 40 minutes, or until the beets are tender when pierced with a fork.

Yield: 4 to 6 servings

ROASTED BUTTERNUT SQUASH WITH SHALLOTS AND GOLDEN RAISINS

Winter squash is a rich source of the carotenoid, beta-cryptoxanthin, which, when consumed, may lower your risk of developing lung cancer. Serve this warming winter vegetable dish with slow roasted organic beef and steamed kale for a balanced meal.

---

1 medium butternut squash, peeled, seeded, and diced
6 small shallots, sliced into halves
½ cup golden raisins

¼ teaspoon ground cardamom
¼ teaspoon sea salt
3 tablespoons extra-virgin olive oil

Preheat the oven to 400°F.

Place all the ingredients into a large baking dish, and stir to coat with the olive oil.

Roast for 35 to 40 minutes, or until the squash is tender.

Yield: 4 to 6 servings

ROASTED YAMS WITH ROSEMARY

Yams, which in the United States are actually sweet potatoes, are an excellent source of beta-carotene, vitamin C, and Vitamin B6. Beta-carotene is a powerful antioxidant, which works in the body to eliminate free radicals. Vitamin B6 is needed to convert homocysteine into the beneficial amino acid cysteine. High homocysteine levels are associated with an increased risk of heart attack and stroke. I like to serve this dish with the Wild Salmon with Ginger-Lime Marinade (page 317).

2 large yams, peeled and cubed
½ to 1 tablespoon finely chopped fresh
   rosemary

2 tablespoons extra-virgin olive oil
½ teaspoon sea salt

Preheat the oven to 425°F.

Put the yam cubes, rosemary, olive oil, and sea salt into a large baking dish and mix well to coat with the oil.

Bake, uncovered, for 35 to 45 minutes, or until the yams are very tender.

Yield: 4 servings

ROASTED ROOT VEGETABLES WITH FRESH HERBS

Make this dish during the bounty of the autumn harvest. It can be served with baked chicken or fish or a bean stew and a wild green salad. You can vary the vegetables according to what you have on hand.

2 to 3 red potatoes, cut into chunks

1 yam, peeled and cut into chunks

2 to 3 Jerusalem artichokes, scrubbed and cut into chunks

2 to 3 carrots, cut into chunks

1 to 2 beets, peeled and cut into chunks

½ teaspoon sea salt or Herbamare

2 to 3 tablespoons fresh herbs (rosemary, thyme, savory)

2 to 3 tablespoons extra-virgin olive oil

chopped fresh parsley, for garnish

Preheat the oven to 400°F.

Place the cut vegetables, sea salt, herbs, and olive oil into a 9 x 13-inch glass baking dish and toss well.

Transfer to the oven and roast, uncovered, for 40 to 45 minutes or until the vegetables are tender.

Garnish with fresh parsley and serve.

Yield: 4 to 6 servings

BAKED WINTER SQUASH

The autumn harvest brings many varieties of winter squash including acorn, butternut, buttercup, delicata, golden turban, hubbard, kabocha, spaghetti, and pie pumpkins. Each has its own unique flavor and an incredible sweetness. Winter squash is an excellent source of beta-carotene, which has very powerful antioxidant and anti-inflammatory properties. Beta-carotene prevents the oxidation of cholesterol in the body. Oxidized cholesterol is the type the builds up on blood vessel walls and contributes to the risk for heart attack or a stroke. Winter squash is also a good source of vitamin C, potassium, and manganese. Try serving baked winter squash with a drizzle of extra-virgin olive oil and a few dashes of cinnamon.

1 winter squash

Preheat the oven to 350°F.

Cut the squash lengthwise in half using a strong, sharp knife. Scoop out the fiber and seeds. Set the seeds aside to roast for another use, if desired.

Place the squash flesh side down into a roasting pan and add ¼ to ½ inch of water. Bake until tender. Smaller squashes may take up to 35 minutes while larger ones, including pie pumpkins, may take 45 to 90 minutes. Test by inserting a fork; it should slide in easily and feel soft.

Yield: 1 baked squash

17

WHOLE GRAINS

You gain strength, courage, and confidence by every experience in which you really stop to look fear in the face.

—*Eleanor Roosevelt*

Whole grains are so versatile that they can be used to make casseroles, salads, pilafs, even meatless burgers. A pot of grains may never turn out the same way twice. The amount of time it takes for the grain to cook, how much water it will absorb, and how fluffy your end product is depends on many factors, including the age of the grain, the conditions under which it was stored, and the temperature in which you cooked it.

The following pages contain information on how to cook whole grains, including basic recipes for each whole grain. Hopefully you will learn to love the flavor and diversity that whole grains can bring to your dinner table.

HOW TO COOK WHOLE GRAINS

Following these basic steps for cooking whole grains you can prepare highly nourishing, plant-rich meals for your family. We cook a few pots of whole grains every week to use in salads, soups, and as part of our main meals.

Sort

Before using, sort through your grains for tiny rocks and other debris. Dry quinoa often contains small stones. Millet and buckwheat can be cross contaminated with gluten grains if not certified gluten-free. Remove them from the rest of the grains before cooking. You can do this by pouring one-third of a cup of grain at a time onto a plate. Simply sort through with your fingers and pick out the rocks or foreign material. This can be a very exciting job for young children to participate in!

Rinse

Some grains need to be rinsed prior to cooking to remove chaff, dust, or other debris. These include millet, quinoa, amaranth, and sometimes brown rice. Quinoa also has a bitter saponin coating that repels insects and birds and, if not rinsed off, may cause digestive upset when consumed. To rinse grains, place them in a fine-mesh strainer and run warm water through them until the water runs clear. You may also place them into a pot with water and swirl the grains around using your hand. Then drain off the water through a fine-mesh strainer.

Soak

To soak grains, measure the desired amount and place it into a bowl. Cover with at least 1 inch of warm water and add 1 to 2 tablespoons of raw apple cider vinegar or raw coconut vinegar to each cup of grain. Soak, uncovered, on your kitchen counter for 12 to 24 hours. Then drain and rinse through a fine-mesh strainer. Follow the guidelines on the following page for water requirements and cooking times.

Add Sea Salt

Adding sea salt brings out the sweetness in grains and helps the grain to open up. Grains cooked without salt will taste flat. We generally use ⅛ to ¼ teaspoon of sea salt per 1 cup of dry grain.

Cook

To cook a whole grain you will need to first bring the pot of grain and water to a boil. Once boiling, immediately lower the heat to a simmer. Start timing when you turn down the heat to a simmer. Grains that have been boiled for too long may turn out tough and chewy. If your grains turn out mushy or clumped together, you may have added too much water, or not brought the heat to a high enough temperature initially. It is also very important to use the proper cookware when cooking whole grains. A stainless steel pot with a thick bottom that contains an aluminum core will distribute the heat evenly and prevent the bottom layer of grains from burning. Use a 1-quart pot for cooking 1 cup of grain, a 2-quart pot for cooking 2 cups of grain, or a 3-quart pot for cooking 3 cups of grain.

No Stirring!

Remember never to stir a pot of cooking grains. Whole grains create their own steam holes so the top layer of grains cooks as evenly as the bottom layer of grains. When you stir a pot of cooking whole grains, the steam holes are destroyed, which causes some of your grain to never fully cook.

Cooking Chart for Soaked Whole Grains

Grains (1 cup dry)	Water (cups)	Cooking Times (minutes)	Yield (cups)
Short-grain Brown Rice	1½	50	3½
Long-grain Brown Rice	1¼ to 1½	45	3
Sweet Brown Rice	1½	50	2½
Wild Rice	1¾	75	4
Buckwheat	1	15	2
Millet	1½	25–30	3½
Quinoa	1¼–1½	12–15	3
Teff	—	—	—
Amaranth	—	—	—

Cooking Chart for Unsoaked Whole Grains

Grains (1 cup dry)	Water (cups)	Cooking Times (minutes)	Yield (cups)
Short-grain Brown Rice	2	55–60	3½
Long-grain Brown Rice	1¾	50	3
Sweet Brown Rice	2	55–60	2½
Wild Rice	2½	75	4
Buckwheat	1½	15–20	2
Millet	2–2½	30–35	3½
Quinoa	1¾	15–20	3
Teff	3	15–20	2½
Amaranth	2½	20–25	2

The following pages contain basic cooking instructions for each grain. The grains in this chapter are all gluten-free, which include amaranth, brown rice, wild rice, buckwheat, millet, and quinoa. Oats are gluten-free only if they are certified gluten-free.

Tip: Many grains that are purchased in bulk bins have a potential for being cross contaminated with flour dust from nearby bins, scoops used for gluten products, or gluten grains that were previously stored in that bin. Some stores respond well to requests to separate gluten-containing grains and flours from the nongluten products by moving the bins to a different location altogether and being aware of these cross contamination issues. Some grains can also be contaminated with gluten during growing and processing—brown rice, wild rice, quinoa, and amaranth are the least likely to be contaminated. Packaged grain products must be labeled gluten-free and produced in a dedicated facility to be considered truly gluten-free.

BASIC AMARANTH

Amaranth is an ancient Aztec grain that is rich in protein and calcium. Amaranth releases a lot of starch while it is cooking, creating a soupier cooked grain rather than a fluffy one. It is best not to add salt to amaranth while it is cooking, or it will not absorb enough water to become tender.

1 cup amaranth	2½ cups water

Place the amaranth and water in a 2-quart pot with a tight-fitting lid and bring to a boil. Reduce the heat to low and simmer for 20 to 25 minutes, or until most of the liquid has been absorbed.

Yield: 2 cups

BASIC BROWN RICE

Rice with just the hull removed is brown rice. Rice with the hull, bran, and germ removed is white rice. There is a wide variety of brown rice to choose from: short grain, long grain, sweet, jasmine, and basmati are just a few.

1 cup brown rice	pinch sea salt
1½ to 2 cups water	

Place the rice, water, and sea salt into a medium pot with a tight-fitting lid and bring to a boil. Reduce the heat to a low simmer and cook for about 45 minutes, or until all of the water has been absorbed. Remember never to stir the rice while it is cooking.

Remove the rice from the heat and let stand in the pot for about 10 minutes.

Yield: 2½ to 3½ cups

BASIC STICKY BROWN RICE

Serve this rice with a hearty bean soup, or use it to make sushi rolls. You may want to make a half batch of this recipe if serving only a small number of people. The amount of water varies in this recipe depending on whether you have soaked the grains overnight—use 4½ cups of water if the rice has been soaked or 6 cups of water for unsoaked rice.

---

2 cups sweet brown rice

1 cup short-grain brown rice

4½ to 6 cups water

½ teaspoon sea salt

Put the rice, water, and sea salt in a medium stainless steel pot over medium-high heat and bring to a boil. Cover, reduce the heat to low, and simmer for about 45 minutes.

Let stand for at least 10 minutes before serving.

Yield: 8 cups

BASIC WILD RICE

Wild rice is a seed of a grass that grows in small lakes and slow-flowing streams, and is native to North America. Native Americans harvested wild rice by canoeing into a stand of plants and bending the ripe grain heads with wooden sticks, called knockers, to get the rice into the canoe. Wild rice is closely related to true rice as both share the same plant tribe, the Oryzeae. Wild rice is higher in protein than regular brown rice and contains a high amount of zinc. Cooked wild rice can be added to soups, made into grain pilafs, or stuffed into cooked winter squash.

---

1 cup wild rice

1¾ to 2½ cups water

pinch sea salt

Rinse the wild rice in a fine-mesh strainer and put into a medium pot with the water and sea salt, cover, and bring to a boil. Reduce the heat to low and simmer for 60 to 75 minutes.

Remove the pot from heat and let the wild rice stand 10 minutes.

Yield: 4 cups

BASIC BUCKWHEAT

Buckwheat can either be found raw or roasted at your local co-op or health food store. The roasted version of buckwheat is called kasha. Both have a strong and hearty flavor that lends well for cold-weather eating.

1 to 1½ cups water	1 cup buckwheat groats
¼ teaspoon sea salt	

In a medium pot, bring the water and sea salt to a boil, add the buckwheat, and cover the pot. Reduce the heat to low and simmer for 15 to 20 minutes.

Yield: 2 cups

BASIC MILLET

Millet is a small, round, yellow grain with a sweet, earthy taste. It is one of the oldest known grains consumed by humans. Millet is easily digested and is also one of the least allergenic grains. Millet is beneficial in destroying harmful yeasts and bacteria in the gut.

1 cup millet	pinch sea salt
1½ to 2½ cups water	

Wash the millet and drain it through a fine-mesh strainer. Place the millet, water, and sea salt into a medium pot with a tight-fitting lid and bring to a boil. Reduce the heat to low, and simmer for 30 to 35 minutes, or until all of the water has been absorbed. Use less water for a fluffy grain, or more water for a creamier grain.

Yield: 3½ cups

BASIC OAT GROATS

Oats, or *Avena sativa*, originated in Asia and have been cultivated throughout the world for over 2,000 years. Oat groats are simply the hulled version of oats. Oats contain a specific fiber known as beta-glucan, which can significantly lower cholesterol levels and help prevent heart disease. Oats contain antioxidant compounds called avenanthramides, which help to prevent free radicals from damaging LDL cholesterol, thus reducing the risk of heart disease. If you are gluten-sensitive, be sure to purchase organic certified gluten-free oats.

1 cup oat groats
2¼ cups water

pinch sea salt

Place the oats, water, and sea salt into a medium pot with a tight-fitting lid and bring to a boil. Reduce the heat to low and simmer for about 1 hour, or until most of the water has been absorbed.

Let stand for 10 minutes.

Yield: 2 to 2½ cups

> **Tip:** Whether or not oats can be consumed by gluten-sensitive people is quite controversial. Research indicates that the majority of oat samples tested in both Europe and the United States are cross contaminated with gluten. Thankfully there are certified gluten-free manufacturers of rolled oats and oat products. However, there are still a good number of gluten-sensitive people who react to the avenin protein in oats. Many people who are gluten-sensitive benefit from leaving oats out of their diet until they can be challenged through an Elimination Diet.

BASIC QUINOA

Quinoa, pronounced "KEEN-wah," comes from the Andes Mountains in South America where it was once a staple food for the Incas. Quinoa contains all eight essential amino acids and has a delicious, light nutty flavor. Quinoa makes wonderful grain salads or is great served with a vegetable and bean stew.

1 cup quinoa   pinch sea salt
1½ to 1¾ cups water

Rinse the quinoa well with warm water and drain through a fine-mesh strainer. Quinoa has a natural saponin coating that repels insects and birds. It has a bitter taste and can cause some digestive upset when consumed. Rinsing with warm water removes the saponin.

Place the rinsed quinoa, water, and sea salt into a medium pot with a tight-fitting lid and bring to a boil. Reduce the heat to low and simmer for 15 to 20 minutes, or until all of the water has been absorbed.

Fluff with a fork before serving.

Yield: 3 cups

BASIC TEFF

Teff is a very tiny grain that is available in three colors—white, red, or brown—each with its own distinct flavor. Teff originated in Africa where it was once a foraged wild grass before it was cultivated as a staple grain for the Ethiopians. It is now grown in the Snake River Valley of Idaho. Teff is very high in minerals, namely iron.

3 cups water   1 cup teff
pinch sea salt

In a medium pot, bring the water and sea salt to a boil. Add the teff and stir briefly. Cook for 15 to 20 minutes, covered, stirring occasionally toward the end of the cooking time. Serve.

Yield: 2½ cups

BUCKWHEAT SOBA NOODLE SALAD

Buckwheat does not contain any gluten even though the name implies so. However, if you are gluten-sensitive, it is difficult to find a brand of noodles that doesn't also process wheat in the same facility. Brown rice noodles can easily replace the buckwheat noodles in this recipe for a true gluten-free salad. This dish is great to take to work or school or bring to a potluck. People are always attracted to this dish because of the beautiful array of colors it contains.

SALAD

1 package buckwheat soba noodles

2 tablespoons hijiki seaweed

1 cup cold water

1 cup grated carrots

1 cup thinly sliced red cabbage

3 green onions, sliced into thin rounds

½ cup chopped fresh cilantro

¼ cup sesame seeds, toasted

DRESSING

3 tablespoons toasted sesame oil

2 tablespoons wheat-free tamari or coconut aminos

2 tablespoons brown rice vinegar or coconut vinegar

1 tablespoon pure maple syrup

1 to 2 teaspoons hot pepper sesame oil

1 to 2 teaspoons grated fresh ginger

2 to 3 garlic cloves, crushed

To prepare the salad, cook the buckwheat noodles according to the package directions. When the noodles are cooked, drain and rinse with cool water, and set aside.

While the noodles are cooking, place the hijiki in a small saucepan with about 1 cup of cold water. Let soak for about 5 minutes. Place the saucepan of hijiki on the stovetop and simmer over medium heat for 20 to 25 minutes. Drain the hijiki in a fine-mesh strainer and set aside.

Place the noodles, hijiki, carrots, cabbage, green onions, cilantro, and toasted sesame seeds into a large bowl.

To make the dressing, whisk together the ingredients in a separate bowl. Pour the dressing over the salad and toss well. Serve.

Yield: 4 servings

RICE NOODLES AND RED CABBAGE IN A SPICY CASHEW SAUCE

Serve this easy-to-make dish with some grilled chicken or fish and steamed broccoli for a complete meal. Brown rice noodles come in a variety of shapes and sizes, any of which can be used in this recipe. You can substitute organic unsalted peanut butter for the cashew butter in the sauce if you wish.

SALAD

1 package brown rice noodles

1½ cups finely sliced red cabbage

4 green onions, sliced into thin rounds

½ cup finely chopped fresh cilantro

SAUCE

2 teaspoons virgin coconut oil

4 garlic cloves, crushed

1 teaspoon grated fresh ginger

½ cup cashew butter

1 cup water

2 tablespoons wheat-free tamari or coconut aminos

1 tablespoon brown rice vinegar or coconut vinegar

1 tablespoon pure maple syrup

1 to 2 teaspoons hot pepper sesame oil

To make the salad, cook the rice noodles according to the package directions.

While the noodles are cooking, prepare the sauce. Heat the coconut oil in a small saucepan over medium heat. Add the garlic and ginger and sauté 30 seconds. Add the cashew butter, water, tamari, vinegar, maple syrup, and hot pepper sesame oil. Simmer over low heat, whisking, until thickened, adding more water if necessary. This should only take a few minutes.

To assemble the salad, place the drained, warm noodles, cabbage, green onions, and cilantro into a large serving bowl. Pour the cashew sauce over the noodles and cabbage mixture and gently toss. Serve warm.

Yield: 4 servings

NORI ROLLS WITH VEGETABLES AND STICKY BROWN RICE

Nori is a sea vegetable that has been dried and made into thin flat sheets. It is what is used to make sushi. Nori can also be crumbled and sprinkled onto salads, cooked vegetables, or soups. It is rich in minerals and lignans. Lignans are compounds that are cancer-protective. Nori rolls typically contain raw fish and white rice, but they can also be made with cooked fish or sautéed tofu and sticky brown rice. A variety of thinly sliced vegetables is usually put into the center, including carrot, green onion, avocado, daikon radish, and red cabbage. These are then rolled together and sliced. Serve with coconut aminos or tamari, wasabi, and pickled ginger if you like.

RICE

2 cups sweet brown rice

1 cup short-grain brown rice

6 cups water

½ teaspoon sea salt

3 tablespoons seasoned brown rice vinegar

VEGETABLES

nori sheets

2 to 3 carrots, cut into thin matchsticks

1 to 2 avocados, sliced into thin strips

3 to 4 green onions, sliced into thin strips

OPTIONAL GARNISHES

wheat-free tamari or coconut aminos

wasabi

To make the rice, place the rice into a pot with the water and sea salt, cover, and bring to a boil. Reduce the heat to low and simmer for 45 minutes. Remove from the heat and let the rice stand for 20 minutes. Transfer the rice to a bowl, drizzle with the vinegar, and mix well.

To assemble the nori rolls, place a sheet of nori, shiny side down, on a clean surface. Spread a thin layer of rice to within 2 inches below the top of the sheet. Place the vegetables at the bottom of the sheet. Tightly roll from the vegetable end. The nori rolls can be sealed by running your finger with a little water along the seam side.

Repeat this process until you have the desired amount of rolls. When ready to serve, slice the nori rolls with a serrated knife that has been dipped in water. Serve with tamari and wasabi if desired.

Yield: 4 to 8 servings

INDIAN FRIED RICE

This tasty rice dish is delicious served with the Curried Vegetables (page 254) and Red Lentil Dal (page 198). If you cannot find brown jasmine rice in your area, then use brown basmati rice instead.

RICE

2 cups brown jasmine rice

3½ cups water

¼ teaspoon sea salt

OTHER INGREDIENTS

2 tablespoons virgin coconut oil

½ cup raw cashews

¼ teaspoon sea salt

1 teaspoon ground cumin

1 teaspoon black mustard seeds

1½ teaspoons ground coriander

1 bunch green onions, sliced diagonally into ½-inch pieces

¼ cup dried currants

½ cup chopped fresh cilantro

To cook the rice, place the rice, water, and sea salt into a 2-quart pot with a tight-fitting lid and bring to a boil. Reduce the heat and simmer for about 40 minutes. Remove the pot from the heat and let the rice stand and cool for about 30 minutes; in fact, it is even better if you let the rice cool completely before sautéing it with the other ingredients.

To prepare the cashew-spice mixture, heat the coconut oil in an 11- or 12-inch skillet over medium heat. Add the cashews, sea salt, and spices and sauté, stirring, for about 1 minute. After the cashews have begun to turn golden and you smell a rich fragrance, add the green onions and currants. Add the rice and continue stirring and keep the mixture moving until all of the rice is well combined.

Stir in the cilantro and serve.

Yield: 6 servings

LENTIL AND RICE SALAD WITH LEMON AND OLIVES

Serve this dish as part of a light summer meal or for a simple lunch. If you cannot find French lentils you can substitute green or brown lentils instead. This salad will keep in a covered container in the refrigerator for up to 5 days.

LENTILS

6 cups water

1½ cups French lentils, rinsed and drained

RICE

1 cup brown basmati rice

1¾ cups water

pinch sea salt

SALAD

2 medium carrots, diced

1 pint cherry tomatoes

1 cup Kalamata olives, pitted and chopped

1 cup chopped fresh parsley

1 small bunch green onions, chopped

½ cup chopped fresh basil

DRESSING

6 tablespoons freshly squeezed lemon juice

4 tablespoons extra-virgin olive oil

2 garlic cloves, crushed

2 teaspoons finely grated lemon zest

1 tablespoon chopped fresh oregano

½ teaspoon sea salt

½ teaspoon freshly ground black pepper

To make the lentils, place the water and lentils into a 3- or 4-quart pot and bring to a boil. Cover, reduce the heat, and simmer for 20 to 25 minutes, or until the lentils are tender. Once the lentils are cooked, drain in a fine-mesh strainer

To make the rice, place the rice, water, and sea salt into a small pot and bring to a boil. Reduce the heat to low and cook, covered, for about 45 minutes. Remove from the heat and let stand at least 20 minutes.

Transfer the lentils and rice to a large serving bowl and add the carrots, tomatoes, olives, parsley, green onions, and basil.

To make the dressing, whisk together all the ingredients in a separate bowl. Pour over the lentil mixture and toss to coat. Serve

Yield: 6 servings

PINE NUT–STUDDED RICE

Serve this Mediterranean-style dish with the Poached Halibut with Tomatoes and Fresh Herbs (page 319) and a few spoonfuls of the Pickled Lemon-Rosemary Cauliflower (page 99) for a complete meal.

RICE

2 cups brown basmati rice

3½ cups water

¼ teaspoon sea salt

OTHER INGREDIENTS

1 tablespoon extra-virgin olive oil

¼ to ½ cup pine nuts

4 green onions, sliced diagonally into ½-inch pieces

⅓ cup dried currants

4 cups baby spinach leaves

1 tablespoon chopped fresh oregano

½ teaspoon freshly ground black pepper

2 to 3 tablespoons freshly squeezed lemon juice

¼ teaspoon sea salt or Herbamare

To cook the rice, place the rice, water, and sea salt in a 2-quart pot with a tight-fitting lid and bring to a boil. Reduce the heat and simmer for about 40 minutes. Remove the pot from the heat and let the rice stand and cool for about 30 minutes.

To make the pine nut mixture, heat the olive oil in an 11- or 12-inch skillet over medium heat. Add the pine nuts and green onions and sauté for a minute or two until the pine nuts begin to change color. Quickly add the currants and spinach and continue to cook, stirring. Add the rice and gently stir the mixture to combine. Add the oregano, pepper, lemon juice, and sea salt and stir to evenly coat. Remove from the heat and serve.

Yield: 6 servings

SPANISH RICE

Serve this grain dish with the Sensuous Vegan Vegetable and Bean Enchiladas (page 310) for a gourmet vegetarian meal or simply serve with some cooked black beans and a fresh green salad for an easy, flavorful meal.

---

2 tablespoons extra-virgin olive oil

1 medium onion, diced

3 garlic cloves, crushed

1 teaspoon sea salt

1 teaspoon ground cumin

½ teaspoon chili powder

1 jalapeño pepper, finely diced

1 small red bell pepper, diced

2 cups brown basmati rice

3¾ cups water

1 cup tomato sauce or 2 to 3 tablespoons tomato paste

Heat the olive oil in a 3-quart pot over medium heat. Add the onion and garlic and sauté until soft, about 5 minutes. Add the sea salt, cumin, chili powder, jalapeño pepper, and bell pepper, stir, and sauté for 2 minutes more.

Stir in the rice, water, and tomato sauce or paste and bring to a boil. Reduce the heat to low and simmer, covered, until all of the liquid has been absorbed, about 50 minutes.

Yield: 6 servings

THAI FRIED RICE

This dish is a fun way to dress up plain brown rice. You may even want to cook the rice a day ahead of time to have on hand for a quick side dish to an evening meal. Use brown basmati rice if you cannot find brown jasmine rice.

RICE
2 cups brown jasmine rice
3½ cups water
¼ teaspoon sea salt

OTHER INGREDIENTS
1 tablespoon virgin coconut oil, plus more if needed
1 bunch green onions, sliced diagonally, ½ inch thick

½ cup raw cashews
5 garlic cloves, crushed
¼ teaspoon ground white pepper
¼ cup raisins
1 medium firm tomato, chopped
1 tablespoon coconut sugar
1 to 2 tablespoons wheat-free tamari or coconut aminos
½ cup chopped fresh cilantro

To cook the rice, place the rice, water, and sea salt into a 2-quart pot with a tight-fitting lid and bring to a boil. Reduce the heat to a low simmer and cook for about 40 minutes, or until done. Remove the pot from the heat and let stand at least 30 minutes.

To make the cashew-vegetable mixture, heat the coconut oil in an 11- or 12-inch skillet, preferably cast iron, over medium heat. Add the green onions and cashews and cook, stirring frequently, for a minute or two, or until the cashews are lightly toasted. Add the garlic and pepper and cook for about 30 seconds more, stirring. Add the raisins and stir to coat with oil.

Add the cooked rice and continue cooking and stirring. Add more coconut oil if needed. Add the chopped tomato, sugar, and tamari and cook a few minutes more, continuing to stir. Remove from the heat and stir in the fresh cilantro.

Yield: 6 servings

WEHANI RICE AND PECAN PILAF

Wehani rice is a light clay-colored aromatic brown rice that has a popcorn-like fragrance when cooked. It splits slightly during cooking much like wild rice does. You can buy it in the bulk section of most health food stores and food co-ops. Serve this rice dish in the fall or winter or as part of a holiday meal. It also makes a great stuffing for turkey, chicken, or baked winter squash.

RICE

2 cups wehani rice

4 cups water

pinch sea salt

PILAF

2 tablespoons extra-virgin olive oil or organic butter

1 medium red onion, diced

2 garlic cloves, crushed

1 teaspoon dried thyme

1 cup coarsely chopped pecans

½ cup dried cranberries or dried cherries

¼ cup freshly squeezed orange juice

½ cup finely chopped fresh parsley

½ teaspoon sea salt or Herbamare

To cook the rice, place the rice, water, and sea salt into a medium pot with a tight-fitting lid and bring to a boil. Reduce the heat to low and simmer for about 45 minutes. Remove from heat and let stand for 10 to 15 minutes.

To make the pilaf, heat the olive oil or butter in an 11- or 12-inch skillet over medium heat. Add the onion and sauté for 5 minutes or until soft. Add the garlic, thyme, and pecans and continue to sauté for 2 to 3 minutes more.

Add the dried cranberries and the cooked rice and stir to coat with the oil. Add the orange juice, parsley, and sea salt and mix gently. Continue to cook for about a minute more. Remove from the heat, taste, and adjust the salt and seasonings if necessary.

Yield: 6 servings

Variation: You can replace the wehani rice with wild rice or black rice.

WILD RICE AND KALE SALAD

This zesty grain salad is very easy to prepare. The combination of the raw kale and red pepper with the cooked wild rice create a nice flavor and texture combination. Serve with roasted organic turkey or a bean and vegetable soup.

RICE
1½ cups wild rice
3¾ cups water
pinch sea salt

SALAD
4 to 5 curly green kale leaves, rinsed and
  chopped

1 small red bell pepper, diced
1 bunch green onions, cut into thin rounds
½ cup freshly squeezed lemon juice
¼ cup extra-virgin olive oil
sea salt
freshly ground black pepper

To cook the rice, place the rice, water, and sea salt into a 2-quart pot, cover, and bring to a boil. Reduce the heat to low and simmer for 50 to 55 minutes. Remove from the heat and let stand for at least 30 minutes to cool.

To make the salad, place the chopped kale, bell pepper, green onions, lemon juice, and olive oil into a large bowl and toss gently. Add the cooked rice. Then season with salt and pepper to taste. Toss again and serve.

Store any extra rice salad in a glass container in the refrigerator for up to 5 days.

Yield: 6 servings

WILD RICE–STUFFED SQUASH

This recipe is great for holiday gatherings or as a warm autumn meal. Try adding some sliced organic sausages to the rice mixture for a little extra flavor and protein.

RICE

½ cup wild rice
½ cup long-grain brown rice
2 cups water
pinch sea salt

SQUASH

3 small acorn squash, cut in half crosswise

STUFFING

1 tablespoon olive oil
1 small leek, chopped
3 garlic cloves, crushed
2 celery stalks, chopped
1 teaspoon dried sage
1 teaspoon dried thyme
½ teaspoon sea salt or Herbamare
½ cup chopped fresh parsley
½ cup organic dried cranberries (fruit-juice sweetened)
¾ cup pecans, chopped

To cook the rice, place the wild rice and long-grain brown rice in a 2-quart pot. Add the water and a pinch of sea salt, cover, and bring to a boil. Reduce the heat to low and simmer for 45 minutes, or until all the water has been absorbed. Remove the pot from the heat and let stand while preparing the other ingredients.

Preheat the oven to 400°F.

To prepare the squash, scoop out the seeds from the squash and place the squash halves, flesh side down, in a glass baking dish filled with ¼ inch of water. Bake, uncovered, for 35 to 40 minutes, or until the squash is fork-tender. Drain any excess water from the baking dish and set aside.

To make the stuffing, heat the olive oil in a 10-inch skillet over medium heat. Add the leek and sauté about 3 minutes. Add the garlic, celery, sage, thyme, and sea salt or Herbamare and sauté for 5 to 6 minutes more. Transfer the leek-celery mixture to a bowl, add the parsley, cranberries, pecans, and cooked rice, and mix well. Taste and adjust the salt and seasonings as desired.

Evenly distribute the stuffing mixture among the squash halves, placing it into the center of each. Place the stuffed squash back into the baking dish and transfer to the oven for 10 to 20 minutes, or until heated through.

Yield: 6 servings

COCONUT QUINOA PILAF

This yummy Thai-style quinoa dish is delicious served on its own, or serve it with the Asian Cabbage Slaw (page 220) and baked wild salmon for a balanced meal.

2 cups quinoa

one 14-ounce can coconut milk

2 cups water

1 bunch green onions, sliced

1 medium red bell pepper, diced

3 to 4 garlic cloves, crushed

¾ teaspoon sea salt

½ to 1 teaspoon crushed red chili flakes

½ cup chopped fresh cilantro

Rinse the dry quinoa in a fine-mesh strainer under warm running water. Quinoa has a natural saponin coating that repels insects and birds and can create a bitter taste. Rinsing the quinoa with warm water removes the saponin; drain well.

Place the rinsed quinoa into a 2- or 3-quart saucepan with the coconut milk, water, green onions, bell pepper, garlic, sea salt, and red chili flakes. Cover and bring to a boil. Reduce the heat to a low simmer and cook for about 20 minutes.

Remove the saucepan from the heat and let the pilaf cool in the pan for about 10 minutes. Add the cilantro and gently fluff with a fork. Serve hot.

Yield: 4 servings

COMPOSED SALAD OF QUINOA, CHICKPEAS, AND TOMATOES

This grain salad makes for an elegant lunch or evening meal. We like to use organic heirloom tomatoes here, which are in season during the summer. We also like to use the bright green, round Castelvetrano olives in the recipe, though any high-quality olive will do. Oftentimes we will steam a large amount of fresh greens, such as chard or kale, and add it to this meal.

QUINOA

2 cups quinoa

3½ cups water

¼ teaspoon sea salt

SALAD

2 to 3 cups cooked chickpeas

2 to 3 tomatoes, chopped

1 small red onion, finely diced

1 cup chopped fresh parsley

1 cup (or more) of your favorite variety of olives

LEMON-TAHINI DRESSING

½ cup sesame tahini

1 tablespoon finely grated lemon zest

½ cup freshly squeezed lemon juice

¼ cup extra-virgin olive oil

3 tablespoons water

2 garlic cloves, crushed

½ to 1 teaspoon sea salt

To cook the quinoa, rinse the dry quinoa in a fine-mesh strainer under warm running water; drain well. Place the rinsed quinoa into a 2-quart pot with the water and sea salt, cover, and bring to a boil. Reduce the heat to a low simmer and cook for about 20 minutes. Remove the pot from heat and let the quinoa cool in the pot for at least 30 minutes.

To assemble the salad, arrange the quinoa, chickpeas, tomatoes, onion, parsley, and olives on a large serving platter or wide, shallow bowl. Do not mix the ingredients together; simply let them sit next to each other on the platter. Place a serving spoon on the platter so each person can create their own salad.

To make the dressing, whisk all of the ingredients in a bowl. Pour some of the dressing into a small bowl and set next to, or on, the platter with a small ladle or spoon. Extra dressing can be stored in a glass jar in the refrigerator for up to 10 days.

Yield: 6 servings

HEIRLOOM TOMATO–BASIL QUINOA SALAD

This salad is best served within an hour of making it, though it will last in your refrigerator for up to 3 days. If you have a smaller family, I suggest making a half batch. If you can't find heirloom tomatoes, use any variety of organic, locally grown tomato. If you can't find sweet onions use 3 to 4 green onions, sliced into thin rounds.

QUINOA

2 cups quinoa

3½ cups water

¼ teaspoon sea salt

SALAD

2 large heirloom tomatoes, diced (about 3 to 4 cups)

1 cup finely diced sweet onion

1 cup chopped fresh basil leaves

6 tablespoons organic red wine vinegar

6 tablespoons extra-virgin olive oil

1 teaspoon sea salt

freshly ground black pepper

To cook the quinoa, rinse the quinoa in a fine-mesh strainer under running water and drain well. Place the quinoa into a 2-quart pot, add the water and sea salt, cover, and bring to a boil. Reduce the heat to low and simmer for about 20 minutes. Remove the pot from the heat and let cool completely before using.

To assemble the salad, place the cooled quinoa into a large bowl and fluff with a fork. Add the remaining ingredients and gently toss together. Serve.

Yield: about 6 servings

MEDITERRANEAN QUINOA SALAD

This grain dish is best eaten right after it has been made. The pumpkin seeds will begin to lose their "crunch" after a while. You may use any white beans, though we prefer to use cannellini beans in this dish.

QUINOA

2 cups quinoa

3½ cups water

¼ teaspoon sea salt

SALAD

½ cup pumpkin seeds

2 to 3 cups cooked white beans

2 medium carrots, chopped

one 14-ounce jar artichoke hearts, cut into quarters

½ to 1 cup Kalamata olives, pitted

½ cup chopped, olive oil-packed, sun-dried tomatoes

4 cups fresh baby spinach leaves

½ cup fresh basil, chopped

DRESSING

⅓ cup extra-virgin olive oil

3 tablespoons red wine vinegar

1 teaspoon finely grated lemon zest

4 tablespoons freshly squeezed lemon juice

2 garlic cloves, crushed

½ teaspoon sea salt or Herbamare

To cook the quinoa, rinse the dry quinoa in a fine-mesh strainer under warm running water and drain well. Place the rinsed quinoa into a 2-quart pot with the water and sea salt, cover, and bring to a boil. Reduce the heat to a low simmer and cook for about 20 minutes. Remove the pot from the heat and let the quinoa cool in the pot for at least 30 minutes.

To assemble the salad, toast the pumpkin seeds by placing them into a small skillet and heating them over medium heat. Keep them moving in the skillet until you hear a "pop" and they are slightly golden. Transfer to a small bowl to cool.

Transfer the cooled quinoa to a large serving bowl. Add the cooked white beans, carrots, quartered artichoke hearts, olives, sun-dried tomatoes, spinach, basil, and toasted pumpkin seeds.

To make the dressing, whisk all the ingredients in a small bowl. Pour the dressing over the quinoa salad and mix thoroughly with a large spoon. Serve as soon as possible after preparing.

Yield: 6 servings

QUINOA AND BLACK BEAN SALAD

This protein-packed dish will keep you going during those days when you need a boost without the heaviness of a large meal. Serve this dish alone or with some steamed winter squash.

QUINOA

2 cups quinoa

3½ cups water

¼ teaspoon sea salt

DRESSING

¼ cup extra-virgin olive oil

½ cup freshly squeezed lime juice

1 teaspoon ground cumin

1 to 1½ teaspoons sea salt or Herbamare

SALAD

1 cup chopped fresh cilantro

2 cups cooked black beans

5 green onions, sliced

1 small jalapeño pepper, finely diced

1 small red bell pepper, diced

To cook the quinoa, rinse the dry quinoa in a fine-mesh strainer under warm running water and drain well. Place the rinsed quinoa into a 2-quart pot with the water and sea salt, cover, and bring to a boil. Reduce the heat to a low simmer and cook for about 20 minutes. Remove the cooked quinoa from the pot, transfer to a large bowl, and let cool.

To make the dressing, whisk together the olive oil, lime juice, cumin, and sea salt in a small bowl. Pour the dressing over cooled quinoa, and toss well with a fork.

To complete the salad, add the cilantro, black beans, green onions, jalapeño, and bell pepper and toss again.

Yield: 6 servings

SUMMER VEGETABLE QUINOA SALAD

This quinoa salad makes a great addition to any summer picnic. Any fresh summer vegetables that you have on hand work well here. Try adding diced summer squash, fresh shelled peas, or thinly sliced kale leaves. You can use either leftover cooked sweet corn or raw corn kernels cut right off the cob. They both work great, but I prefer the taste and texture of the raw corn.

QUINOA
2 cups quinoa

3½ cups water

¼ teaspoon sea salt

SALAD
2 carrots, diced

1 cup whole cherry tomatoes

2 ears organic sweet corn, kernels cut from the cob

1 cup chopped fresh parsley

½ cup sunflower seeds, toasted

DRESSING
½ cup freshly squeezed lemon juice

6 tablespoons extra-virgin olive oil

2 to 3 garlic cloves, crushed

1½ teaspoons sea salt or Herbamare

To cook the quinoa, rinse the dry quinoa in a fine-mesh strainer under warm running water; drain well. Place the rinsed quinoa into a 2-quart pot with the water and sea salt, cover, and bring to a boil. Reduce the heat to a low simmer and cook for about 20 minutes. Remove the pot from the heat and let the quinoa cool in the pot for at least 30 minutes.

Transfer the cooled quinoa to a large bowl and add the carrots, tomatoes, corn kernels, parsley, and toasted sunflower seeds.

To make the dressing, whisk together all the ingredients in a separate small bowl. Pour the dressing over the quinoa and vegetables and toss to coat. Serve immediately, or chill for later use.

Yield: 6 servings

WINTER QUINOA SALAD

This flavorful grain salad is perfect for the holidays. It can be made up to a day ahead of time; just wait to add the pecans until ready to serve.

QUINOA

2 cups quinoa
3½ cups water
¼ teaspoon sea salt

SALAD

1 tablespoon extra-virgin olive oil
1 medium red onion, finely diced
2 teaspoons dried thyme
¼ teaspoon sea salt or Herbamare
1 cup pecans

½ cup dried cranberries
1 cup chopped fresh parsley
freshly ground black pepper
sea salt or Herbamare

DRESSING

1 teaspoon finely grated orange zest
½ cup freshly squeezed orange juice
⅓ cup extra-virgin olive oil
1 tablespoon white wine vinegar

Preheat the oven to 350°F.

To cook the quinoa, rinse the dry quinoa in a fine-mesh strainer under warm running water; drain well. Place the rinsed quinoa into a 2-quart pot with the water and sea salt, cover, and bring to a boil. Reduce the heat to a low simmer and cook for about 20 minutes. Remove the pot from the heat and let the quinoa cool in the pot for at least 30 minutes.

To prepare the salad ingredients, heat the olive oil in a 10-inch skillet over medium heat. Add the onion, thyme, and sea salt and sauté for 5 to 6 minutes, or until the onion is soft and beginning to turn color but not brown.

Place the pecans in a small pie plate or other ovenproof dish and lightly roast for about 15 minutes. Watch carefully as they can burn easily.

To assemble the salad, transfer the cooked quinoa to a large serving bowl. Add the sautéed onion, roasted pecans, cranberries, and parsley to the bowl and mix together.

To make the dressing, whisk together the orange zest, orange juice, olive oil, and white wine vinegar to the quinoa mixture and gently mix.

Season the salad with sea salt or Herbamare and pepper to taste.

Yield: 6 servings

LEMON MILLET PATTIES

You will need a food processor to make these. You can make the patties up to 3 days ahead of time and store them in between pieces of waxed paper in a storage container in your refrigerator. Serve with the Navy Beans in a Homemade Barbecue Sauce (page 307) and the Cabbage Salad with Cilantro Vinaigrette (page 226).

MILLET

1 cup millet

2 cups water

pinch sea salt

PATTIES

2 small carrots, chopped

1 to 2 green onions, chopped

1 small handful fresh parsley

2 to 3 teaspoons finely grated lemon zest

3 to 4 tablespoons freshly squeezed lemon juice

¼ teaspoon sea salt or Herbamare

3 to 4 tablespoons virgin coconut oil, for sautéing

To cook the millet, rinse the dry millet in a fine-mesh strainer under warm running water. Place the rinsed millet, water, and sea salt into a medium pot with a tight-fitting lid and bring to a boil. Reduce the heat to low and cook for 30 minutes.

To make the patties, place the carrots, chopped green onions, parsley, lemon zest, lemon juice, and sea salt in a food processor and pulse a few times. Add the cooked millet and continue to pulse until just mixed.

Form the millet mixture into patties. Heat the coconut oil in a large skillet over medium heat. Add the patties and lightly sauté on both sides.

Yield: 4 servings

MILLET WITH SUMMER VEGETABLES

Serve this vegetable-rich dish with the Fresh Garden Salad with Herbal Vinaigrette (page 231) for a simple summer meal.

MILLET

1½ cups millet

3 cups water

¼ teaspoon sea salt

VEGETABLES

2 to 3 tablespoons extra-virgin olive oil

1 medium sweet onion, chopped

2 garlic cloves, crushed

1 large red bell pepper, diced

2 medium zucchini, diced

2 to 3 ears fresh corn, kernels cut off cob

½ to 1 cup chopped fresh parsley

¼ cup finely chopped fresh basil

2 tablespoons fresh thyme leaves

½ to 1 teaspoon sea salt or Herbamare

fresh lemon wedges, for garnish

To cook the millet, rinse the millet in a fine-mesh strainer and place into a 3-quart pot with the water and sea salt. Cover the pot and bring to a boil. Reduce the heat to low and simmer for about 30 minutes. Remove lid and set aside to cool.

To prepare the vegetables, heat the olive oil in an 11- or 12-inch skillet over medium heat. Add the onion and sauté until soft, 5 to 7 minutes. Add garlic, bell pepper, zucchini, and corn kernels and sauté until the vegetables are crisp-tender, another 5 to 7 minutes.

Add the cooked millet to the vegetable mixture and sauté for a minute more, breaking up the millet with the back of a spoon to incorporate it into the vegetables. Remove the skillet from the heat, add the fresh herbs and sea salt, and mix well. Taste and adjust the salt and seasonings if necessary. Serve with the fresh lemon wedges.

Yield: 6 servings

EASY POLENTA

Polenta is made from coarsely ground cornmeal. It can be served with fish or chicken dishes or simply with a red sauce on top of it. You can also double this batch, pour it into a 9 x 13-inch pan, and then use it as an alternative gluten-free pizza crust. Simply top the polenta with pizza sauce, your favorite sautéed vegetables, and some organic grated cheese if you wish. Follow the directions for baking below.

3 cups water

1 teaspoon sea salt

1 tablespoon extra-virgin olive oil, coconut oil, or organic butter, plus more for the pie plate

1 cup organic polenta

Preheat the oven to 350°F. Oil a 9-inch pie plate.

In a 3-quart pot, bring the water to a boil. Add the sea salt and oil. Slowly add the polenta, stirring continuously with a whisk. Lower the heat and continue to cook, stirring with a wooden spoon, for 10 to 15 minutes.

Pour the polenta into the prepared pie plate. Bake in the oven for 25 minutes. Let cool for 5 to 10 minutes, and then serve.

Yield: 4 servings

Tip: Always buy organic corn! Over 90% of corn in the United States is genetically engineered. Genetically modified food has never been proven safe for human consumption. Nonorganic corn is also heavily sprayed with herbicides that, when consumed in food, can contribute to a die-off of friendly bacteria, leading to increased inflammation and a higher risk for food allergies and sensitivities.

18

VEGETARIAN MAIN DISHES

Within each of us lies the power of our consent to health and sickness, to riches and poverty, to freedom and to slavery. It is we who control these, and not another.

—*Richard Bach*

Vegetarian dishes, by their very nature, are rich in nutritious plant-based ingredients. When in their whole form, plant foods provide valuable fibers that feed beneficial intestinal bacteria. Science has been demonstrating how integral bacteria are to our overall health—they help to lower systemic inflammation, reduce the risk of food allergies, and supply us with essential nutrients.

The potent antioxidant phytochemicals found in plant foods fight free radical damage and support our bodies in staying healthy and balanced.

Enjoy the following vegetarian main-dish recipes on a regular basis and hopefully some of them will become your weekly staples.

SUNNY SUNFLOWER SEED BURGERS

Serve these tasty meatless burgers with your favorite organic condiments, sliced avocado, lettuce, tomatoes, and Gluten-Free Hamburger Buns (page 164). Serve with Oven Fries (page 256) and a fresh green salad for a balanced meal.

1 cup short-grain brown rice	½ teaspoon dried oregano
2 cups water	½ teaspoon ground cumin
pinch sea salt	½ teaspoon Herbamare
2 cups raw sunflower seeds	1 small carrot, coarsely chopped
1 teaspoon garlic powder	1 small handful fresh parsley
½ teaspoon dried thyme	extra-virgin olive oil, for cooking

Place the rice into a 1-quart pot with a tight-fitting lid, add the water and sea salt, cover, and bring to a boil. Reduce the heat to a low simmer and cook for 45 minutes. Remove from the heat and let stand for at least 20 minutes to cool.

In a food processor, process the sunflower seeds, garlic powder, thyme, oregano, cumin, and Herbamare until finely ground. Add the carrot and parsley and pulse a few times. Add the rice and pulse a few more times to combine all of the ingredients. Be sure not to overprocess the mixture or it will get very gooey.

Form the mixture into patties. The uncooked patties can be stored in a glass container in between pieces of waxed paper in the refrigerator for up to a week.

When ready to cook, heat a skillet over medium heat and add about 1 tablespoon of extra-virgin olive oil. Add the burgers and cook on both sides for 3 to 5 minutes.

Yield: 6 burgers

TOFU WITH GARLIC-GINGER-KUDZU SAUCE

This is a quick and easy tofu recipe that can be served with brown rice and steamed vegetables for a simple meal. Or try it served with the Lemon Millet Patties (page 288) and a large green salad.

---

one 16-ounce package firm or extra-firm tofu
¼ cup wheat-free tamari
2 tablespoons seasoned brown rice vinegar

virgin coconut oil, for sautéing
Garlic-Ginger-Kudzu Sauce (page 357)

Slice the tofu into 1-inch-thick squares, then slice each square in half to form a triangle. Place the tofu triangles into a medium square glass baking dish. Drizzle with the tamari and vinegar, and mix gently by turning the tofu pieces until they are all covered with the marinade. Marinate on the countertop for about 20 minutes.

Heat a few tablespoons of coconut oil in a skillet over medium-high heat. Place the triangles of tofu in the skillet. If your skillet is too small you will have to do this in two batches. Sauté the tofu for a few minutes on each side.

Remove the tofu from skillet and transfer to a serving dish or plate. Pour the sauce over the tofu triangles and serve immediately.

Yield: 3 to 4 servings

> **Tip:** When you open a package of tofu and only use part of it, the unused portion needs to be stored properly to keep it from spoiling. Rinse the tofu under cool water then place it into a container and fill the container with filtered water to cover the tofu. Change the water every day until you use the remaining tofu.

BLACK BEAN, RICE, AND YAM WRAPS

If you are new to eating whole foods, or would just like a really easy meal to prepare then this recipe is for you. It is simple, flavorful, and can be made ahead of time for a quick meal on the go.

RICE

1½ cups short-grain brown rice

½ cup sweet brown rice

4 cups water

¼ teaspoon sea salt

WRAPS

1 large yam, cut into large chunks

6 gluten-free tortillas, organic corn tortillas, or collard greens

3 cups cooked black beans

1 large avocado, mashed

½ cup salsa

2 cups mixed organic salad greens

Preheat the oven to 425°F.

To cook the rice, put the short-grain rice, sweet rice, water, and sea salt into a 2-quart pot, cover, and bring to a boil. Reduce the heat and simmer for about 45 minutes. Remove the pot from the heat and let stand for at least 10 to 15 minutes.

While the rice is cooking, place the yam chunks into a small casserole dish and fill with about ½ inch of water. Place the lid on the casserole dish and bake in the oven for 40 to 45 minutes, or until the yam chunks are very tender. Remove the skins from the yams and slightly mash them with a fork.

To assemble a wrap, lay a tortilla flat onto a plate and place a small amount of rice in the middle of it, add some cooked black beans, some mashed yam, mashed avocado, salsa, and some mixed greens. Fold the ends in and roll up. Continue to make wraps with the remaining ingredients.

Yield: 6 wraps

> **Tip:** Gluten-free flour tortillas are best warmed before you use them to prevent cracking and breaking. An easy way to warm any type of tortilla is to place it on top of steaming hot food, either in the oven, in a pot, or on your plate. We usually use this approach when making burritos or some kind of wrap with gluten-free tortillas.

HUMMUS AND CARAMELIZED ONION WRAPS

These wraps are made using collard greens instead of tortillas. I've also made them with large broccoli leaves! Serve these tasty wraps alongside a bowl of vegetable bean soup for a light, nutritious meal.

CARAMELIZED ONIONS

2 large red onions

2 tablespoons extra-virgin olive oil

¼ teaspoon sea salt

WRAPS

4 collard greens

1 cup hummus (page 344)

1 small carrot, grated

1 small zucchini, grated

1 cup finely sliced romaine lettuce

1 small avocado, sliced

To make the caramelized onions, remove the skins from the onions, cut the onions in half, and then thinly slice into half-moons. Heat the olive oil in an 11- or 12-inch stainless steel or cast-iron skillet over medium heat. Add the onions and pinch of the sea salt and sauté onions for 15 to 20 minutes, or until very soft and caramelized. Remove from the heat and allow to cool. The onions can be stored in an airtight container in the refrigerator for up to a week.

To assemble a wrap, place a collard green onto a flat surface or a plate. Spread ¼ cup of the hummus evenly over one side of the collard green. Place a few spoonfuls of caramelized onions over the hummus. Then add some grated carrot, grated zucchini, romaine lettuce, and avocado over the onions.

Tightly roll and then cut in half. Serve immediately, or place, seam side down, in a small glass or stainless steel to-go container and store in the refrigerator for up to 2 days. Continue to make wraps with the remaining ingredients.

Yield: 4 wraps

> **Tip:** If your collard greens are large or not very tender, you can blanch them first in a pot of boiling water for 60 seconds before using them as a wrap.

MEXICAN PINK BEAN BURRITOS

Pink beans have a smooth creamy texture similar to pinto beans. You can buy pink beans in bulk at your local co-op or health food store. We often make this recipe and serve it without any tortillas, opting instead to pile mounds of brown rice, pink beans, and a ton of fixings on our plates! Serve with the Live Hot Pepper Relish (page 103) for added spice and a dose of enzymes to help digest the meal.

BEANS
2 cups dry pink beans (soaked for 8 to 24 hours)

1 tablespoon extra-virgin olive oil

1 large onion, chopped

6 garlic cloves, crushed

2 to 3 teaspoons ground cumin

1 tablespoon Mexican seasoning

8 cups water

sea salt

RICE
2 cups short-grain brown rice

4 cups water

¼ teaspoon sea salt

OTHER INGREDIENTS
gluten-free tortillas

sliced avocado or guacamole

salsa

mixed baby greens or thinly sliced lettuce

To cook the beans, place the beans in a medium bowl and cover with water; soak at room temperature for 8 to 24 hours. When ready to cook, drain the beans in a colander and rinse thoroughly.

Heat the olive oil in a 6- to 8-quart pot over medium heat. Add the onion and sauté for about 5 minutes, or until tender. Add the garlic, cumin, and Mexican seasoning and sauté for another minute or two. Add the soaked beans and water; make sure water is at least 2 inches above the beans. Bring to a boil, then reduce the heat to a simmer. Cook, uncovered, for about 1 hour. When the beans are cooked, season to taste with sea salt. Continue to simmer, uncovered, over low heat until the onions fall apart and most of the liquid evaporates, 20 to 30 more minutes.

Start cooking the rice just after you put the beans on the stovetop. Put the rice into a 2-quart stainless steel pot, add the water and sea salt, cover, and bring to a boil. Reduce the heat to low and simmer for about 45 minutes.

To assemble the burritos, place a tortilla on a flat surface. Spread ¼ to ½ cup rice down the center of the tortilla, add about ¼ to ½ cup beans, and your favorite fixings. Fold in each end of the tortilla then roll the burrito away from you, creating a firm wrap.

Yield: 6 servings

RAW THAI WRAPS WITH CILANTRO–PUMPKIN SEED PÂTE

When making these wraps, I usually just use up whatever vegetables I have in my refrigerator. Try thin slices of bell peppers, sunflower sprouts, radish slices, sliced avocado, fresh basil, sliced red cabbage, or even fresh mango! If your collard greens are not young and tender, you might want to blanch them to make them easier to roll (see Tip on page 296). If you don't have raw cashew butter on hand for the dipping sauce, try sunflower seed butter or almond butter instead!

PÂTE

2 cups raw pumpkin seeds (soaked for about 8 hours)

½ cup packed fresh cilantro

1 garlic clove

3 to 4 tablespoons freshly squeezed lime juice

3 to 4 tablespoons water

¾ teaspoon sea salt

WRAPS

8 to 10 small collard greens

2 carrots, cut into strips

1 large cucumber, cut into strips

mung bean sprouts

fresh chives or green onions

fresh mint leaves

DIPPING SAUCE

½ cup water

6 tablespoons raw cashew butter

1 serrano or Thai chile, stem removed (I leave the seeds in)

1 small garlic clove

one 1-inch piece fresh ginger

1 to 2 tablespoons freshly squeezed lime juice

1 tablespoon coconut aminos or wheat-free tamari

To make the pâte, start by adding the pumpkin seeds to a medium bowl and cover with an inch of filtered water. Let them soak for about 8 hours on the countertop. Drain through a colander and rinse with cold running water; drain well. Transfer the seeds to a food processor fitted with the "s" blade. Pulse a few times, then add the remaining ingredients and process until you have a fairly smooth pâte.

To make the wraps, cut the thick bottom part of the stems off the collards. Spread a few tablespoons of pâte down the center of each leaf. Add some carrot strips, cucumber strips, bean sprouts, chives, mint leaves, and whatever other veggies you desire. Fold over the edges and set on a plate, seam side down.

To make the sauce, add all ingredients to a high-powered blender and blend until smooth and creamy. Pour into small bowls for dipping, and serve.

Yield: 8 to 10 wraps

SMASHED YAM AND BLACK BEAN QUESADILLAS

Serve these child-friendly quesadillas with a mild salsa for dipping and a small green salad on the side. Other fun things to serve with these are freshly made guacamole or plain organic yogurt for dipping. Use a pizza cutter to slice into wedges to making dipping easy for little hands. Use the Quinoa Tortillas (page 169) or your favorite gluten-free tortilla.

1 large yam, peeled and cut into chunks

1 tablespoon extra-virgin olive oil

1 small onion, diced

2 teaspoons ground cumin

½ teaspoon chili powder

2 to 3 cups cooked black beans, well drained

¼ teaspoon sea salt

6 to 8 gluten-free tortillas or organic corn tortillas

1 to 2 cups spinach or arugula leaves

½ cup grated organic raw cheese (optional)

Place the yam chunks into a steamer basket in a pot filled with about 2 inches of water, cover, and steam over medium-high heat until fork-tender, 15 to 20 minutes.

To make the beans, heat the olive oil in a large skillet over medium heat. Add the onion and sauté for 5 to 7 minutes, or until very tender.

Add the cumin, chili powder, black beans, and sea salt. Using a fork or a potato masher, smash the black beans as you heat them with the onion. Continue turning and smashing until the desired consistency has been reached. Transfer to a bowl and set aside.

In a clean 10-inch skillet, add a tortilla and spread a layer of black beans, spinach leaves, and cheese if desired. Add a few chunks of yams and smash them with the back of a fork. Top with another tortilla. Heat over medium heat for about 2 minutes then flip the quesadilla and heat the other side for another 2 minutes. Continue to make quesadillas with the remaining ingredients. The trick to making these is to make sure you don't add too much filling!

Transfer the quesadillas to a plate and cut into slices with a pizza cutter.

Yield: 3 to 4 quesadillas

TEMPEH FAJITAS

This tempeh dish is a favorite of ours and will definitely keep you coming back for more. If you are serving this to more than two adults you may want to double the recipe.

TEMPEH

one 8-ounce package tempeh, cut into thin strips

freshly squeezed juice of 1 small lime

2 tablespoons wheat-free tamari

1 to 2 garlic cloves, crushed

1 teaspoon extra-virgin olive oil, plus 1½ tablespoons for sautéing

2 teaspoons ground cumin

¼ to ½ teaspoon chipotle chile powder

VEGETABLES

1 tablespoon extra-virgin olive oil

1 small red onion, cut into half-moons

2 small zucchini, cut into strips

1 red bell pepper, cut into strips

OTHER INGREDIENTS

4 gluten-free tortillas, organic corn tortillas, or collard greens

1 ripe avocado, cut into strips

2 to 3 cups baby arugula or lettuce leaves

½ cup organic salsa

½ cup shredded raw organic Jack cheese (optional)

To prepare the tempeh, place the tempeh slices in a small dish, add the lime juice, tamari, garlic, 1 teaspoon of olive oil, and spices and toss together to coat the tempeh. Let the tempeh marinate for at least 30 minutes. Longer marinating times will produce deeper flavors.

To cook the vegetables, heat 1 tablespoon of olive oil in an 11- or 12-inch cast-iron skillet over medium-high heat. Add the onion and sauté for 5 to 7 minutes. Add the zucchini and bell pepper and sauté about 5 minutes more, or until tender. Remove the skillet from the heat.

To cook the tempeh, heat the remaining 1½ tablespoons olive oil in a separate skillet over medium heat. Add the tempeh strips and sauté on each side for 3 to 4 minutes, being careful not to burn the tempeh.

Fill each tortilla with a few strips of tempeh, some vegetables, a few pieces of avocado, arugula, about 2 tablespoons of salsa, and cheese if using; roll up and enjoy.

Yield: 4 servings

COCONUT VEGETABLE CURRY
WITH CHICKPEAS

This quick curry can be made in a snap! Serve over brown jasmine rice for an easy weekday meal.

2 tablespoons virgin coconut oil

1 tablespoon finely chopped fresh ginger

1½ teaspoons whole cumin seeds

1 teaspoon black mustard seeds

3 small red potatoes, cut into cubes

3 medium carrots, diced

½ teaspoon ground turmeric

2 teaspoons ground coriander

1 teaspoon curry powder

1 tablespoon tomato paste

one 14-ounce can coconut milk

¼ to ½ cup water

1 small zucchini, diced

1 cup frozen peas

2 cups cooked chickpeas

1 to 2 teaspoons sea salt

½ cup chopped fresh cilantro

Heat a 4- to 6-quart pot over medium heat and add the coconut oil. Add the ginger, cumin seeds, and mustard seeds and cook for 1 to 2 minutes, or until the seeds begin to "pop."

Add the potatoes, carrots, turmeric, coriander, and curry powder and stir well. Continue to cook for another minute or so. Add the tomato paste, coconut milk, and water and stir well to combine. Simmer, covered, for 5 to 10 minutes, or until the potatoes and carrots are almost done but still a little crisp.

Add the zucchini, peas, chickpeas, and sea salt, cover, and simmer until the vegetables are tender, another 6 to 7 minutes. Remove from the pot from the heat and stir in the cilantro.

Yield: 4 servings

CUBAN BLACK BEAN AND YAM STEW
WITH AVOCADO SALSA

This hearty stew makes a great weeknight meal! Serve with the Avocado Salsa below and the Cabbage Salad with Cilantro Vinaigrette (page 226).

SOUP

2 cups dry black beans (soaked for 8 to 24 hours)

6 to 8 cups water

2 bay leaves

1 tablespoon extra-virgin olive oil or virgin coconut oil

1 large onion, chopped

6 to 8 garlic cloves, crushed

1 jalapeño pepper, finely diced

2 teaspoons ground cumin

2 teaspoons dried oregano

1 teaspoon chili powder

pinch cayenne pepper

1 large yam, peeled and diced

2 to 4 tablespoons freshly squeezed lime juice

2 to 3 teaspoons sea salt

AVOCADO SALSA

2 large avocados, diced

½ small red onion, finely diced

2 to 3 tablespoons freshly squeezed lime juice

¼ cup chopped fresh cilantro

To cook the beans, drain off the soaking water from the beans and rinse well. Place the beans, water, and bay leaves into a 6- or 8-quart pot and bring to a boil. Cover, reduce the heat to low, and simmer for about 1½ hours, or until the beans are cooked.

When the beans are close to being done, begin to prepare the other ingredients for the stew. Heat the oil in a large skillet over medium heat. Add the onion and sauté until soft, about 5 minutes. Add the garlic, jalapeño pepper, cumin, oregano, chili powder, cayenne, and diced yam and sauté a minute or so more. Transfer the mixture to the pot of cooked black beans and simmer for 15 to 20 minutes, or until the yams and beans are tender. Remove and discard the bay leaves. Add the lime juice and sea salt, and mix well. Taste and adjust the salt and seasonings if necessary.

To make the salsa, place all the ingredients into a small bowl and mix gently. To serve, ladle the stew into serving bowls and top with a few spoonfuls of the salsa.

Yield: 6 servings

CURRIED CHICKPEA AND SQUASH STEW

Serve this flavorful stew over cooked brown jasmine rice, with a dollop of Coconut Milk Yogurt (page 104) on top. You can vary the recipe by replacing the squash with potatoes or yams if desired.

2 tablespoons virgin coconut oil	pinch cayenne pepper
1 medium onion, chopped	2 delicata squash, cut into chunks
4 to 5 garlic cloves, crushed	2 cups diced tomatoes
2 teaspoons curry powder	3 to 4 cups chopped kale or spinach
1 teaspoon ground cumin	3 cups cooked chickpeas
1 teaspoon ground coriander	1 cup reserved bean cooking liquid or water
½ teaspoon ground turmeric	1 to 2 teaspoons sea salt or Herbamare
½ teaspoon ground cinnamon	

Heat the coconut oil in an 11-inch skillet or 6-quart pot over medium heat. Add the onion and sauté for about 5 minutes, or until soft. Add the garlic and spices and sauté for 1 minute more.

Add the squash and tomatoes, cover, and simmer over low to medium-low heat until the squash is tender, about 15 minutes.

Add the kale, cooked chickpeas, bean cooking liquid or water, and sea salt and gently stir to combine. Simmer for 5 minutes more, or until the kale is tender. Taste and add more salt and seasonings if desired.

Yield: 4 to 6 servings

FALL VEGETABLE STEW WITH MOROCCAN SPICES

This is a wonderful warming dish that celebrates the flavors of autumn. Serve this stew over cooked quinoa with a fresh green salad or lightly steamed broccoli on the side.

---

2 tablespoons extra-virgin olive oil

1 large onion, chopped

6 garlic cloves, minced

2 teaspoons ground cardamom

2 teaspoons curry powder

1 to 2 teaspoons sea salt

½ teaspoon freshly ground black pepper

pinch cayenne pepper

3 large carrots, diced

3 medium red potatoes, diced

1 small delicata squash, cut into chunks

½ cup dried currants or raisins

2 cups tomato sauce

2 cups cooked chickpeas

1 cup water

¾ cup almonds

½ cup dried figs, chopped

chopped fresh mint, for garnish

Heat the olive oil in a 6-quart pot over medium heat. Add the onion and sauté until tender, about 5 minutes.

Add the garlic, cardamom, curry powder, sea salt, black pepper, and cayenne and sauté a few minutes more.

Add the carrots and potatoes and stir well to coat with the oil and spices. Sauté the potatoes and carrots for about 5 minutes, then add the squash and stir to combine. Add the currants, tomato sauce, chickpeas, and water. Place a lid on the pot and continue to cook until the vegetables are tender, stirring occasionally, 25 to 30 minutes, adding more water if necessary.

Preheat the oven to 350°F. Spread the almonds out in a glass baking dish. Roast in the oven for about 10 minutes. Transfer to a plate to cool. When completely cooled, chop the almonds.

Just before serving, sprinkle the figs and almonds on top of the stew, and garnish with the chopped mint leaves.

Yield: 4 to 6 servings

LENTIL AND SPINACH DAL

Here is a simple, easy recipe that is delicious served over cooked brown basmati rice with a dollop of Raita (page 353) on top.

1 tablespoon virgin coconut oil	pinch cayenne pepper
1 medium onion, diced	2 cups green or brown lentils, rinsed
2 teaspoons grated fresh ginger	5 to 6 cups water
1 teaspoon ground cumin	3 to 4 cups chopped fresh spinach
1 teaspoon garam masala	1 teaspoon sea salt
½ teaspoon ground turmeric	

Heat the coconut oil in a 4- or 6-quart pot over medium heat. Add the onion and sauté until soft, about 5 minutes. Stir in the ginger, cumin, garam masala, turmeric, and cayenne and sauté for 30 to 60 seconds more.

Add the lentils to the pot with the onions and spices, and stir in the water. Cover and simmer for about 40 minutes, or until the lentils are cooked through.

Add the spinach and sea salt. Taste and add more cayenne if you prefer a spicier dal. Simmer for a few minutes more and serve.

Yield: 4 to 6 servings

LUSCIOUS LENTIL AND BROWN RICE CASSEROLE

I like making casseroles once the weather cools down in autumn. Serve with the Beet, Kale, and Walnut Salad (page 224) and a spoonful of Cultured Vegetables (page 90) for a nourishing, balanced meal.

1 tablespoon extra-virgin olive oil

1 medium red onion, chopped

1 to 2 garlic cloves, crushed

2 large carrots, diced

½ teaspoon dried thyme

1 teaspoon garam masala

1 teaspoon sea salt

2 cups frozen chopped spinach

2 tablespoons red wine vinegar

¾ cup green lentils

½ cup brown basmati rice

4½ cups water

Preheat the oven to 350°F.

Heat the olive oil in an ovenproof pot or 3-quart Dutch oven over medium heat. Add the onion and garlic and sauté, stirring frequently, for about 3 minutes, Add the carrots, thyme, garam masala, and sea salt and stir to coat with the oil. Sauté for a few minutes more, then add the chopped spinach and stir to combine.

Cook until the spinach has thawed and the mixture is sizzling again, then add the vinegar and stir to loosen up any browned bits from the bottom of the pot. Quickly add the lentils, rice, and water and mix well.

Cover, transfer to the oven, and bake for about 90 minutes. Serve.

Yield: 4 servings

NAVY BEANS IN A HOMEMADE BARBECUE SAUCE

Serve these scrumptious beans for a summer meal with the Lemon Millet Patties (page 288) and a large garden salad for a balanced meal. If you do not want to cook your own beans for this, or are pinched for time, you can use 3 cans of navy beans in place of the dry navy beans, water, and garlic cloves. This is adapted from a recipe of Bastyr University instructor, Mary Shaw.

BEANS

1½ cups dry navy beans (soaked for 8 to 24 hours)

6 cups water

4 garlic cloves, peeled

BARBECUE SAUCE

1 tablespoon extra-virgin olive oil

1 small onion, finely chopped

4 garlic cloves, crushed

¼ cup tomato paste

¼ cup apple cider vinegar

¼ cup pure maple syrup

1 tablespoon blackstrap molasses

1 teaspoon sea salt or Herbamare

¼ to ½ teaspoon chipotle chile powder, plus more if desired

½ cup bean cooking liquid or water

To prepare the beans, soak the beans in a large bowl on your kitchen counter for 8 to 24 hours. Drain off soaking water and rinse well. Transfer the beans to a 3-quart pot, add the water and garlic cloves, and bring to a boil. Reduce the heat to a simmer and cook the beans for about 1 hour, or until soft and cooked through. Drain the beans, reserving the cooking liquid, and set aside.

To make the sauce, heat the olive oil in a 6-quart pot over medium heat. Add the onion and crushed garlic and sauté for 5 to 7 minutes.

In a small bowl, mix together the tomato paste, vinegar, maple syrup, molasses, sea salt, chipotle chile powder, and bean cooking liquid or water.

Add the drained beans and tomato mixture to the onion-garlic mixture and mix thoroughly to combine. Simmer, covered, for 20 to 25 minutes, stirring occasionally and adding more water or bean cooking liquid if necessary. Taste and add more sea salt and chipotle chile powder if desired.

Yield: 4 to 6 servings

SPICY BLACK-EYED PEA STEW

Black-Eyed Pea stew, oftentimes called Hoppin John, is a typical southern dish. Serve this stew over brown rice or Easy Polenta (page 290) with a side of Apple-Spiced Collard Greens (page 246) for a balanced, colorful meal!

---

2 cups dry black-eyed peas, rinsed

2 bay leaves

6 cups water

1 tablespoon extra-virgin olive oil

1 medium onion, chopped

8 garlic cloves, minced

2 to 3 tablespoons chopped fresh thyme or 1 tablespoon dried

½ teaspoon crushed red chili flakes

¼ teaspoon freshly ground black pepper

2 large carrots, chopped

2 to 3 celery stalks, chopped

1 medium red bell pepper, diced

½ cup fresh or frozen organic corn kernels

2 teaspoons sea salt or Herbamare

2 to 3 tablespoons brown rice vinegar or apple cider vinegar

Place the black-eyed peas into a 3-quart stainless steel pot with the bay leaves and water, and bring to a boil. Reduce the heat to a simmer and cook for about 45 minutes, or until the peas are cooked. Drain off the peas over a bowl, reserving the cooking liquid to add to the stew if needed. Remove and discard the bay leaves.

Heat the olive oil in an 11- or 12-inch deep skillet, or a 6-quart pot, over medium heat. Add the onion and garlic and sauté for about 5 minutes. Add the thyme, red chili flakes, black pepper, carrots, celery, bell pepper, and corn kernels and sauté for 5 to 7 minutes more, or until the vegetables begin to get tender.

Add the cooked beans and sea salt and simmer, covered, until the vegetables are tender, about 10 minutes more, adding a little of the reserved bean cooking liquid if necessary. Stir in the vinegar. Taste and adjust the salt and seasonings if necessary.

Yield: 4 to 6 servings

WHITE BEAN AND VEGETABLE STEW

Serve this scrumptious stew with the Italian Greens Salad with Red Wine Vinaigrette (page 234) and the Herbed Focaccia Bread (page 163) for a balanced meal. If you don't have cannellini beans on hand, try cooking with another white bean such as navy or Great Northern.

BEANS

3 cups dry cannellini beans (soaked for 8 to 24 hours)

1 strip kombu

8 cups water

STEW

2 tablespoons extra-virgin olive oil

1 large onion, chopped

4 to 5 garlic cloves, crushed

1 tablespoon dried thyme

2 teaspoons dried rosemary, crushed

2 teaspoons dried tarragon

3 celery stalks, chopped

3 large carrots, peeled and diced

4 cups bean cooking liquid, chicken stock, or water

2 medium zucchini, diced

1 to 2 teaspoons sea salt or Herbamare

½ cup finely chopped fresh parsley

OPTIONAL GARNISHES

chopped fresh parsley

sliced Kalamata olives

crumbled organic feta cheese

To cook the beans, drain and rinse the soaked beans, place them into a 6-quart pot with the kombu and water, and bring to a boil. Reduce the heat and simmer for about 1 to 1½ hours. Drain the beans through a colander over a bowl, reserving the bean cooking liquid. Set aside.

To make the stew, heat the olive oil in a 6-quart pot over medium heat. Add the onion and sauté for about 5 minutes. Add the garlic, thyme, rosemary, and tarragon and sauté for 1 minute more. Add the celery and carrots and sauté for about 3 minutes more.

Add the cooked beans and bean cooking liquid, stock, or water. Add extra liquid for a thinner stew. Simmer, covered, for about 15 minutes, or until carrots and celery are slightly tender but not completely soft. Add the zucchini and continue to simmer until the zucchini is tender, 5 to 10 minutes more.

Season with sea salt or Herbamare to taste and stir in the parsley. Ladle into bowls and top each bowl with chopped parsley, olive slices, and crumbled cheese if desired.

Yield: 6 servings

SENSUOUS VEGAN VEGETABLE AND BEAN ENCHILADAS

This recipe does take some time to prepare, but you are rewarded with a large batch of enchiladas that are bursting with flavor. The enchiladas can easily be frozen before they are baked for another night's quick meal. Serve with the Arugula Salad with Lime Vinaigrette (page 218).

SAUCE

2 large dried ancho chiles, seeded

2 small dried chipotle chiles, seeded

1½ cups boiling water

¼ cup extra-virgin olive oil

6 garlic cloves, crushed

1 small onion, finely diced

2 teaspoons sea salt

2 tablespoons ground cumin

2 tablespoons raw cacao powder

1 tablespoon coconut sugar

2 cups organic tomato sauce

½ cup tapioca flour or arrowroot powder

2 cups cold water

ENCHILADAS

1 tablespoon extra-virgin olive oil, plus more for greasing the dishes

1 large onion, diced

4 garlic cloves, crushed

2 teaspoons sea salt

1 tablespoon ground cumin

2 teaspoons dried oregano

½ teaspoon ground cinnamon

2 large yams, peeled and diced

2 medium zucchini, diced

1 medium red bell pepper, diced

2 tablespoons freshly squeezed lime juice

6 cups cooked black beans

1 cup reserved bean cooking liquid or water

16 to 20 organic corn tortillas or collard greens

To make the sauce, place the seeded ancho and chipotle chiles in a small bowl and pour the boiling water over them; let stand for 15 minutes.

In a 2- or 3-quart saucepan over medium heat, heat the olive oil. Add the garlic, onion, and sea salt and sauté until tender. Add the ground cumin, cacao powder, and sugar and sauté for a few minutes more. Add the tomato sauce and soaked chile peppers with their soaking water and simmer for about 10 minutes.

Mix the tapioca flour and cold water in a small bowl and stir to dissolve. Pour the sauce mixture and the dissolved tapioca flour into a blender and blend on high until smooth.

To make the enchiladas, heat the olive oil in an 11- or 12-inch skillet over medium heat. Add the onion and garlic and sauté for 3 to 5 minutes. Add the sea salt, cumin, oregano, and cinnamon and sauté for 1 minute.

Add the diced yams and sauté for about 5 minutes. Then add the diced zucchini and diced bell pepper and sauté for about 5 minutes more, or until the zucchini begins to get tender. Turn off heat and add the fresh lime juice, cooked black beans, and the 1 cup reserved cooking liquid or water. Taste and adjust the salt and seasonings if necessary.

Preheat the oven to 400°F.

This recipe makes about 16 large enchiladas; enough to fill two 9 x 13-inch baking dishes. You may either bake them all at once in two baking dishes or bake just one dish and freeze the other half of the enchiladas in two 8 x 8-inch food storage containers before baking (see Tip).

To assemble the enchiladas, coat one or two 9 x 13-inch baking dishes with olive oil. Warm each corn tortilla in a skillet with oil or dip each in the warm sauce. Take a warmed corn tortilla and fill it with the bean and vegetable mixture, roll, and place in the prepared baking dish with the seam side down. Repeat this until all of the filling has been used. Cover the enchiladas evenly with the sauce. (At this point, if you are not planning to bake all the enchiladas at once, cover and freeze some of them in food storage containers.)

Place a lid or baking sheet over the 9 x 13-inch baking dish and bake the enchiladas for 45 to 50 minutes.

Yield: 10 to 12 servings

> **Tip:** To bake frozen enchiladas, place the container under hot running water to release. Then transfer the frozen enchiladas to an appropriate-size, oiled baking dish and bake as directed above. It will take at least an additional 20 minutes to bake frozen enchiladas.

SAVORY ADZUKI BEAN AND MUSHROOM SHEPHERD'S PIE

Serve this nourishing, hearty meal on a chilly winter evening along with a few spoonfuls of Garlic Kale Kraut (page 91) and steamed broccoli.

FILLING

2 cups dry adzuki beans, rinsed

6 cups water

1 strip kombu

1 tablespoon extra-virgin olive oil, plus more for greasing the dish

1 medium onion, diced

1 to 2 teaspoons dried thyme

1 teaspoon dried oregano

3 to 4 carrots, chopped

3 to 4 celery stalks, chopped

2 to 3 cups chopped cremini mushrooms

1 to 2 cups Homemade Vegetable Stock (page 186) or Homemade Beef Stock (page 184)

½ cup chopped fresh parsley

sea salt

freshly ground black pepper

TOPPING

3 large baking potatoes or yams, peeled and cut into large chunks

¼ cup extra-virgin olive oil or organic butter

sea salt or Herbamare

To cook the adzuki beans, rinse the beans and place them into a 3-quart pot, add the water and kombu, and bring to a boil. Reduce the heat to a simmer and cook for 1 hour, or until the beans are tender. Remove the kombu.

Preheat the oven to 375°F. Oil a 3-quart casserole dish.

To make the filling, when the beans are almost done, heat the olive oil in an 11-inch skillet over medium heat. Add the onion and sauté until soft, about 5 minutes. Then add the dried herbs, carrots, celery, and mushrooms and sauté for another 5 to 7 minutes, or until the vegetables are barely tender but not soft.

Add the stock and chopped parsley, and season to taste with sea salt and black pepper. Add the cooked beans and mix well to combine. Simmer for a few minutes, and then transfer the mixture to the oiled casserole dish.

To make the topping, put the potatoes or yams (or a combination of both) into a 3-quart pot, cover with water, and boil for 7 to 10 minutes, or until soft and cooked through. Drain off most of the water, reserving some.

Transfer the potatoes to a glass mixing bowl, add the olive oil or butter and sea salt, and beat with an electric mixer until light and fluffy, adding some of the reserved cooking water if necessary. Spoon the potato topping onto the bean and vegetable mixture in the casserole dish and spread it out with the back of the spoon. Bake for 30 to 35 minutes. Serve piping hot.

Yield: 6 servings

19

FISH, POULTRY, AND MEAT

There is no higher religion than human service. To work for the common good is the greatest creed.
—Woodrow Wilson

Animal foods can play a very healthful role in the diet. In fact, animal foods contain essential nutrients for proper cognitive development in children and in utero—omega-3 fatty acids, zinc, B vitamins, Vitamin A, and essential amino acids. Replacing refined, processed foods with wholesome meals based on animal foods nourishes a depleted body, as animal foods are dense sources of so many nutrients.

Remember to always purchase organic pastured chicken, organic grass-fed meats, and wild Alaskan fish to be sure you are getting the safest and most nutritious forms of these foods. For more information on this please refer to pages 68–69.

Use the recipes in this chapter to create healthy meals for you and your family. It's important to remember that animal foods are digested and utilized by the body best when served with vegetables—try a raw, lacto-fermented recipe in "Get Cultured!" (chapter 11) or any of the recipes in the Fresh Salads and Vegetables chapter (chapter 16).

BASIL-BALSAMIC WILD SALMON WITH PLUM TOMATO TOPPING

Serve this flavorful salmon dish with the Balsamic Roasted Beets (page 257) and a large garden vegetable salad. Always remember to purchase wild salmon from the Pacific coast—preferably from Alaska. Avoid consuming farmed salmon as it is a dangerous risk to your health. Research shows that most farmed salmon contains chemicals that damage mitochondrial function in the body, which changes how you process blood sugar, leading to an increased risk for diabetes.

2 pounds wild Alaskan salmon fillets

MARINADE

1 cup tightly packed fresh basil leaves
freshly squeezed juice of 1 lemon
¼ cup balsamic vinegar
¼ cup extra-virgin olive oil
3 garlic cloves, peeled
1 teaspoon sea salt
1 to 2 teaspoons finely grated lemon zest

TOPPING

1 cup chopped fresh plum tomatoes
½ cup Kalamata olives, pitted and chopped
½ cup crumbled organic feta cheese (optional)
1 tablespoon extra-virgin olive oil
2 to 3 tablespoons finely chopped fresh basil

Rinse the salmon fillets under cool running water and place them, skin side up, in a shallow baking dish.

To make the marinade, place all the ingredients for the marinade into a blender and blend on high until completely puréed and smooth. Pour the marinade over the salmon fillets, cover, and let marinate in the refrigerator for 1 to 4 hours.

Preheat the oven to 400°F. Drain off the marinade from the fish and flip the fillets so that the skin side is down. Bake the salmon for 10 minutes per inch of thickness. Drizzle some of the remaining marinade over the salmon halfway through the baking. Discard the remaining marinade.

While the salmon is baking, prepare the topping. Place all the ingredients for the topping into a small bowl and gently mix to combine. To serve, let each person spoon some of the topping over his or her piece of salmon.

Yield: 4 to 6 servings

SPICED CITRUS SALMON

This salmon recipe contains a bouquet of citrus flavors and pairs well with the Steamed Vegetables with Lemon-Garlic Dressing (page 255) and cooked quinoa. Try topping the baked salmon with the Fresh Mango Salsa (page 354).

---

2 pounds wild Alaskan salmon fillets

MARINADE

½ cup freshly squeezed orange juice

¼ cup freshly squeezed lime juice

¼ cup freshly squeezed lemon juice

¼ cup extra-virgin olive oil

2 tablespoons minced shallots

2 garlic cloves, crushed

1 to 2 teaspoons sea salt

½ to 1 teaspoon crushed red chili flakes

Rinse the salmon under cool running water and place the fillets, skin side up, in a shallow baking dish.

To make the marinade, in a separate dish, whisk together all the ingredients. Pour the marinade over the salmon fillets, cover, and let marinate in the refrigerator for 2 to 4 hours.

Preheat the oven to 400°F. Drain off the marinade from the fish and flip the fillets so that the skin side is down. Bake, uncovered, for 10 minutes per inch of thickness. To avoid overcooking, it is best to take the salmon out just before it is cooked through as it will continue to cook after you take it out of the oven.

Yield: 4 to 6 servings

WILD SALMON WITH GINGER-LIME MARINADE

Wild salmon is a good source of vitamin D, protein, omega-3 fatty acids, selenium, and vitamins B12 and B3. Serve this dish with Roasted Yams with Rosemary (page 258), and the Autumn Harvest Salad with Balsamic Vinaigrette (page 221).

2 pounds wild Alaskan salmon fillets

MARINADE
½ cup tamari or coconut aminos
freshly squeezed juice of 1 lime

2 tablespoons pure maple syrup
1 teaspoon grated fresh ginger
2 to 4 garlic cloves, crushed
few dashes hot pepper sesame oil

Rinse the salmon under cool running water and place the fillets, skin side up, in a glass baking dish.

To make the marinade, mix all the ingredients in a small bowl and pour over the salmon. Cover the baking dish and marinate in the refrigerator for 30 minutes to 2 hours.

Preheat the oven to 400°F. Drain off the marinade from the fish and flip the fillets so that the skin side is down. Cook 10 minutes per inch of thickness, 15 to 25 minutes, or until done.

Yield: 4 to 6 servings

WILD SALMON WITH LEMON, GARLIC, AND THYME

Baking is a great and easy way to prepare salmon. Serve salmon with Baked Winter Squash (page 260) and the Pear and Hazelnut Salad with Creamy Cranberry Dressing (page 235).

---

2 pounds wild Alaskan salmon fillets

¼ teaspoon sea salt or Herbamare

2 teaspoons dried thyme

½ teaspoon freshly ground black pepper

3 to 5 garlic cloves, crushed

2 tablespoons extra-virgin olive oil

1 lemon, cut into slices

Preheat the oven to 400 F.

Rinse the salmon under cool running water and pat dry. Place the fillets, skin side down, in a glass baking dish. Sprinkle with sea salt, dried thyme, and pepper. Rub in the crushed garlic then drizzle with the olive oil. Place the lemon slices on top of the salmon.

Bake for 10 minutes per inch of thickness. To avoid overcooking, it is best to take the salmon out just before it is cooked through because it will continue to cook after you take it out of the oven.

Yield: 4 to 6 servings

POACHED HALIBUT WITH TOMATOES AND FRESH HERBS

Serve this simple fish dish over brown rice noodles or Pine Nut–Studded Rice (page 275) and a fresh green salad. If halibut is unavailable, you can use wild salmon instead—it's equally delicious!

2 pounds fresh halibut fillets, skin removed
¼ cup freshly squeezed lemon juice
½ teaspoon sea salt
1 tablespoon extra-virgin olive oil
1 small red onion, chopped
1 teaspoon Italian seasoning
2 garlic cloves, crushed

2 small zucchini, chopped
½ cup Kalamata olives, pitted
2 cups chopped plum tomatoes
½ cup chopped fresh basil
2 teaspoons chopped fresh oregano
1 tablespoon sherry vinegar

Cut the skin from halibut with a very sharp knife, then place halibut fillets in a shallow dish and cover with the lemon juice and sea salt. Let the fillets marinate for about 10 minutes while preparing the other ingredients.

Heat the olive oil in an 11-inch, deep skillet over medium heat. Add the onion and sauté for 5 to 7 minutes, or until it begins to turn golden. Add the Italian seasoning, garlic, zucchini, and olives and sauté for 1 minute more.

Move vegetables to the side of the skillet and add the halibut fillets. Cook for 3 minutes then flip. Add the tomatoes, basil, and oregano, and a little water if needed. Move the vegetables so they surround the halibut fillets. Cover and simmer on low until the halibut is done and flakes easily, about 10 minutes. Add the vinegar and serve.

Tip: When you purchase your fish at the market, have the fishmonger cut the skin off the fish.

Yield: 4 to 6 servings

FISH TACOS WITH FRESH TOMATO-PEACH SALSA

These soft tacos are easy to make and delicious served with the peach salsa. If peaches are out of season, or you do not want to take the extra time to prepare the salsa, then use an organic store-bought tomato salsa instead.

1 pound fresh wild Alaskan salmon or halibut
    fillets, skin removed

virgin coconut oil, for sautéing

MARINADE

3 tablespoons freshly squeezed lime juice

2 garlic cloves, crushed

2 teaspoons ground cumin

¼ teaspoon chipotle chile powder

½ teaspoon sea salt

OTHER INGREDIENTS

organic sprouted corn tortillas or gluten-free
    tortillas

thinly sliced avocado

thinly sliced Napa cabbage or romaine lettuce

1 recipe Fresh Tomato-Peach Salsa (page 355)

grated raw organic Jack cheese (optional)

Cut the skin off the fish fillets, then cut the fish into 1-inch cubes. Place the cubes into a small bowl or shallow dish.

To make the marinade, mix all the ingredients in a small bowl. Pour the marinade over the fish and mix gently with a spoon. Transfer to the refrigerator and let marinate for about 30 minutes.

While the fish is marinating, prepare the other ingredients.

To cook the fish, heat about 1 tablespoon of virgin coconut oil in an 11- or 12-inch skillet over medium-high heat. Add the cubed fish and sauté gently for 5 to 6 minutes, or until the fish is cooked through.

Fill each tortilla with some of the cooked fish, avocado, cabbage, salsa, and the cheese if desired. Serve immediately.

Yield: 4 servings

CHICKEN FRICASSEE

A stew made by frying the meat first and then cooking it with vegetables and a liquid is called a fricassee. There are many different fricassee recipes using all sorts of different ingredients and herbs. This recipe is made gluten-free by replacing the traditional white flour for dredging with arrowroot powder. Serve this dish over polenta or brown rice noodles along with a large green salad.

¼ cup arrowroot powder

½ teaspoon sea salt or Herbamare

½ teaspoon freshly ground black pepper

1 teaspoon dried thyme

1 to 1½ pounds organic skinless, boneless chicken breasts, cut into pieces

1 tablespoon extra-virgin olive oil

10 to 12 garlic cloves, crushed

2 cups chopped tomatoes

3 tablespoons white wine vinegar

2 tablespoons tomato paste

¼ to ½ cup water

one 14-ounce jar artichoke hearts, drained and rinsed

½ cup pitted Kalamata olives

¼ cup tightly packed chopped fresh basil

2 tablespoons chopped fresh oregano

6 cups baby spinach

sea salt

freshly ground black pepper

chopped fresh basil, for garnish

chopped fresh oregano, for garnish

In a shallow dish gently mix together the arrowroot powder, sea salt or Herbamare, pepper, and thyme with a fork. Add the chicken pieces and stir around to coat with arrowroot mixture.

Heat the olive oil in an 11-inch, deep skillet over medium heat. Add the chicken pieces and sauté lightly for about 5 minutes, turning the chicken to cook on all sides. Add the garlic and continue to cook for 1 minute more, keeping everything moving in the skillet. Add the tomatoes, vinegar, tomato paste, and water and stir to combine. Add the artichoke hearts, olives, basil, and oregano and mix well. Cover and simmer for 25 to 35 minutes over low heat, stirring occasionally.

Add the spinach and cook for 5 minutes more. Remove from the heat and season with salt and pepper to taste. Garnish with chopped fresh basil and oregano.

Yield: 4 to 6 servings

CHICKEN VERDE ENCHILADAS

Sometimes I like to boil a whole chicken and use the broth to make a soup, and the chicken for a variety of other dishes, this one being one of them. Remember to save some of the broth for making this recipe. These enchiladas can easily be frozen in serving-size containers before baking. This way you will have a homemade meal ready to go in the oven for another night. Serve the enchiladas with cooked brown basmati rice and the Cabbage Salad with Cilantro Vinaigrette (page 226).

SAUCE

1 pound fresh tomatillos, husks removed

1 small onion, peeled and ends trimmed off

4 to 5 garlic cloves, peeled

2 jalapeño peppers, seeded

2 to 3 serrano chiles, seeded

¼ cup tightly packed fresh cilantro

1 tablespoon extra-virgin olive oil

1 cup organic chicken broth

½ to 1 teaspoon sea salt

ENCHILADAS

1 tablespoon extra-virgin olive oil, plus more for greasing the pan

1 small onion, finely diced

3 garlic cloves, crushed

2 teaspoons ground cumin

½ teaspoon sea salt

2 small zucchini, diced

4 cups chopped fresh spinach

½ cup chopped fresh cilantro

2 to 3 cups shredded cooked organic chicken

1 cup grated organic Pepper Jack cheese (optional)

organic corn tortillas, warmed

To make the sauce, place the tomatillos, onion, garlic, jalapeño and serrano chile peppers, and cilantro in a blender and blend on high until smooth. Heat a 3-quart pot over medium heat and add the olive oil. Add the blended green sauce and cook the sauce, stirring, for about 5 minutes, or until darkened and thickened. Add the chicken broth and sea salt to taste.

To make the enchiladas, heat the olive oil in an 11- or 12-inch skillet over medium heat. Add the onion and sauté for 5 minutes, or until soft. Add the garlic, cumin, and sea salt and sauté for 1 minute more. Add the zucchini and spinach and sauté for about 5 minutes more, or until tender. Transfer the filling to a large bowl along with the chopped cilantro, shredded chicken, and Pepper Jack cheese if using. Mix well.

Preheat the oven to 375°F. Oil a 9 x 13-inch pan or similar-size casserole dish with a lid.

To assemble the enchiladas, place about ½ cup of the filling in a corn tortilla and roll tightly. Place the tortilla, seam side down, in the oiled dish. Repeat this process until all of the filling has been used. Pour the sauce over the enchiladas.

You may want to place some enchiladas into a small rectangular food storage container with some sauce on top and freeze for later use.

Sprinkle the grated cheese over the sauce, if desired. Place the lid over the dish and transfer to the preheated oven. Bake for about 40 minutes, or until the sauce is bubbly.

Yield: 6 servings

> **Tip:** To warm tortillas for rolling, cook them one at a time in a skillet over low heat with a little coconut or olive oil, adding more oil with each one. Alternatively, you can dip the tortillas in the warm sauce to soften.

SIMPLE CHICKEN NUGGETS

If you are in a quandary as to what to make for dinner, try this recipe and serve it alongside steamed potatoes and green beans. The ingredients below give two versions, with eggs or egg-free; choose one or the other. Serve the nuggets with organic honey mustard for dipping, Oven Fries (page 256), and a steamed or raw vegetable for a quick, nutritious, child-friendly meal.

1 to 1½ pounds organic skinless, boneless chicken breasts

virgin coconut oil, for cooking

EGG-FREE BOWL #1

½ cup arrowroot powder

6 tablespoons water

WITH EGGS BOWL #1

2 large organic eggs, whisked

BOWL #2:

1 cup chickpea (garbanzo bean) flour
1 teaspoon Herbamare

freshly ground black pepper

Cut the chicken breasts into 1½-inch cubes.

For an egg-free version, whisk together the arrowroot and water in a small bowl and set aside. If you are using eggs, then whisk the eggs together in a separate small bowl and set aside.

In another mixing bowl, whisk together the chickpea (garbanzo bean) flour, Herbamare, and pepper.

Dip the chicken pieces into bowl #1 and then dredge in the flour mixture (bowl #2). Transfer the nuggets to a plate as you dredge them.

Heat a large 11- or 12-inch skillet over medium heat, then add about ¼ cup coconut oil to the hot pan. Add the nuggets, being careful not to crowd the skillet, and cook them in batches if needed. Cook for 3 to 4 minutes on each side; the timing will depend on the size of the nuggets and the heat of your skillet. Transfer to a plate lined with a paper towels. Serve immediately.

Yield: 4 servings

> **Tip:** I use Sprouted Garbanzo Bean Flour in my cooking because it's easier to digest and tastes better. You can order gluten-free sprouted flours online. See the Resources section in the back of the book.

COCONUT-LIME CHICKEN WITH ALMOND DIPPING SAUCE

This quick-to-prepare meal is always a crowd-pleaser. Try serving it with brown rice and steamed vegetables for an easy weeknight dinner. The chicken can also be replaced with tofu or tempeh for equally delicious results.

CHICKEN

1 to 1½ pounds organic skinless, boneless chicken breasts, cut into 1-inch cubes

virgin coconut oil, for sautéing

MARINADE

2 tablespoons coconut milk

2 tablespoons freshly squeezed lime juice

2 tablespoons wheat-free tamari or coconut aminos

ALMOND-LIME DIPPING SAUCE

6 tablespoons almond butter

¼ cup freshly squeezed lime juice

¼ cup coconut milk

1 to 2 tablespoons wheat-free tamari or coconut aminos

1 tablespoon honey or pure maple syrup

1 to 2 garlic cloves, crushed

Place the chicken breast pieces in a bowl.

To make the marinade, mix together the coconut milk, lime juice, and tamari or coconut aminos in a small bowl. Cover the chicken with the marinade. Stir the chicken and marinade together with a spoon to evenly distribute. Let the chicken marinate in the refrigerator for 20 to 30 minutes.

Heat about 1 tablespoon of virgin coconut oil in a 10-inch skillet over medium-high heat. Add the chicken pieces and sauté, stirring frequently, for 3 to 5 minutes, or until cooked through. The cooking time will vary depending on the size of the chicken pieces.

To make the dipping sauce, whisk together all the ingredients in a bowl until well combined. The sauce can also be warmed on the stovetop in a small pot over low heat if desired.

To serve, divide the dipping sauce equally among four small serving bowls and serve with the chicken.

Yield: 4 servings

HOME-STYLE CHICKEN AND VEGETABLE STEW

This hearty stew is great for a chilly evening. It is quick to prepare, so it works well for a weeknight dinner. A large green salad is always a nice accompaniment to this meal.

1 to 2 tablespoons extra-virgin olive oil

1 medium onion, diced

3 to 4 garlic cloves, crushed

1 teaspoon dried thyme

1 to 1½ pounds organic skinless, boneless chicken breasts, cut into pieces

2 to 3 large carrots, diced

3 to 4 celery stalks, diced

2 large red or yellow potatoes, diced

2½ to 3 cups Homemade Chicken Stock (page 185)

¼ cup arrowroot powder

1 teaspoon sea salt or Herbamare

1 cup fresh or frozen peas

½ cup chopped fresh parsley

Heat the olive oil in an 11-inch, deep skillet over medium heat. Add the onion and sauté until soft, about 5 minutes. Add the garlic, thyme, and chicken pieces and sauté a few minutes more. Add the carrots, celery, and potatoes and sauté 1 minute more.

Combine the stock and arrowroot powder and whisk well to combine. Transfer this mixture to the skillet. Season the mixture with the sea salt or Herbamare, cover, and simmer for 20 to 25 minutes.

Add the peas and parsley, cover, and simmer for 5 minutes more. Taste and adjust the salt and seasonings if necessary.

Yield: 4 servings

INDIAN CHICKEN CURRY

This dinner makes for a quick, easy weeknight meal. Serve the curry over cooked brown jasmine rice with a large green salad on the side. Try eating a spoonful of Cultured Vegetables (page 90) with this meal to maximize digestion.

1 tablespoon virgin coconut oil

1 medium onion, diced

4 garlic cloves, crushed

2 teaspoons ground cumin

1 teaspoon ground coriander

1 teaspoon curry powder

½ teaspoon ground turmeric

½ teaspoon ground cinnamon

pinch cayenne pepper

1 to 1½ pounds organic skinless, boneless chicken breasts, cut into pieces

3 large carrots, peeled and sliced

one 14-ounce can coconut milk

1 tablespoon tomato paste

4 cups thinly sliced kale or Swiss chard

1 to 2 teaspoons sea salt or Herbamare

Heat the coconut oil in a 4 to 6-quart pot over medium heat. Add the onion and sauté until soft, about 5 minutes. Add the garlic, cumin, coriander, curry powder, turmeric, cinnamon, and cayenne and sauté for 2 minutes more. Add the chicken pieces and sauté in the spices and onion for another 5 minutes. Add the carrots, coconut milk, and tomato paste and stir well to combine. Cover and simmer on low heat for 15 to 20 minutes, stirring occasionally.

Add the kale, stir well, and simmer for an additional 5 minutes. Turn off the heat and season with sea salt or Herbamare to taste.

Yield: 4 servings

MUSTARD-TARRAGON ROASTED CHICKEN

Use the extra sauce in the baking dish to drizzle over steamed red potatoes or cooked quinoa. I usually make a double batch of this recipe so I can have leftovers for chicken salad.

---

2 pounds organic chicken thighs, bone in, skin on

SAUCE

½ cup fresh tarragon leaves

¼ cup Dijon mustard

2 tablespoons honey

¼ cup water

½ teaspoon sea salt

Preheat the oven to 425°F. Set out an 8 x 8-inch baking dish.

Place the chicken thighs into the baking dish and set aside.

To make the sauce, place all the ingredients into a blender and blend until smooth.

Pour the sauce over the chicken in the dish. Roast the chicken for about 40 minutes. Serve.

Yield: 4 to 6 servings

ROASTED CHICKEN WITH GARLIC AND HERBS

Serve this quick-and-easy dish with cooked brown rice and sautéed kale or a large green salad for dinner. Use the drippings from the chicken to drizzle over the chicken and brown rice on your plate.

2½ to 3 pounds bone-in chicken breasts and legs

¼ cup white wine

2 tablespoons extra-virgin olive oil or organic butter

2 heads garlic

4 to 5 sprigs fresh thyme

4 to 5 sprigs fresh rosemary

1 teaspoon coarse sea salt

freshly ground black pepper

Preheat the oven to 400°F. Set out a 9 x 13-inch rectangular baking dish.

Rinse the chicken and place it into the baking dish. Pour the white wine over it, then drizzle with the olive oil. Break the heads of garlic into cloves and place them around the chicken. Add the fresh thyme and rosemary sprigs to the baking dish, then sprinkle the chicken with the sea salt and pepper.

Bake for 40 to 50 minutes, or until the chicken juices run clear. Remove the baking dish from the oven and let the chicken rest for about 10 minutes before serving.

Yield: 4 to 6 servings

WHOLE ROASTED ORGANIC CHICKEN WITH LEMON AND HERBS

You will need to plan in advance in order to roast a whole chicken because of the long cooking time. Serve roasted chicken with mashed Yukon gold potatoes or baked sweet potatoes, steamed broccoli, and a fresh salad for a complete meal.

---

1 whole organic chicken (3½ to 5 pounds)

1 small onion, chopped

3 garlic cloves, chopped

2 celery stalks, chopped

1 small lemon, cut into chunks

1 handful fresh parsley, chopped

¼ cup chopped fresh herbs (rosemary, thyme, marjoram)

1 tablespoon extra-virgin olive oil or organic butter

2 teaspoons sea salt or Herbamare

freshly ground black pepper

2 tablespoons arrowroot, for the gravy

Preheat the oven to 450°F.

Place the chicken in a clean sink and rinse, inside and out. Transfer to a 9 x 13-inch glass baking dish.

In a small bowl, mix together the onion, garlic, celery, lemon chunks, parsley, fresh herbs, 1 tablespoon olive oil, and 2 teaspoons sea salt or Herbamare, and pepper. Place some of the mixture into the cavity of the chicken and sprinkle the rest around the chicken in the dish. Add about ½ inch of water to the bottom of the baking dish. Sprinkle the top of the chicken with additional sea salt or Herbamare, pepper, and a bit of olive oil.

Roast the chicken for 25 minutes to seal in the juices. Reduce the heat to 325°F and continue to roast for 1 to 1½ hours, or until the chicken juices run clear. Baste the chicken throughout the roasting time to keep the chicken moist.

To test for doneness, pull the thigh away and check for clear juices. If they are still little pink, then the chicken needs more roasting time. You can also use a meat thermometer to test for doneness. Insert it into the thickest part of the thigh; it should register about 165°F when fully cooked. When the chicken is done, transfer it to a platter to rest for about 10 minutes before carving.

Pour the juices from the baking dish through a fine-mesh strainer into a small saucepan. Whisk about 2 tablespoons of arrowroot powder mixed with a little cold water in a small bowl and stir to dissolve. Add to the juices in the saucepan and whisk together. Simmer over low heat, whisking constantly, until the gravy thickens. Season to taste with salt and pepper.

Carve the chicken and serve with the hot gravy.

Yield: 6 to 8 servings

APRICOT AND FIG ROASTED TURKEY BREAST

Serve this festive dish at your next holiday gathering or for just a comfy home cooked family meal on a chilly evening. Try serving it with Baked Winter Squash (page 260), and the Pear and Hazelnut Salad with Creamy Cranberry Dressing (page 342). Dried figs can replace the fresh ones here; just soak them in water for about 30 minutes before using.

1 organic turkey breast (2½ to 3 pounds) bone in, skin on

¼ cup apricot jam

¼ cup balsamic vinegar

¼ cup water

2 tablespoons extra-virgin olive oil

1 tablespoon finely chopped fresh oregano

1 teaspoon sea salt

1 small leek, chopped

8 to 10 fresh black mission figs

Rinse the turkey breast and place it in a baking dish.

In a small bowl, whisk together the apricot jam, balsamic vinegar, water, olive oil, oregano, and sea salt and pour over the turkey breast. Place the leek and figs on the bottom of the dish around the turkey. Cover the dish and refrigerate for 1 to 4 hours, or overnight.

Preheat the oven to 325°F. Transfer the baking dish with the turkey and marinade to the preheated oven and roast for 1½ to 2 hours, or until the juices run clear. A meat thermometer inserted into thickest part of meat should read approximately 170°F. I have also baked this at 200°F for 3 to 4 hours, which makes the meat much more tender. Remove from oven and let rest for about 10 minutes before carving.

To serve, cut the turkey into slices and transfer to a serving platter. Place the figs and leeks on the platter, and pour the juices over the turkey slices.

Yield: 4 to 6 servings

GREEN CURRY LAMB STEW

Use this recipe in your slow cooker, or cook it on the stovetop over low heat. Meat becomes more tender and easier to digest when it's cooked at a low temperature for a long period. Use any vegetables you have on hand in this stew. The key is to add them later in the cooking process so that they don't turn to mush. If you can't find Thai basil then use regular basil instead.

SAUCE

one 14-ounce can coconut milk
½ cup chopped fresh cilantro
4 garlic cloves
one ½-inch piece fresh ginger
1 serrano or Thai chile pepper, stemmed
1 tablespoon freshly squeezed lime juice
1 teaspoon sea salt

STEW

2 pounds lamb stew meat
1 small sweet onion, cut into half-moons
¼ pound green beans, cut into 3-inch pieces
1 medium zucchini, chopped
1 yellow bell pepper, chopped
6 to 8 cremini mushrooms, quartered
1 handful fresh Thai basil leaves

To make the sauce, place all the ingredients into a blender and blend on high until smooth. Pour the sauce into a 3- or 4-quart slow cooker.

To assemble the stew, add the lamb stew meat and onion to the sauce in the slow cooker, cover, and cook on low for 5 hours or on high for 2½ hours.

Add the remaining vegetables, stir, and continue to cook for another 1 to 1½ hours on low; or an additional 30 minutes on high. You may want to add the green beans first because they take longer to cook than the other vegetables; let them cook for about 10 minutes, then add remaining vegetables.

If you don't have a slow cooker, simmer the sauce, meat, and onions in a covered pot on the stovetop on the lowest heat for 1½ to 2 hours. Then add the remaining vegetables and continue to simmer until tender, about 20 minutes more.

> **Tip:** Don't remove the seeds in the hot peppers—they add a little spice to the stew!

Yield: 6 to 8 servings

BEEF AND BROCCOLI RED CURRY

I use my slow cooker to make this—it takes me all of about 5 minutes to toss together! Serve this hearty, nourishing stew with cooked rice or quinoa and a few spoonfuls of Cultured Vegetables (page 90).

2 pounds organic beef stew meat

one 14-ounce can coconut milk

1 tablespoon red curry paste

1 tablespoon peanut butter, cashew butter, or sunflower seed butter

1 to 2 garlic cloves, crushed

1 teaspoon sea salt

1 medium red bell pepper, chopped

1 small head broccoli, cut into florets

1 handful fresh Thai basil leaves

Place the beef, coconut milk, red curry paste, peanut butter, garlic, and sea salt into a 3-quart slow cooker and stir to combine. Cook on low for about 6 hours, or on high for about 3 hours. Add the bell pepper and broccoli and continue to cook until tender, 15 to 20 minutes on high.

If you don't own a slow cooker, place all the ingredients except for the bell peppers and broccoli into a pot and simmer on low on the stovetop for 45 to 60 minutes. Add the vegetables and cook for another 10 to 15 minutes or until tender.

Add the Thai basil leaves and serve.

Yield: 6 servings

BEEF STEW WITH SWISS CHARD

It is best to buy organic grass-fed beef if you are going to eat meat. If you cannot find it locally then you can order it online and have it shipped to you. Serve this stew over cooked quinoa. The juices from the stew will seep down into the quinoa creating a luxurious combination. Use the Homemade Beef Stock (page 184) in this recipe rather than store-bought canned or packaged stock.

2 tablespoons extra-virgin olive oil

1 medium onion, chopped

3 shallots, minced

4 garlic cloves, minced

2 teaspoons dried thyme

1 teaspoon dried rosemary, crushed

2 cups cremini mushrooms, quartered

2 large carrots, sliced ½ inch thick

1 pound organic beef stew meat

2 cups chopped fresh tomatoes

1 cup Homemade Beef Stock (page 184)

1 to 2 teaspoons sea salt or Herbamare

¼ to ½ teaspoon freshly ground black pepper

4 cups thinly sliced Swiss chard

1 tablespoon red wine vinegar

Heat the olive oil in a 4-quart pot over medium heat. Add the onion, shallots, and garlic; sauté for 5 to 7 minutes, or until soft and beginning to turn golden.

Add the thyme, rosemary, mushrooms, and carrots; sauté for an additional 5 minutes. Add the beef stew meat and continue to sauté for about 5 minutes more.

Add the tomatoes, beef stock, sea salt, and black pepper, cover, and simmer over low heat for 60 to 90 minutes, stirring occasionally. Add the chard and vinegar; simmer for a few minutes more, or until the chard is tender. Taste and adjust the salt and seasonings if necessary.

Yield: 4 servings

FALL VEGETABLE BEEF ROAST

This recipe was passed down to me from my mother and makes a great hearty meal when the weather is beginning to get cold. Serve with raw sauerkraut and Baked Winter Squash (page 260) for a balanced meal.

1 tablespoon extra-virgin olive oil or ghee

1 organic beef roast (2 to 3 pounds)

1 teaspoon sea salt

1 teaspoon freshly ground black pepper

2 teaspoons dried thyme

1 medium onion, cut into chunks

2 cups organic vegetable juice cocktail or tomato purée

2 cups Homemade Beef Stock (page 184)

3 to 4 large carrots, peeled and cut into 3-inch pieces

4 to 5 red potatoes, cut into large chunks

1 rutabaga or 1 yam, cut into large chunks

3 celery stalks, cut into 3-inch pieces

sea salt or Herbamare

Preheat the oven to 325°F.

Heat the olive oil in a large Dutch oven over medium-high heat. Rub the salt and pepper into the roast on all sides. Add the roast to the Dutch oven and sear for a few minutes on all sides. Add the thyme, onion, vegetable juice, and beef stock.

Cover, transfer to the preheated oven, and braise for 2 hours. Remove the pot from the oven and add the remaining vegetables. Return the pot to the oven and continue to cook for 1 to 2 more hours, or until the roast begins to fall apart and the vegetables are tender.

Season to taste with sea salt or Herbamare.

Yield: 6 to 8 servings

SUMMER VEGETABLE SPAGHETTI

I like to make this sauce toward the end of summer when there is an abundance of vegetables need-ing to be used. You can freeze the sauce in pint-size jars for future use. I prefer to serve the sauce over baked spaghetti squash, but my children prefer brown rice noodles—either way it's a nutrient-dense meal! Serve with a large green salad.

1 tablespoon extra-virgin olive oil

1 medium onion, diced

3 to 4 garlic cloves, crushed

1 tablespoon Italian seasoning

2 teaspoons sea salt

1 pound ground organic beef

3 carrots, diced

2 red bell peppers, diced (about 1½ cups)

1 large zucchini (about 2 cups diced)

2½ cups tomato sauce (one 24-ounce jar)

¾ cup tomato paste (one 7-ounce jar)

1 to 2 cups chopped kale

½ cup packed fresh basil leaves, chopped

½ cup fresh parsley, chopped

freshly ground black pepper

pinch crushed red chili flakes (optional)

baked spaghetti squash or brown rice noodles, for serving

Heat the olive oil in an 11- or 12-inch, deep skillet over medium heat. Add the onion and sauté for about 5 minutes. Add the garlic, Italian seasoning, sea salt, and ground beef and sauté for another 5 to 7 minutes, or until the beef is no longer pink. Add the carrots, bell peppers, and zucchini and sauté for 5 minutes more.

Stir in the tomato sauce and paste, cover, and cook for about 20 min-utes, or until the vegetables are tender. Stir in the kale, basil, parsley, black pepper, and red chili flakes if using and simmer for few minutes more. Taste and adjust the salt and seasonings if necessary. Serve over baked spaghetti squash or brown rice noodles.

Yield: 6 servings

> **Tip:** We use strained tomatoes (similar to tomato sauce) and tomato paste preserved in glass jars from the company Bionaturae. You can order them online or find them at your local health food store.

20

DRESSINGS, DIPS, AND SAUCES

Laughter is the tonic, the relief, the surcease for pain.
—*Charlie Chaplin*

Having fresh salad dressings ready to go in your fridge will be an invaluable asset to your health. Simply drizzle your favorite dressing over some fresh, organic mixed greens and you'll have a vital, nutrient-packed snack or meal. Stored in a glass jar, all of the following dressings will keep for 7 to 10 days in the refrigerator. Since the olive oil in these dressings will harden slightly at cold temperatures, simply place the jar under warm running water to thin out before using.

Eating raw vegetables with a bean dip or nut pâte is a wonderful way to get more raw vegetables into your diet. Raw vegetables provide the desirable "crunch" that people crave, and dips provide a slightly salty flavor and a creamy consistency that we all love.

Sauces are indispensable for spicing up cooked grains, whole-grain noodles, or steamed vegetables. Some sauces may also be easily frozen for later use.

Enjoy the healthy whole foods recipes in this chapter in place of salad dressings, sauces, and condiments you would buy at the store—they are much healthier for you!

SALAD DRESSINGS

BALSAMIC VINAIGRETTE

¼ cup extra-virgin olive oil

3 tablespoons balsamic vinegar

1 tablespoon pure maple syrup

2 teaspoons Dijon mustard

¼ teaspoon sea salt

Whisk together all the ingredients in a small bowl. Store the vinaigrette in a covered glass jar in the refrigerator.

ORANGE VINAIGRETTE

¼ cup extra-virgin olive oil

1 teaspoon finely grated orange zest

¼ cup freshly squeezed orange juice

1 tablespoon balsamic vinegar

1 tablespoon chopped fresh fennel tops

¼ teaspoon sea salt

¼ teaspoon ground cinnamon

Whisk together all the ingredients in a small bowl. Store the vinaigrette in a covered glass jar in the refrigerator.

HONEY–POPPY SEED VINAIGRETTE

¼ cup extra-virgin olive oil

3 tablespoons red wine vinegar

1 to 2 tablespoons honey

1 tablespoon poppy seeds

¼ teaspoon sea salt

Whisk together all the ingredients in a small bowl. Store the vinaigrette in a covered glass jar in the refrigerator.

CILANTRO VINAIGRETTE

¼ cup chopped fresh cilantro

¼ cup extra-virgin olive oil

3 tablespoons brown rice vinegar or coconut vinegar

¼ teaspoon sea salt

pinch cayenne pepper

Place all the ingredients into a blender and blend until smooth. Store the vinaigrette in a covered glass jar in the refrigerator.

HERBAL VINAIGRETTE

freshly squeezed juice of 1 small lemon

⅓ cup extra-virgin olive oil

2 tablespoons balsamic vinegar

2 teaspoons Dijon mustard

1 tablespoon pure maple syrup

2 tablespoons chopped fresh basil

2 tablespoons chopped fresh chives

1 tablespoon chopped fresh oregano

½ teaspoon sea salt

Whisk together all the ingredients in a small bowl. Store the vinaigrette in a covered glass jar in the refrigerator.

RED WINE VINAIGRETTE

¼ cup extra-virgin olive oil

¼ cup red wine vinegar

1 teaspoon Dijon mustard

1 teaspoon pure maple syrup

½ teaspoon sea salt

1 teaspoon Italian seasoning

1 garlic clove, crushed

Whisk together all the ingredients in a small bowl. Store the vinaigrette in a covered glass jar in the refrigerator.

LIME VINAIGRETTE

¼ cup extra-virgin olive oil

1 to 2 teaspoons finely grated lime zest

¼ cup freshly squeezed lime juice

1 tablespoon brown rice vinegar or apple cider vinegar

1 garlic clove, crushed

¼ teaspoon sea salt

¼ teaspoon ground cumin

pinch ground cardamom

Whisk together all the ingredients in a small bowl. Store the vinaigrette in a covered glass jar in the refrigerator.

WHITE NECTARINE VINAIGRETTE

½ ripe white nectarine

6 tablespoons extra-virgin olive oil

¼ cup white wine vinegar

1 small garlic clove

¼ to ½ teaspoon sea salt

1 to 2 tablespoons finely chopped fresh parsley

Place all the ingredients except for the parsley into a blender and blend on high until puréed. Add the parsley and blend on low speed just until incorporated; if you blend the parsley too long it will turn the dressing green. Store the dressing in a glass jar in the refrigerator.

CREAMY GINGER DRESSING

⅓ cup sesame seeds

½ cup chopped celery

3 to 4 tablespoons chopped fresh ginger

½ cup extra-virgin olive oil

3 tablespoons brown rice vinegar or coconut vinegar

3 tablespoons wheat-free tamari or coconut aminos

2 tablespoons water

1 tablespoon pure maple syrup

⅛ teaspoon ground white pepper

Heat a small skillet over medium-low heat, add the sesame seeds, and toast for about 3 minutes. Be sure to keep seeds moving in the skillet to prevent burning.

Remove from the heat and transfer the seeds to a blender with the remaining ingredients; blend on high until smooth. Store the dressing in a glass jar in the refrigerator.

CREAMY CRANBERRY DRESSING

2 teaspoons extra-virgin olive oil, plus ¼ cup

2 shallots, peeled and thinly sliced

1 cup fresh cranberries

1 teaspoon finely grated orange zest

¼ cup freshly squeezed orange juice

¼ cup extra-virgin olive oil

2 tablespoons balsamic vinegar

3 to 4 tablespoons pure maple syrup

½ teaspoon sea salt or Herbamare

Heat a small skillet over medium heat. Add the 2 teaspoons of olive oil and the shallots and sauté for 3 to 5 minutes, or until soft. Add the cranberries and continue to sauté until the cranberries are soft and have "popped."

Transfer the mixture to a blender along with the orange zest, orange juice, ¼ cup olive oil, vinegar, maple syrup, and sea salt and blend on high until smooth. For a thinner consistency, add a few more tablespoons of water and blend again. Store the dressing in a glass jar in the refrigerator for up to 10 days.

HOMEMADE KETCHUP

Use this healthier, homemade recipe for ketchup as a dip for roasted potato wedges, spread onto burgers, or wherever you would use store-bought ketchup! I use organic tomato paste sold in glass jars from the company Bionaturae.

1½ cups tomato paste (two 7-ounce jars)
¼ cup water
¼ cup raw apple cider vinegar
3 to 4 tablespoons coconut sugar
1½ teaspoons sea salt or Herbamare
¼ teaspoon dry mustard powder

¼ teaspoon garlic powder
⅛ teaspoon celery salt
⅛ teaspoon ground cloves
⅛ teaspoon ground allspice
pinch cayenne pepper

Whisk all the ingredients together in a small saucepan and cook over very low heat for 2 to 3 minutes to help dissolve the coconut sugar and meld the spices with the tomato paste. Taste and adjust the salt and seasonings if necessary. Pour into a clean glass jar, cover, and store in the refrigerator where it will keep for months.

Yield: 2 cups

QUICK ALMOND MAYO

Use this simple egg-free, soy-free mayonnaise to spread onto bread for sandwiches or use it to make dips and salad dressings.

1½ cups slivered almonds
¾ to 1 cup warm water
⅓ cup raw apple cider vinegar

1½ teaspoons sea salt or Herbamare
1 tablespoon Dijon mustard
⅔ cup unrefined avocado oil

Place the slivered almonds, water, vinegar, sea salt, and mustard into a blender and blend until smooth. With the motor running on a low speed, slowly add the oil. Keep blending until combined; it should thicken up quickly.

Store the mayo in a glass jar in the refrigerator for up to 3 weeks.

Yield: about 2 cups

HUMMUS

Hummus is a traditional Middle-Eastern dish made from chickpeas, also called garbanzo beans, and tahini. It makes an excellent dip for fresh vegetables or a great spread for sandwiches or wraps.

3 cups cooked chickpeas

½ cup sesame tahini

½ cup freshly squeezed lemon juice

¼ cup extra-virgin olive oil

2 teaspoons garlic powder or 2 cloves, crushed

1 teaspoon ground cumin

1 to 2 teaspoons sea salt or Herbamare

¼ cup bean cooking liquid or water to reach desired consistency

Place all the ingredients into a food processor and process until smooth and creamy.

You will want to taste the hummus to see if it needs more lemon, tahini, garlic, or salt. For a thinner consistency, add more water and process again. Hummus freezes very well.

Yield: 4 cups

WHITE BEAN AND ROASTED RED PEPPER DIP

This bean dip is a great alternative to hummus for people with sesame seed allergies. Try putting some into a gluten-free tortilla along with some chopped cucumbers, tomatoes, olives, and lettuce. Use navy, Great Northern, or cannellini beans in this recipe.

3 cups cooked white beans

1 small red bell pepper, roasted (see Tip)

½ cup almond butter

¼ cup freshly squeezed lemon juice

3 tablespoons extra-virgin olive oil

1 teaspoon garlic powder or 2 garlic cloves, crushed

½ to 1 teaspoon chili powder

1 teaspoon sea salt or Herbamare

bean cooking liquid or water

Place all the ingredients into a food processor and process until smooth and creamy.

Taste the bean dip to see if it needs more lemon, garlic, or salt. For a thinner consistency, add bean cooking liquid or water and process again.

Yield: 4 cups

Tip: To roast red bell peppers, place them in a baking dish under the broiler until the skin is charred, turning frequently, for 8 to 10 minutes. Remove the peppers from the baking dish and transfer to a paper bag or a covered glass bowl; let steam at room temperature for about 10 minutes. Remove the peppers and peel off the charred skins. Cut the peppers and remove the seeds.

SPICY BLACK BEAN DIP

Not only are black beans good in soup, but they are also wonderful as a dip. If you would like an even spicier dip, try adding one additional jalapeño pepper and some crushed red chili flakes. You may freeze some of this dip as long as you keep the fresh tomato out of the portion you will freeze.

1 tablespoon extra-virgin olive oil

1 small onion, chopped

1 small jalapeño pepper, chopped

3 garlic cloves, crushed

1 tablespoon ground cumin

1 teaspoon chili powder

3 cups cooked black beans, drained

1 to 2 tablespoons raw apple cider vinegar

½ teaspoon sea salt

1 to 2 plum tomatoes, diced

Heat the olive oil in a large skillet over medium heat. Add the onion, jalapeño pepper, and garlic and sauté until the soft, about 5 minutes. Add the cumin and chili powder and sauté 1 minute more, stirring often.

Add the cooked beans and mix in thoroughly, making sure you scrape up all of the spices from the bottom of the skillet.

Transfer the bean and spice mixture to a food processor and process until smooth. Add the vinegar and sea salt to taste and process again. Taste and season with more salt if necessary.

Scrape the dip from the processor into a medium bowl. Stir in the diced tomatoes.

Yield: 3 cups

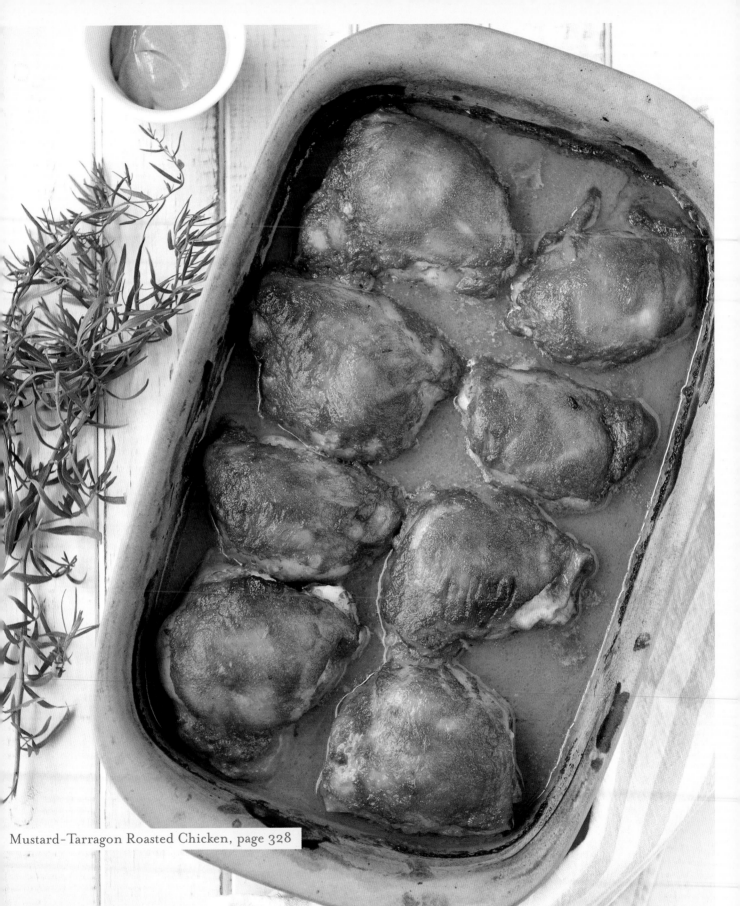
Mustard-Tarragon Roasted Chicken, page 328

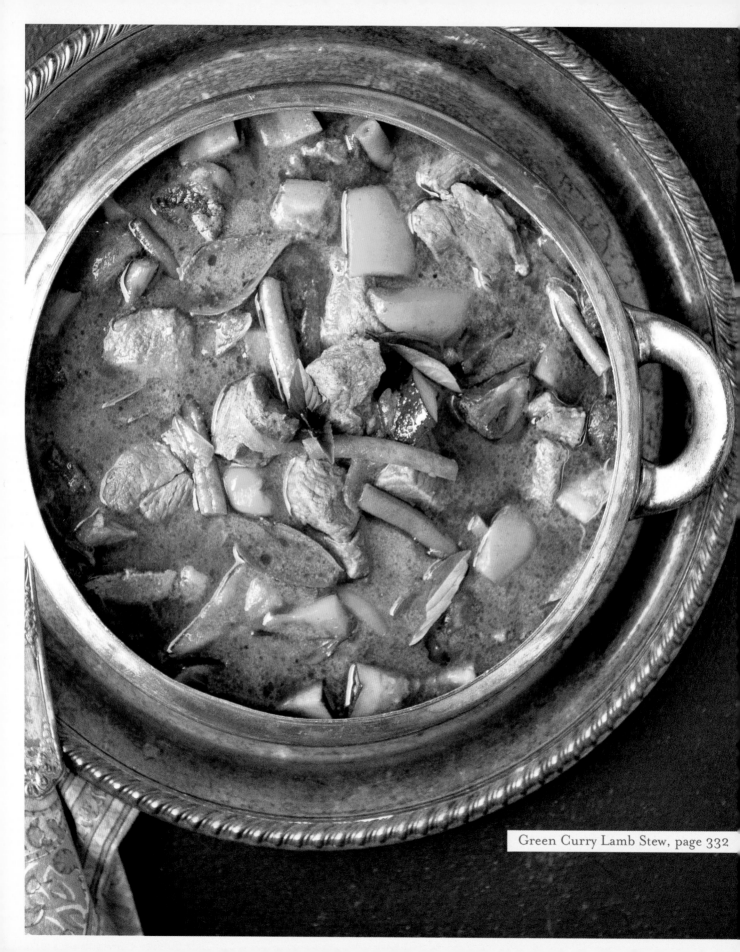

Green Curry Lamb Stew, page 332

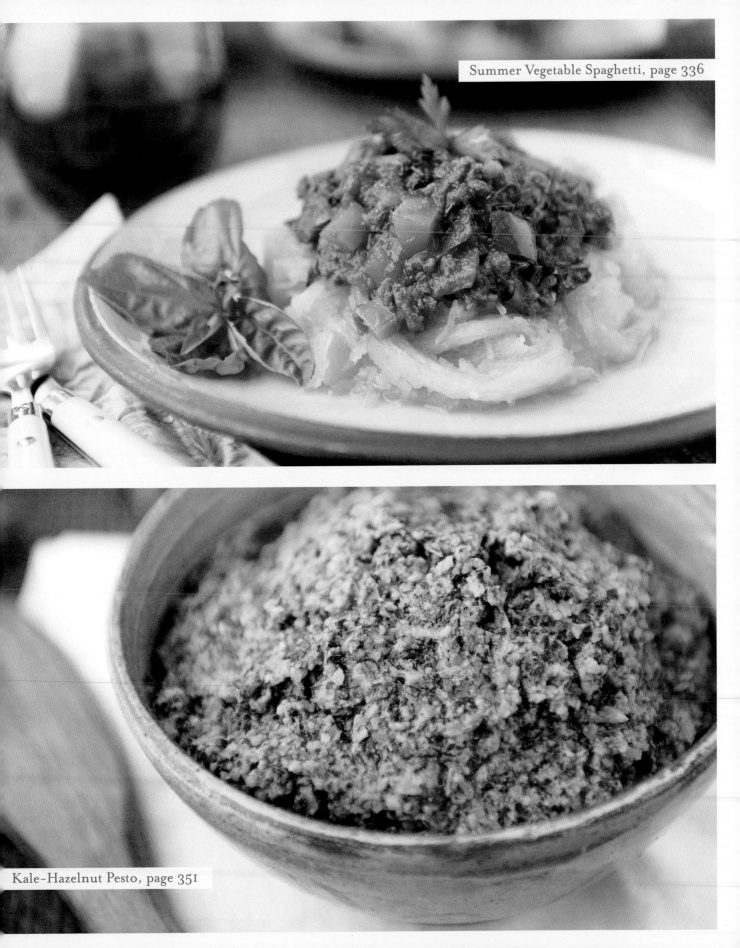

Summer Vegetable Spaghetti, page 336

Kale–Hazelnut Pesto, page 351

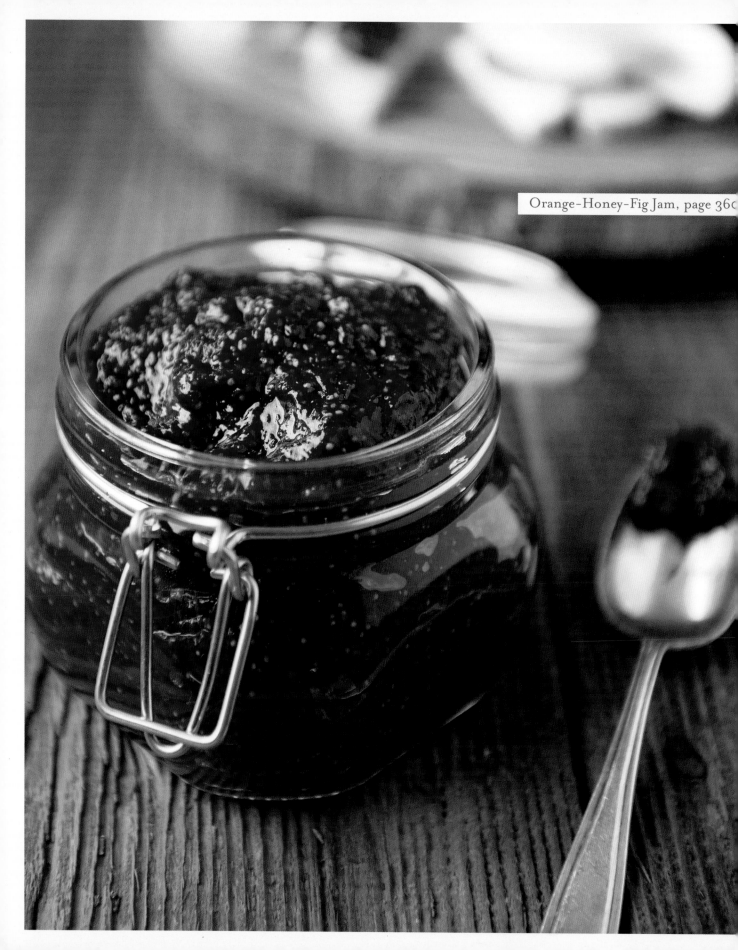

Orange-Honey-Fig Jam, page 360

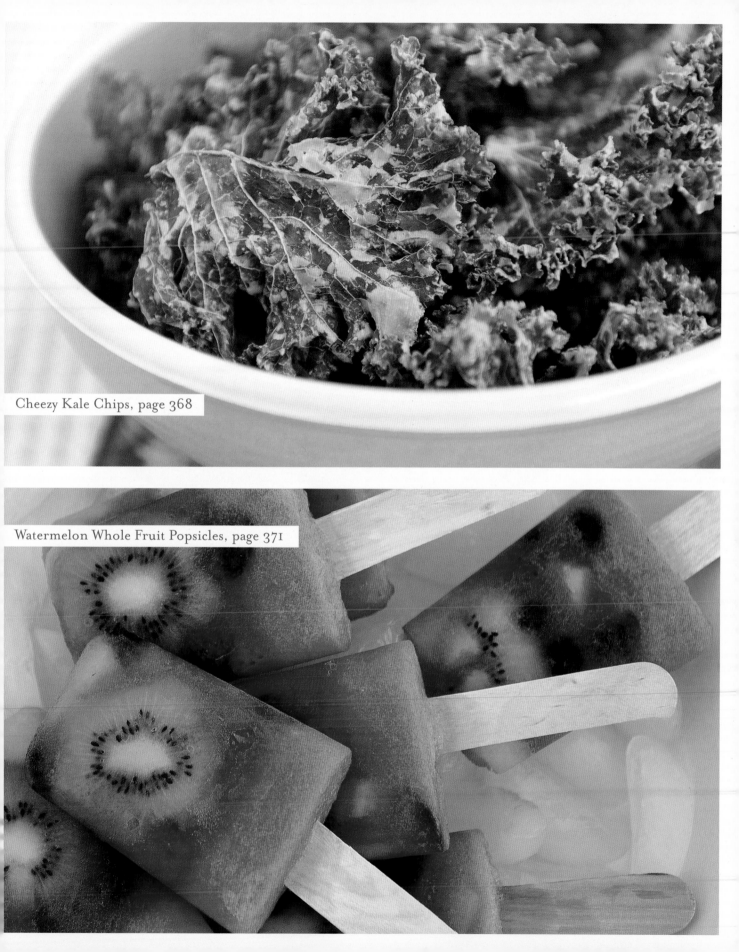

Cheezy Kale Chips, page 368

Watermelon Whole Fruit Popsicles, page 371

Raw Chocolate–Avocado Pudding, page 381

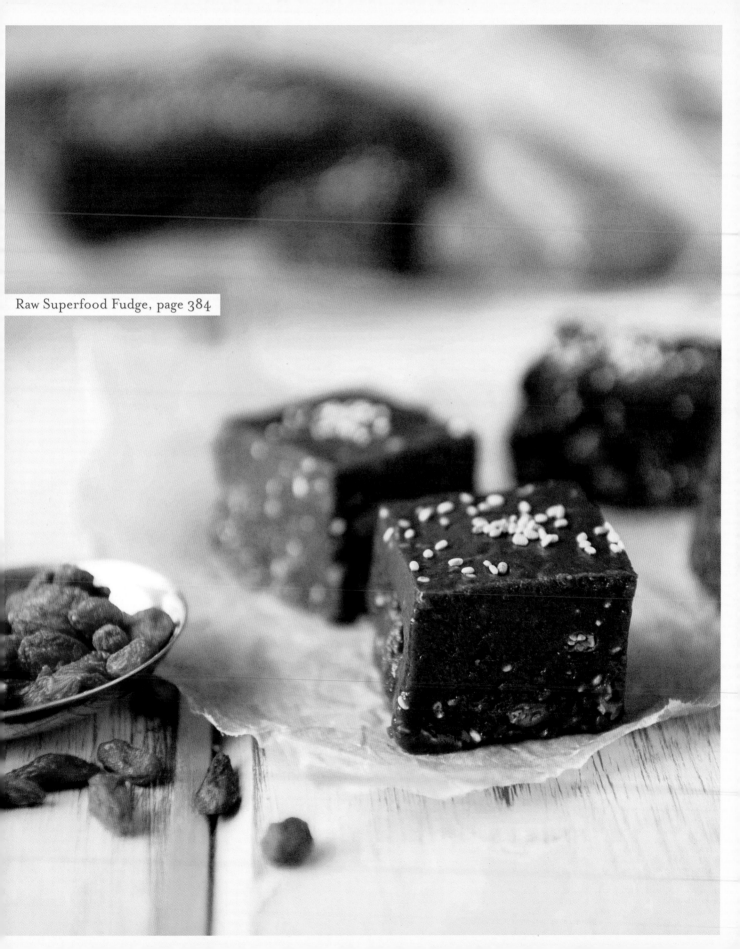
Raw Superfood Fudge, page 384

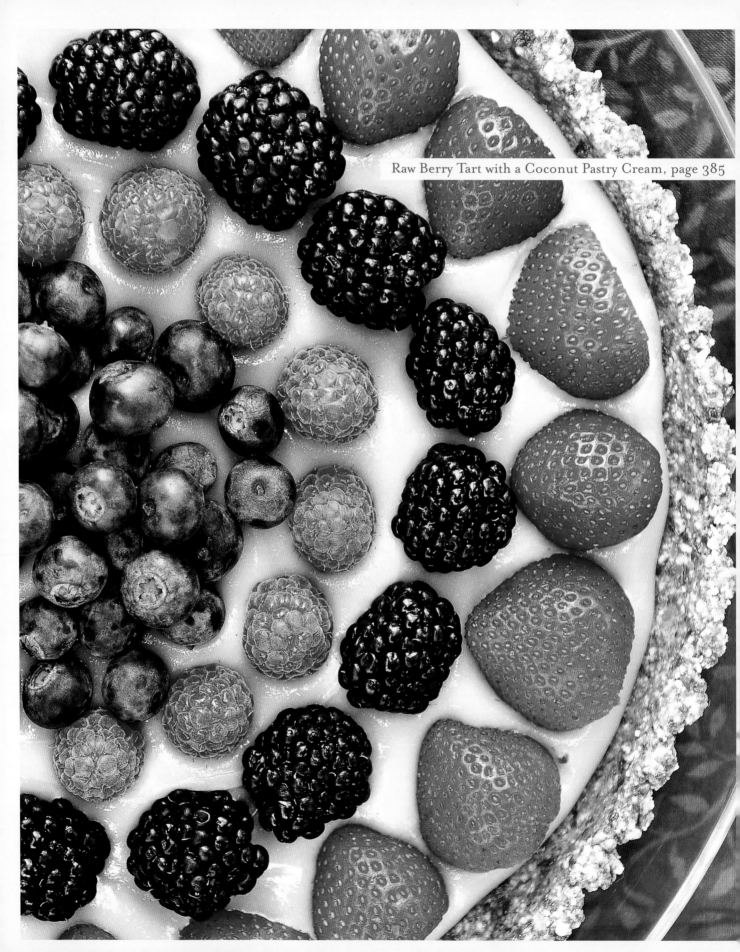
Raw Berry Tart with a Coconut Pastry Cream, page 385

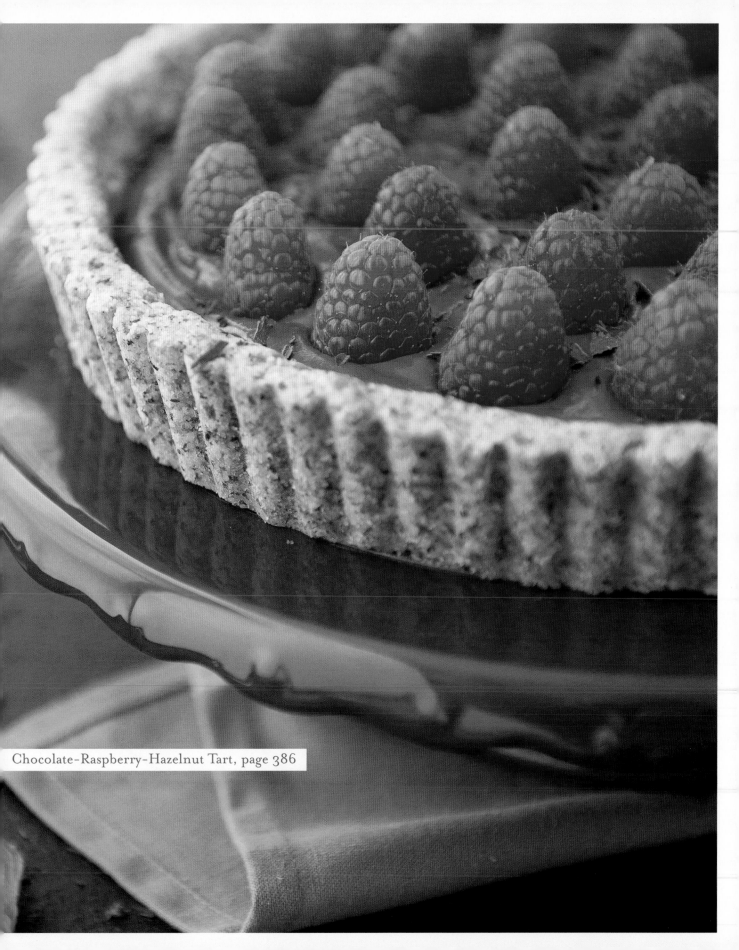

Chocolate-Raspberry-Hazelnut Tart, page 386

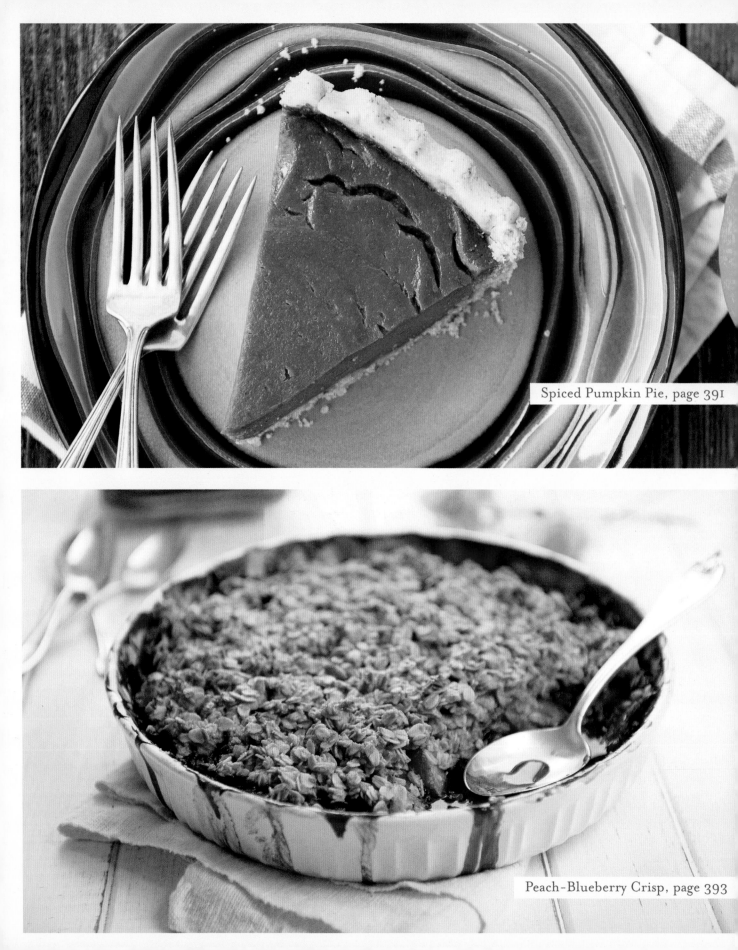

Spiced Pumpkin Pie, page 391

Peach-Blueberry Crisp, page 393

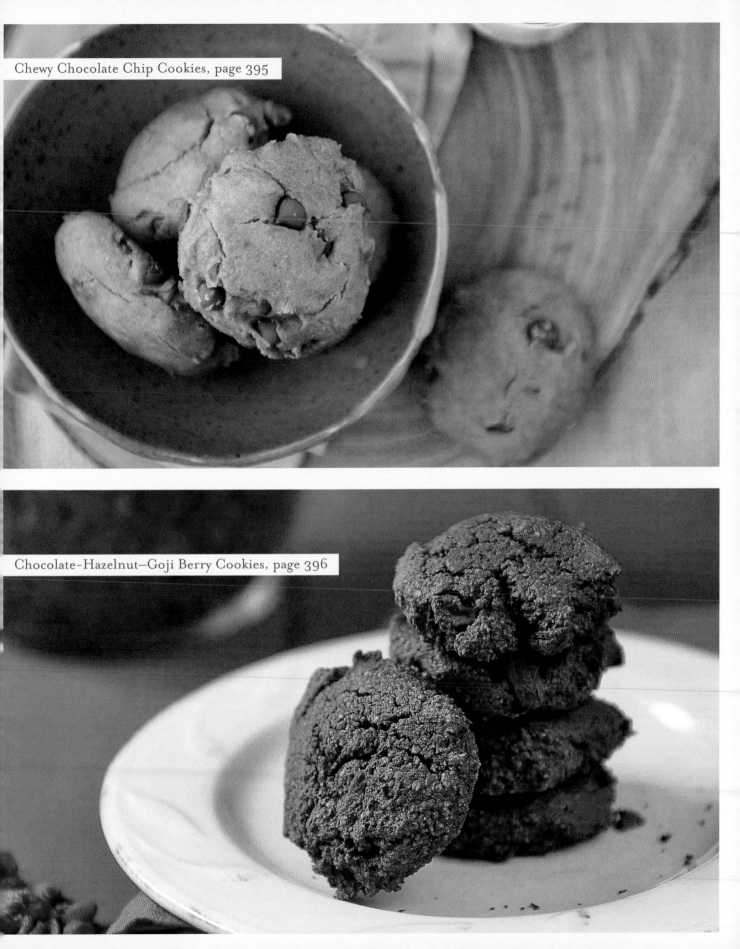

Chewy Chocolate Chip Cookies, page 395

Chocolate–Hazelnut–Goji Berry Cookies, page 396

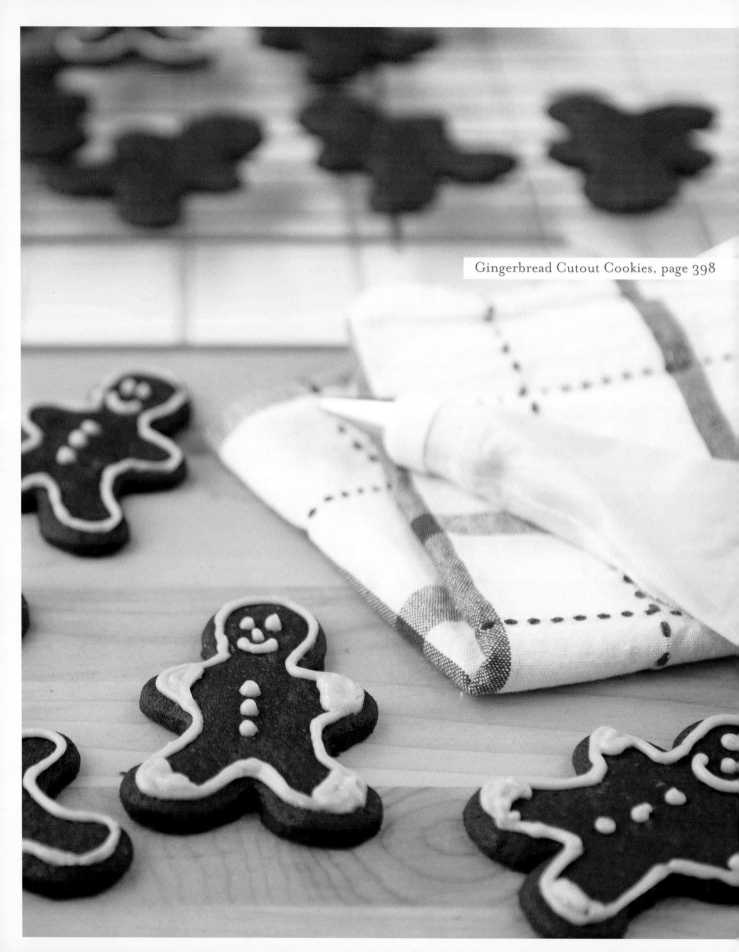

Gingerbread Cutout Cookies, page 398

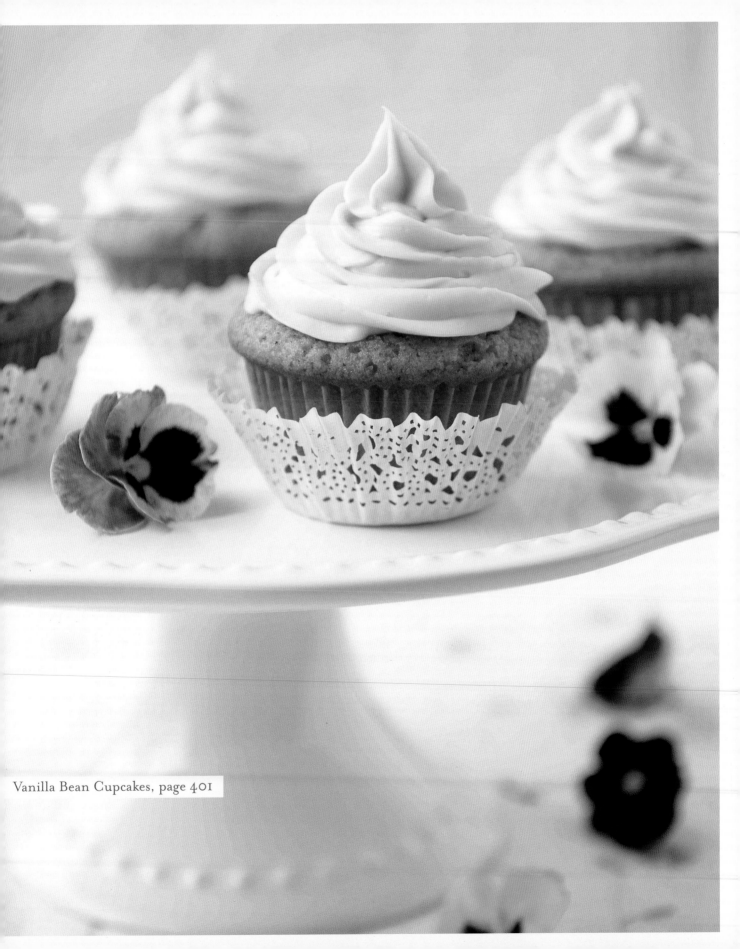

Vanilla Bean Cupcakes, page 401

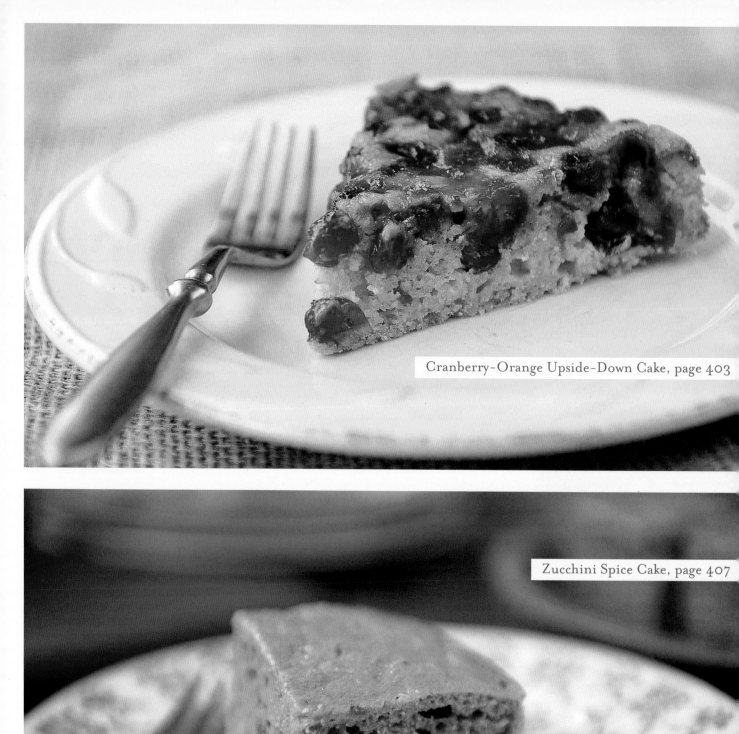

Cranberry-Orange Upside-Down Cake, page 403

Zucchini Spice Cake, page 407

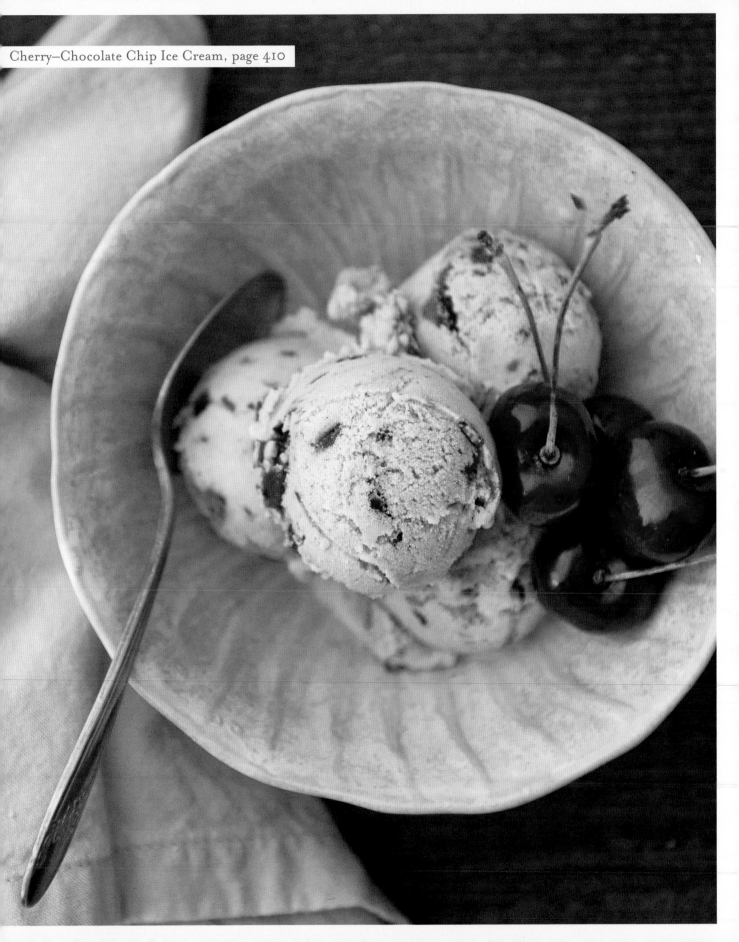
Cherry–Chocolate Chip Ice Cream, page 410

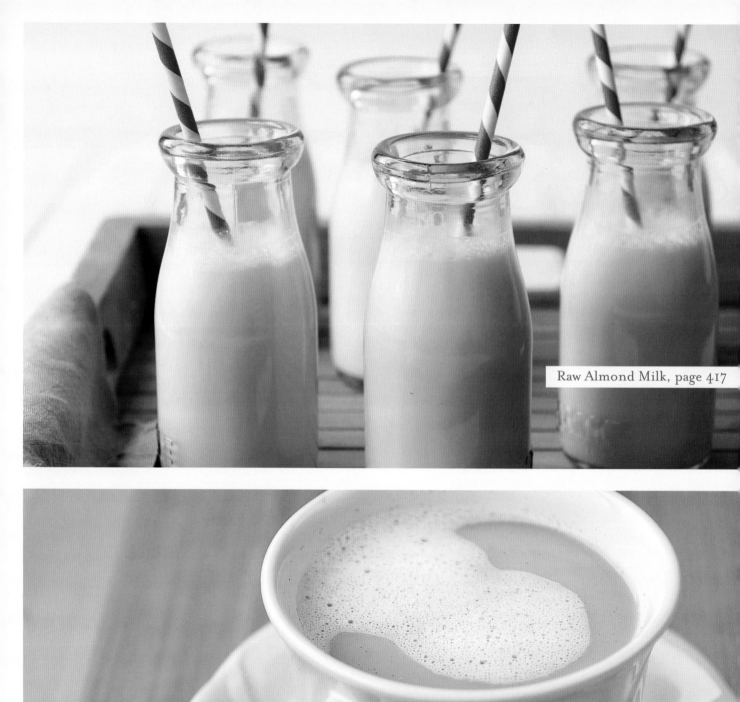

Raw Almond Milk, page 417

Dandelion Root Chai Tea, page 425

ARTICHOKE AND ALMOND PÂTE

This delightful pâte is wonderful served in a bowl next to a platter of raw vegetables, or you can try rolling into romaine lettuce leaves for a snack. You can use jarred artichoke hearts for this recipe or you can use about 1½ cups freshly cooked artichoke hearts.

1 cup raw almonds (soaked overnight)

one 14-ounce jar of artichokes, drained and rinsed

¼ cup extra-virgin olive oil

¼ cup freshly squeezed lemon juice

½ small red onion, coarsely chopped

2 tablespoons organic capers

1 small garlic clove, peeled

½ teaspoon sea salt

Soak the almonds in a medium bowl with water to cover. Set on the countertop overnight, or for 8 to 12 hours. When ready to use drain off the soaking water and rinse well.

Place all the ingredients into a food processor fitted with the "s" blade and process until the mixture is smooth.

Yield: 4 to 6 servings

RAW ALMOND AND VEGETABLE PÂTE

Serve this tasty and nourishing pâte with a platter of fresh organic vegetables and flax crackers. We like to use a gluten-free cracker called Mary's Gone Crackers, which are available at most health food stores and food co-ops. Wakame is a sea vegetable that gives this recipe added flavor while providing an abundance of trace minerals; look for it in the bulk section or macrobiotic section of your local food co-op or health food store.

1½ cups raw almonds (soaked overnight)

¼ to ½ cup wakame pieces, soaked

1 cup coarsely chopped carrots

1 cup coarsely chopped celery

½ cup coarsely chopped red bell pepper

2 to 3 garlic cloves, chopped

½ cup chopped fresh parsley

5 Medjool dates, pitted

1 to 2 tablespoons wheat-free tamari or 1 teaspoon sea salt

Soak the almonds in a medium bowl with water to cover. Set on the countertop overnight, or for 8 to 12 hours. When ready to use drain off the soaking water and rinse well.

Soak the wakame pieces in a small bowl with some filtered water for about 10 minutes. Drain off the soaking water and place the wakame in a food processor fitted with the "s" blade.

Add the drained, soaked almonds, carrots, celery, bell pepper, chopped garlic, parsley, and dates and pulse until well combined, being careful not to overprocess.

Add the tamari or sea salt to taste and pulse again. Store in the refrigerator until ready to serve.

Yield: 4 to 6 servings

OLIVE TAPENADE

Olive tapenade is delicious when used as a dip with carrot sticks, flax crackers, or spread onto baked fish. You can also use it as a garnish for the White Bean and Vegetable Stew (page 309).

---

1 cup Kalamata olives, pitted

¼ cup pine nuts

¼ cup coarsely chopped roasted red bell peppers (see Tip, page 345)

¼ cup tightly packed fresh basil leaves

¼ cup fresh parsley

2 tablespoons capers

1 tablespoon freshly squeezed lemon juice

1 to 2 garlic cloves

¼ teaspoon freshly ground black pepper

2 tablespoons extra-virgin olive oil

Place all the ingredients except for the olive oil into a food processor fitted with the "s" blade and pulse a few times. While still pulsing, slowly add the olive oil through the feed tube. Make sure not to overprocess, as the mixture can quickly turn into a paste. You will want it to be a rather coarse mixture.

Yield: 1½ cups

LEMON-BASIL PESTO

Make this pesto in the summer when fresh basil is in season and freeze in small containers for later use. This pesto is delicious served over cooked brown rice noodles or baked fish. It also works well tossed with lightly steamed vegetables, or spread onto a baked gluten-free pizza crust.

½ cup pine nuts

2 garlic cloves, peeled

1 to 2 teaspoons finely grated lemon zest

¼ to ½ teaspoon sea salt or Herbamare

3 cups tightly packed fresh basil leaves

¼ cup extra-virgin olive oil

3 to 4 tablespoons freshly squeezed lemon juice

Place the pine nuts, garlic cloves, lemon zest, and sea salt in a food processor fitted with the "s" blade and pulse a few times until the mixture is coarsely ground.

Add the basil leaves and, with the food processor running, slowly add the olive oil and lemon juice through the feed tube. Continue to process until the pesto is the desired consistency. For a thinner consistency, add water, one tablespoon at a time.

Yield: 1 cup

KALE-HAZELNUT PESTO

Kale and hazelnuts are signature foods of the Pacific Northwest—where we live—so it would make sense to use them in as many ways possible. Kale Pesto is one! Serve a dollop of this pesto over baked organic chicken or grilled salmon, or toss with steamed vegetables and cooked brown rice noodles.

¾ cup hazelnuts

4 cups chopped kale

1 to 2 garlic cloves, crushed

freshly squeezed juice of 1 lemon

½ teaspoon sea salt

½ cup extra-virgin olive oil

Preheat the oven to 350°F. Spread the hazelnuts out in a baking dish and roast in the oven for 15 to 18 minutes. Remove from oven and let cool. Transfer the roasted hazelnuts to a food processor fitted with the "s" blade and pulse to grind coarsely.

Add the kale, garlic, lemon juice, and sea salt and process until finely ground. With the processor running, slowing add the olive oil though the feed tube and process until combined. Taste and add more salt and lemon juice if desired and pulse again.

Scrape the pesto out of the food processor with a rubber spatula and transfer to a jar. Refrigerate until ready to serve.

Yield: about 1½ cups

GUACAMOLE

Guacamole is delicious served with many of the recipes in this cookbook. Try it with the Mexican Pink Bean Burritos (page 297) or dolloped onto bowls of Spicy Black Bean Soup (page 199), or simply serve as a dip for fresh cucumber slices.

3 small ripe avocados (1 pit reserved)
freshly squeezed juice of 1 lime
¼ cup finely diced red onion
1 small plum tomato, diced
¼ cup finely chopped fresh cilantro
¼ teaspoon sea salt

OPTIONAL ADDITIONS
finely diced fresh jalapeño pepper
cayenne pepper

Place the avocados into a medium bowl and mash with a fork to the desired consistency. For a smoother dip you may place the avocados into a blender and blend until creamy.

Mix the mashed or blended avocados with the remaining ingredients in a bowl. Taste and add more salt and lime juice if necessary.

For a spicier dip, try adding a finely diced jalapeño pepper and a pinch or so of cayenne.

If not serving right away, place the reserved pit into center of the dip, cover, and refrigerate until ready to serve.

Yield: 2 to 4 servings

RAITA

Raita is a classic Indian condiment that provides a cooling accompaniment to many spicy dishes. Try serving a dollop of raita atop a serving of Lentil and Spinach Dal (page 305) or Curried Vegetables (page 254). Use the Coconut Milk Yogurt (page 104) if you are dairy-free.

1 cup organic plain yogurt (cow, goat, or coconut)

1 small cucumber, seeded and finely diced

1 tablespoon finely chopped fresh mint

½ teaspoon whole cumin seeds

pinch sea salt

Combine all the ingredients in a small bowl and chill until ready to serve.

Yield: 1½ cups

AVOCADO SALSA

This salsa tastes great atop spicy bean stews, wrapped inside burritos, or as a garnish to any enchilada recipe. It is best eaten the day it is made.

2 large avocados, diced

½ small red onion, finely diced

2 to 3 tablespoons freshly squeezed lime juice

¼ cup chopped fresh cilantro

sea salt or Herbamare

Place all the ingredients except for the sea salt in a small bowl and mix gently. Season to taste with sea salt or Herbamare. Serve immediately, or refrigerate for up to 2 hours.

Yield: about 2 cups

FRESH TOMATO SALSA

Serve this fresh salsa with the Mexican Pink Bean Burritos (page 297), or as a dip for the Smashed Yam and Black Bean Quesadillas (page 299).

4 plum tomatoes, diced
½ small red onion, finely diced
¼ cup chopped fresh cilantro
1 small jalapeño pepper, minced
1 to 2 tablespoons apple cider vinegar

1 small garlic clove, minced
¼ teaspoon sea salt
¼ teaspoon ground cumin
pinch cayenne pepper

Place all the ingredients into a small bowl and mix gently. Taste and adjust the salt and seasonings if necessary. Store the salsa in a covered glass container in the refrigerator for up to 3 days.

Yield: 2 cups

FRESH MANGO SALSA

Serve this salsa over the Spiced Citrus Salmon (page 316), or atop fresh baby arugula greens for a light, refreshing salad.

2 mangos, peeled and diced
1 small red onion, finely diced
½ red bell pepper, finely diced

1 small jalapeño pepper, minced
2 to 3 tablespoons freshly squeezed lime juice
sea salt or Herbamare

Place all the ingredients except for the sea salt into a small bowl and gently mix. Season to taste with sea salt or Herbamare. Store the salsa in a covered glass container in the refrigerator for up to 3 days.

Yield: 1½ cups

FRESH TOMATO-PEACH SALSA

Serve this salsa with the Fish Tacos (page 320), or with your favorite spiced bean and grain combination.

2 firm plum tomatoes, diced
1 ripe firm peach, diced
½ small red onion, finely diced
1 small jalapeño pepper, finely diced

½ cup chopped fresh cilantro
1 to 2 tablespoons freshly squeezed lime juice
sea salt or Herbamare

Place all ingredients except for the salt into a small bowl and mix gently. Season with sea salt or Herbamare to taste. Store the salsa in a covered glass container in the refrigerator for up to 3 days.

Yield: 1½ cups

FRESH MARINARA SAUCE

This sauce is fun to make with children—they love to help pick the fresh herbs and stir the sauce. Blending the sauce makes the flavors meld together perfectly, also making it suitable for young children who sometimes like things smoother.

---

3 to 4 tablespoons extra-virgin olive oil

1 small onion, chopped

4 to 5 garlic cloves, crushed

1 teaspoon sea salt or Herbamare

3 to 4 tablespoons fresh herbs (thyme, oregano, parsley, basil, rosemary)

6 cups chopped fresh plum tomatoes

¼ cup organic tomato paste

1 tablespoon coconut sugar

1 to 2 tablespoons red wine vinegar

Heat the olive oil in an 11- or 12-inch, deep skillet over medium heat. Add the onion and sauté for about 5 minutes, or until softened. Add the garlic and sea salt and sauté about 2 minutes more.

Add the herbs, tomatoes, tomato paste, sugar, and vinegar and simmer, uncovered, over low heat for 20 to 30 minutes.

Spoon the sauce mixture into blender and blend on high until smooth.

Yield: 1 quart

ALMOND-LIME DIPPING SAUCE

This sauce is delicious served with sautéed chicken or tofu for dipping or over steamed vegetables or a cooked whole grain. You can also use other nut butters in place of the almond butter. Try cashew butter, peanut butter, or sunflower seed butter for some tasty alternatives.

6 tablespoons almond butter
¼ cup freshly squeezed lime juice
¼ cup coconut milk

1 to 2 tablespoons wheat-free tamari or coconut aminos
1 tablespoon honey or pure maple syrup
1 to 2 garlic cloves, crushed

Place all the ingredients into a bowl and whisk together until the mixture is thickened and well combined. For a thinner consistency, add water.

Yield: 1 cup

GARLIC-GINGER-KUDZU SAUCE

Serve this sauce over sautéed broccoli, tofu, chicken, or baked fish. It is also wonderful served over the **Lemon Millet Patties (page 288)**.

1 cup water
2 tablespoons kudzu
3 to 4 tablespoons wheat-free tamari or coconut aminos
2 to 3 tablespoons brown rice vinegar or coconut vinegar

1 tablespoon pure maple syrup or honey
2 to 3 teaspoons hot pepper sesame oil
1 garlic clove, crushed
1 to 2 teaspoons grated fresh ginger

Place all the ingredients into a small saucepan and mix well to dissolve the kudzu.

Place the pan over medium heat and bring to a gentle simmer. Reduce the heat to low and simmer for about 5 minutes, stirring constantly, or until the sauce has thickened and is clear.

Remove the sauce from the heat. Taste and adjust ingredients as necessary.

Yield: 1½ cups

LEMON-TAHINI SAUCE

Tahini is made from ground sesame seeds and is very high in calcium. Serve this creamy and light sauce over steamed vegetables—it's especially good over asparagus. You can also add more water and use it as a salad dressing.

½ cup sesame tahini

2 to 3 teaspoons finely grated lemon zest

½ cup freshly squeezed lemon juice

¼ cup extra-virgin olive oil

3 to 4 tablespoons water

2 garlic cloves, crushed

½ to 1 teaspoon sea salt

Place all the ingredients into a small bowl and whisk together with a fork. Taste and add more salt if necessary. For a thinner consistency, add more water.

Yield: 1½ cups

MISO SAUCE

Serve this sauce over steamed vegetables, baked fish, or a cooked whole grain. We use gluten-free, soy-free miso from the South River Miso Company.

¼ cup gluten-free miso

3 tablespoons water

2 tablespoons toasted sesame oil

1 tablespoon honey

2 to 3 teaspoons brown rice vinegar or coconut vinegar

dash hot pepper sesame oil

Whisk together all the ingredients in a small bowl. For a thinner consistency, add more water.

Yield: ¾ cup

WARM BERRY SAUCE

Serve this scrumptious sauce over pancakes for breakfast, or with chocolate cake for dessert. The sauce can be made with only one fruit or a combination of a few—try blueberries, raspberries, strawberries, or blackberries.

---

1 to 2 tablespoons kudzu
1 cup organic apple or berry juice

2 cups fresh or frozen organic berries

Place the kudzu, juice, and berries into a blender and purée until very smooth. Use 1 tablespoon kudzu for a thinner sauce or 2 tablespoons for a thicker sauce.

If using raspberries or blackberries, you may want to strain the purée through a fine-mesh strainer to remove the seeds.

Add the purée to a small saucepan over medium heat. Bring to a simmer, whisking continuously until the mixture has thickened and is translucent. Serve warm.

Yield: 2 cups

ORANGE-HONEY-FIG JAM

If you want a beautiful dark, ruby-colored jam, use a darker-colored fig for this recipe, such as black mission or brown turkey figs. Serve a dollop of the jam on buttered toast. This jam also makes a great accompaniment to an appetizer plate with sliced tart apples and hard cheeses.

6 cups chopped fresh figs (about 3 pints)
½ cup honey
1 teaspoon finely grated orange zest

¼ cup freshly squeezed orange juice
1 cinnamon stick

Place the figs in a blender or food processor and blend on low until you reach a slightly chunky purée. Pour the fig purée into a 4- to 6-quart pot and add the honey, orange zest, orange juice, and cinnamon stick and bring to a boil, stirring constantly (I use a silicone spatula). Reduce the heat to low and simmer for 25 to 30 minutes, stirring occasionally. Watch carefully; you will need to keep your heat low enough so that the jam doesn't burn, yet still maintain a gentle simmer. Keep stirring to help release some of the moisture. Remove and discard the cinnamon stick. Scoop the cooked jam into four clean ½-pint jars, screw on the lids, and store in the refrigerator.

> **Tip:** It is best to use a wide pot for this, or even a deep skillet, so that the moisture can easily escape and the jam can reduce.

Yield: 4 cups

RAW BLUEBERRY-CHIA JAM

I love making jam in the summertime, and with all of the organic blueberries our family picks, I do both canned and raw versions. This raw jam recipe captures all of the amazing flavors and bright colors found in blueberries, not to mention the protective polyphenols. Spread it onto whole-grain toast for breakfast, raw crackers as a snack, or dollop over your favorite breakfast porridge.

2 cups fresh blueberries

1 tablespoon whole chia seeds

2 tablespoons raw honey

2 teaspoons freshly squeezed lemon juice

Place all the ingredients into a high-powered blender and blend until completely smooth, scraping down the sides and blending again as needed.

Pour the jam into a clean glass jar, cover, and place into the refrigerator to thicken for about 4 hours before using. The jam will last in the refrigerator for up to 1 week.

Yield: 1½ cups

21

HEALTHY SNACKS

The first wealth is health.
—*Ralph Waldo Emerson*

Snacking in between meals on wholesome food is a great way to keep blood sugar levels stable, energy levels high, and can even help you from overeating at a single meal. Snacking is very important for children, pregnant and lactating women, and endurance athletes as their energy demands are very high.

This chapter provides a few nutritious snack recipes, most of which can be packaged to take with you during the day or packed in your child's lunch box.

QUICK NUTRITIOUS SNACK IDEAS

✓ Hummus spread onto flax crackers such as Mary's Gone Crackers
✓ Wild Alaskan salmon jerky
✓ Organic celery sticks dipped in raw almond butter
✓ Nori Rolls (page 272)
✓ Organic Popcorn (page 369) cooked in virgin coconut oil on the stovetop
✓ Raw kale chips and a glass of kombucha
✓ A handful of raw walnuts and sliced organic apples
✓ Trail mix made from raw nuts and dried fruit
✓ Raw assorted organic vegetables (cauliflower, carrots, red bell pepper) dipped in Lemon-Tahini Sauce (page 358) or Hummus (page 344)
✓ Fresh organic seasonal fruit
✓ Frozen fruit, such as cherries, blueberries, raspberries, and peaches. This is a great snack for children to enjoy any time of day.
✓ Steamed yams
✓ Sliced avocado and sprouted pumpkin seeds

AUTUMN HARVEST TRAIL MIX

Walnuts have essential fatty acids and melatonin for improving mood. Pumpkin seeds are an excellent source of zinc, and provide lignan compounds that assist in balancing our intestinal organisms. Figs are a great source of fiber and potassium. Raisins are one of the top sources of the trace mineral, boron, which helps to provide protection against osteoporosis.

1 cup raw walnuts

1 cup raw pumpkin seeds

1 cup dried figs

1 cup raisins

2 cups dried apple slices

Place all the ingredients into a large glass jar and shake gently to combine. Store in a cool, dry place.

Yield: 5 cups

Tip: To make the trail mix more digestible, and its nutrients more bioavailable, soak the nuts and seeds in filtered water in a small bowl for 8 to 24 hours. Then drain, rinse, and dehydrate at 105 to 115°F until crispy, 12 to 24 hours.

SUPER ANTIOXIDANT TRAIL MIX

The antioxidants in this trail mix are indeed "super." Antioxidants are chemicals that have been shown to fight cancer, heart disease, and aging. The almonds provide the antioxidant vitamin E; in fact, ¼ cup of almonds provides nearly half of your daily need for this vitamin. Scientific research has demonstrated that eating almonds daily can significantly lower your risk of heart disease. Dried apricots contain significant amounts of the powerful antioxidant beta-carotene. This vitamin quenches free radical damage to cells and tissues. Dark chocolate is high in plant phenols, specifically called cacao phenols. These antioxidants work to reduce free radical damage in the body. In fact, dark chocolate has the highest ORAC (oxygen radical absorbance capacity) value per 100 grams when compared to other foods such as raisins, kale, spinach, and broccoli. Blueberries' famed antioxidant power comes from phytochemicals called anthocyanidins, which also gives them their dark bluish-purple color. These antioxidants neutralize free radical damage to the collagen matrix of cells and tissues. Remember to always purchase organic, unsulphured dried fruit and organic dark chocolate.

---

1 cup raw sprouted almonds	½ cup dried blueberries
1 cup dried apricots	½ cup organic dark chocolate chips or raw cacao nibs

---

Place all the ingredients into a large glass jar and shake gently to combine. Store in a cool, dry place.

Yield: 3 cups

BROWN RICE CRISPY TREATS

Serve these tasty and nutritious treats to children for an after-school snack. They are also great to take with you on a camping or hiking trip. We like to use Erewhon's Gluten-Free Crispy Brown Rice Cereal, which can be found at most health food stores.

---

2 to 3 tablespoons virgin coconut oil, plus more for greasing the pan
1 cup brown rice syrup or coconut nectar
¾ cup almond butter or unsalted peanut butter
1 teaspoon vanilla extract
6 cups Brown Rice Crispy Cereal

OPTIONAL ADDITIONS
¼ cup sesame seeds
½ cup pumpkin or sunflower seeds
½ cup chopped nuts (cashew, almond, walnut)
½ to ¾ cup raisins or dried cranberries

OPTIONAL TOPPING
¾ cup organic dark chocolate chips
3 tablespoons virgin coconut oil

Grease a 9 x 13-inch glass baking pan with coconut oil and set aside.

To make the rice crispy treats, heat the coconut oil in a medium saucepan over medium heat. Add the brown rice syrup and nut butter and heat until tiny bubbles form, stirring constantly with a wire whisk. Immediately take the pan off the heat and stir in the vanilla.

Place the cereal into a large bowl and add any of the optional additions. Pour the hot syrup mixture over it and immediately mix together with a wooden spoon.

Pour the mixture into the prepared pan and press the mixture flat. You may need to place a little coconut oil or water on your hands so the mixture won't stick to them.

If you would like to add the chocolate topping, place the dark chocolate in a heavy-bottomed saucepan over very low heat, stirring occasionally, until completely melted. Pour over the top of the crispy treats, spreading it evenly with the back of a spoon. Sometimes I top half of the pan with chocolate and leave the other half plain. Cool completely before slicing into bars.

Yield: 15 squares

> **Tip:** If you are gluten-sensitive then be sure to use a rice crispy cereal that is gluten-free, as some brands do contain barley malt, which contains gluten.

RAW ENERGY BALLS

This is a great snack to take with you on a long hike or a long day at work. You can also add one to your child's lunch box for a sweet, nutritious treat.

1 cup raw sprouted almonds or walnuts

1 cup Medjool dates, pitted

¼ cup raisins

¼ teaspoon ground cinnamon

¼ teaspoon ground cardamom

¼ cup raw almond butter

½ cup shredded organic coconut

In a food processor fitted with the "s" blade, process the almonds until finely ground. Add the dates, raisins, and spices and grind to a fine meal. Add the almond butter and process again until thoroughly mixed.

Form the mixture into balls and roll in shredded coconut.

Store in a sealed container on the countertop for up to 3 days, or refrigerate for up to 3 weeks.

Yield: 1 dozen balls

CHEEZY KALE CHIPS

Craving something salty and crunchy? Instead of reaching for a bag of potato chips, try making these. You can bake them at a low temperature or use a food dehydrator. I prefer to dehydrate them, which keeps all of the nutrients intact.

---

2 large bunches green curly kale

SAUCE
1 cup raw cashews
1 cup water
½ cup chopped red bell pepper

2 tablespoons freshly squeezed lemon juice
¼ cup nutritional yeast
2 garlic cloves
½ to 1 teaspoon sea salt or Herbamare

Rinse the kale and remove the tough rib that runs down the center of each leaf. Tear the kale leaves into big pieces and place into a large bowl or 8-quart pot.

Place all the sauce ingredients into a high-powered blender and blend on high until ultrasmooth and creamy. Pour the sauce over the kale and massage it in, making sure that it covers all of the leaves. Place the kale into 4 to 5 trays of a food dehydrator and set to 115°F. Dehydrate for 6 to 8 hours, or until crispy.

If you don't have a dehydrator, place the kale onto 2 to 3 large baking sheets lined with unbleached parchment paper and bake for about 2 hours at 200°F, or until crispy. Flip the kale chips part way through baking time using a spatula. Watch carefully and remove the kale chips as soon as they have crisped up.

Yield: 4 servings

POPCORN

Once you begin to make your own popcorn, you won't ever want to go back to eating microwave popcorn! Popcorn makers are another popular way of making popcorn, but unfortunately the combination of the heat and the plastic can cause highly toxic plastic compounds to leach into the popcorn. We prefer to use the age-old method of cooking the kernels in a large pot on the stovetop. Once cooked, the popcorn can be seasoned in a variety of ways. You can use plain sea salt, Herbamare, nutritional yeast, dried herbs, or even a combination of a little organic butter and maple syrup!

3 to 4 tablespoons virgin coconut oil   1 to 2 cups organic popcorn kernels
½ teaspoon sea salt

Heat an 8-quart stainless steel pot over medium-high to high heat, then add the coconut oil and sea salt.

Once the oil has melted, quickly add the popcorn kernels, cover the pot with a lid, and shake the pot continuously to prevent burning.

The popcorn is done once you hear very few popping sounds. Immediately remove the pot from the heat source and pour the popcorn into a large glass bowl. Add your favorite seasonings to taste.

Yield: 4 to 6 servings

FRESH FRUITSICLES

This is a great way to use and store fresh fruit from the summer harvest. I like to have many Popsicle molds on hand and make all sorts of different flavor combinations. Using the whole fruit makes for a healthful snack alternative to the sugary Popsicles you buy at the store. Below are a few different ideas. Try some, then create your own combinations. Use stainless steel Popsicle molds or small paper or glass drinking cups with a wooden Popsicle stick inserted to avoid exposure to plasticizing chemicals like BPA and phthalates.

STRAWBERRY-BANANA-COCONUT

1 to 2 cups fresh strawberries, trimmed	½ cup coconut milk
1 ripe banana, peeled and cut into chunks	1 to 2 tablespoons raw honey

STRAWBERRY-PEACH-ORANGE

1 to 2 cups fresh strawberries, trimmed	½ cup freshly squeezed orange juice
1 ripe peach or nectarine, cut into chunks	1 to 2 tablespoons raw honey

BLUEBERRY-CHERRY-APPLE

1 cup fresh blueberries	½ cup organic apple juice
1 cup fresh cherries, pitted	1 to 2 tablespoons raw honey

Place all the ingredients for the fruitsicles into a blender and blend until smooth.

Pour the mixture into Popsicle molds, insert sticks, and freeze for 6 to 8 hours, or overnight.

To release the fruitsicles from the mold simply run under hot water for about 30 seconds.

Yield: 6 fruitsicles

WATERMELON WHOLE FRUIT POPSICLES

I love making these healthy Popsicles full of fresh antioxidant-rich fruits. All of the children I've served these to have loved them. The colors of the fruit are so vibrant and beautiful—no toxic food dyes needed! Use any fresh organic fruit you have on hand. I like using contrasting colors because it makes the Popsicles look so pretty! Don't forget to use seedless watermelon!

3 cups watermelon purée (about ¼ to ½ of a watermelon)

½ cup fresh blueberries

½ cup fresh cherries, pitted and chopped

½ cup chopped fresh strawberries

1 kiwi, peeled and sliced

1 peach or nectarine, diced

Cut the watermelon into chunks and purée it in a blender until smooth. Set aside.

Set out about 1 dozen Popsicle molds (the amount needed will vary depending on size of molds). Fill each one halfway with the blueberries and chopped fresh fruit, then pour in the watermelon purée until each mold is filled to the top. Place a Popsicle stick into each one, and then freeze for 6 to 8 hours.

When ready to serve, run the Popsicle molds under warm water for a few seconds to release from the mold.

Yield: about 1 dozen

Variation: Use puréed honeydew melon or cantaloupe in place of the watermelon.

22

NUTRITIOUS DESSERTS

Sharing food with another human being is an intimate act that should not be indulged in lightly.
—M. F. K. Fisher

Removing refined sugar from your diet is a big step toward improving your overall health and vitality. This type of sugar has been stripped of all of its natural vitamins and minerals, and when consumed, leaves the body susceptible to large spikes in blood sugar, mood swings, lowered immunity, and a host of other short- and long-term health problems. Eating a healthy balanced diet full of vegetables, meats, whole grains, beans, and fresh fruits usually eliminates the cravings for refined sweets. However, sweetness is an important flavor to have in the diet and need not be eliminated completely. It balances other flavors in the diet including bitter, salty, pungent, and sour. Your overall diet will be much more satisfying with the occasional consumption of natural sweets. By wisely adding these, you will find that cravings for junk food will wane and bingeing will disappear. The following recipes contain natural sweeteners combined with other wholesome ingredients such as fresh or dried fruit and nuts, whole-grain flours, and healthy fats to create a satisfying yet nutrient-packed way to round out your meals.

FRESH STRAWBERRIES WITH HONEY-LEMON-CASHEW SAUCE

Serve this dessert in late spring or early summer when the strawberries are in peak season. In mid-summer, try pouring the cashew sauce over a bowl of fresh raspberries, blueberries, peaches, or apricots for a delicious, seasonal dessert.

1 pound fresh organic strawberries

SAUCE
1 cup raw cashews
½ teaspoon finely grated lemon zest
¼ cup freshly squeezed lemon juice

¼ cup honey or pure maple syrup
1 to 2 tablespoons water, or as needed
1 to 2 teaspoons nonalcoholic vanilla extract
pinch sea salt

Rinse and trim the strawberries and place into a serving bowl.

To make the sauce, place all of the ingredients into a high-powered blender and blend until creamy and smooth, adding more water if necessary.

Drizzle the cashew sauce over the fresh strawberries and serve.

Yield: 4 servings

SPRING RHUBARB AND GINGER COMPOTE

Tart and tangy rhubarb is the quintessential "fruit" of spring. Of course rhubarb is not a fruit, but rather a vegetable, though its culinary use is much like a fruit. In most climates it comes up before any other fruits are available making it the perfect component of a spring dessert. Serve compote over homemade ice cream, or topped with the Cashew Cream recipe (page 377), sliced strawberries, and a sprig of fresh mint if desired.

½ pound fresh rhubarb stalks, cut into 1-inch pieces

¼ to ½ cup honey

2 tablespoons freshly squeezed orange juice

1 tablespoon arrowroot powder

1 teaspoon finely grated orange zest

½ to 1 teaspoon grated fresh ginger

pinch sea salt

Place the rhubarb pieces and honey into a 2-quart pot.

In a small bowl, whisk together the 2 tablespoons of the orange juice and arrowroot powder and add it to the pot with the rhubarb. Add the remaining ingredients and stir gently.

Place the pot over medium heat on the stovetop. Simmer, uncovered, for 5 to 6 minutes. Be very careful not to overcook the rhubarb, as it will get very mushy if cooked for too long.

Transfer the compote to a glass bowl and cool in the refrigerator. To serve, spoon the chilled compote into individual serving bowls, top with cashew cream, strawberries, and mint sprigs if desired.

Yield: 4 to 6 servings

DRIED FRUIT COMPOTE WITH CASHEW CREAM

This recipe makes for a wonderful winter dessert when fresh fruit is not in season. I like to dehydrate fresh apples, pears, and plums in the fall when they are abundant and falling off the trees. We store our dried fruit in glass jars in our pantry to use during the winter months. If you are sensitive to nuts, top the compote with a dollop of organic Greek yogurt or Coconut Milk Yogurt (page 104) mixed with a little raw honey.

FRUT COMPOTE

½ cup dried apricot halves

½ cup dried apples

½ cup dried pear halves

½ cup prunes

¼ cup dried cherries

2 cinnamon sticks

2 cups water

½ cup raisins

¼ cup honey

freshly squeezed juice of 1 small lemon

fresh mint leaves, for garnish

CASHEW CREAM

½ cup raw cashews

2 to 3 tablespoons pure maple syrup

2 to 3 tablespoons water

1 to 2 teaspoons nonalcoholic vanilla extract

To make the compote, place the dried fruit into a large pot with the cinnamon sticks and water and heat gently until almost boiling. Cover the pot, lower the heat, and simmer gently for 12 to 15 minutes, or until the fruit has softened.

Remove the pot from the heat, add the raisins and honey, and stir to combine. Cover the pot with the lid and let cool.

To make the cashew cream, add the cashews, maple syrup, water, and vanilla to a high-powered blender and blend until smooth and creamy.

Once the compote has cooled, remove and discard the cinnamon sticks and stir in the lemon juice. Serve in small containers at room temperature with a dollop of cashew cream. Garnish with fresh mint leaves.

Yield: 4 to 6 servings

CHERRY-APPLE PUDDING WITH ALMOND CREAM

Serve this easy-to-make pudding at the peak of cherry season when fresh cherries are in abundance. You can also use frozen cherries if fresh are not available. Serve this pudding to older babies or toddlers without the almond cream for a healthy treat.

PUDDING

4 tablespoons kudzu

2 to 3 tablespoons water

1 cup organic apple juice

2 cups fresh or frozen pitted cherries

2 to 4 tablespoons pure maple syrup

ALMOND CREAM

1 cup raw cashews

¼ cup honey or pure maple syrup

2 to 3 tablespoons water

1 to 2 teaspoons nonalcoholic vanilla extract

½ to 1 teaspoon organic almond extract

GARNISH

fresh cherries, stems attached

finely chopped raw almonds (optional)

To make the pudding, place the kudzu and water in a small saucepan, stir with a fork, and let stand for 2 to 4 minutes until the kudzu has completely dissolved.

Place the juice, cherries, and maple syrup into a blender and blend on high until very smooth. Pour the cherry juice mixture into the pan with the kudzu slurry.

Place the saucepan over medium heat and cook, stirring continuously with a wire whisk, until thick and clear, 5 to 10 minutes. Remove from the heat and pour the pudding into parfait glasses or small, individual serving bowls. Transfer to the refrigerator to set; it will take about 30 minutes to 1 hour.

To make the almond cream, place all the ingredients into a high-powered blender and blend on high until thick and creamy. Taste and adjust sweetness if necessary.

To serve, place a large dollop of almond cream atop each dish of cherry pudding. Place a whole cherry in the middle of the cream and sprinkle with chopped raw almonds if desired.

Yield: 6 servings

LEMON-BLUEBERRY PUDDING

Children will love this rich yet nutritious dessert. Tapioca is the starch from the root of the cassava plant—a shrubby tropical plant that is grown for its large, tuberous, starchy roots.

1½ cups water	¾ cup freshly squeezed lemon juice
½ cup small pearl tapioca	½ teaspoon sea salt
1 cup raw cashews	1½ cups fresh or frozen blueberries
1 cup pure maple syrup	1 tablespoon vanilla extract
2 cups water	½ teaspoon organic lemon flavoring

Place the water and tapioca pearls in a 3- or 4-quart pot and soak for 1 hour.

Place the cashews, maple syrup, water, lemon juice, and sea salt into a high-powered blender and blend on high for 1 to 2 minutes until smooth and creamy. Add the blueberries, vanilla, and lemon flavoring and blend on high again for 1 to 2 minutes more, or until very smooth and creamy.

Add this mixture to the pot of soaked tapioca pearls, stir well, and bring to a boil. Reduce the heat to a low simmer, stirring frequently, for about 15 minutes, or until the pudding has thickened and tapioca pearls are translucent.

Pour the pudding into small serving bowls and chill in the refrigerator; the pudding will thicken as it cools.

Yield: 6 servings

PUMPKIN PUDDING

This recipe is another version of our Lemon-Blueberry Pudding. It is delicious served in the fall and wintertime when pumpkins and other winter squash are in abundance. See page 260 for directions on baking pumpkins and other winter squash.

1½ cups water

½ cup small pearl tapioca

1 cup raw cashews

2 cups water

½ cup pure maple syrup

2 cups baked sugar pie pumpkin or other winter squash

1 tablespoon freshly squeezed lemon juice

2 teaspoons vanilla extract

½ teaspoon sea salt

½ teaspoon ground cinnamon

¼ teaspoon ground ginger

¼ teaspoon ground nutmeg

pinch ground cloves

Place the water and tapioca pearls in a 3- or 4-quart pot and let soak 1 hour.

Place cashews, water, and maple syrup in a blender and blend on high for 1 to 2 minutes or until smooth and creamy. Add the pumpkin, lemon juice, vanilla, sea salt, and spices and blend for 1 to 2 minutes more, or until very smooth and creamy.

Transfer this mixture to the pot of soaked pearl tapioca and whisk together and bring to a boil while stirring. Reduce the heat to low and simmer, stirring frequently, for about 15 minutes, or until the pudding has thickened and the tapioca pearls are translucent.

Pour the pudding into small serving bowls and chill in the refrigerator; the pudding will thicken as it cools.

Yield: 6 servings

RAW CHOCOLATE–AVOCADO PUDDING

When our second daughter was 2 years old she spent a lot of time with our friends who were raw foodists. Chocolate avocado pudding was one of the treats she would get at their house. It is such a delicious way to have children eat avocados! Top each serving of pudding with goji berries, shredded coconut, hemp seeds, or chopped sprouted almonds if desired.

½ cup packed Medjool dates, pitted

3 large avocados (about 2 heaping cups mashed)

6 tablespoons raw cacao powder

2 tablespoons pure maple syrup

1 tablespoon nonalcoholic vanilla extract

Put the dates into a small bowl and cover with warm water. Let soak for about 30 minutes, then drain.

Place the mashed avocados, dates, cacao powder, maple syrup, and vanilla into a high-powered blender or food processor and blend until supersmooth and creamy; you may need to stop the machine multiple times and scrape down the sides. Taste and add more maple syrup if desired.

Transfer the pudding to a glass container to chill or serve immediately. The pudding will keep in the refrigerator for up to 3 days.

Yield: six ½-cup servings

HEALTHY FRUIT GEL

Using agar flakes or gelatin and organic fruit juice creates a nutritious dessert without all of the sugar, artificial flavors, and dyes found in packaged Jell-O mixes. This recipe makes for a light, nutritious dessert or snack that children will love. Try pouring it into parfait glasses with sliced cherries at the bottom. Sprinkle the top with shredded organic coconut for a deliciously simple dessert.

---

4 cups organic fruit juice

2 tablespoons agar flakes or unflavored gelatin

virgin coconut oil, for the pan

sliced fresh fruit (optional)

Pour the juice into a 2-quart saucepan and stir in agar flakes or gelatin. Set aside for 15 minutes so the agar flakes or gelatin can soften. Bring to a boil, then reduce the heat and simmer gently, stirring constantly, for 5 to 10 minutes, or until the agar flakes have completely dissolved.

Lightly grease a 9 x 13-inch pan with coconut oil. Place any sliced fresh fruit you would like on the bottom of the pan. Pour the juice mixture into the pan.

> **Tip:** Look for kosher gelatin that comes from grass-fed cows. I buy it online from www.GreatLakesGelatin.com.

Chill in the refrigerator for about 1 hour. Before serving let pan sit at room temperature for 10 to 15 minutes. Cut into squares or spoon into small bowls. Store in the refrigerator for up to a week.

Yield: 6 to 8 servings

RAW CHOCOLATE–WALNUT TRUFFLES

These healthful and easy-to-make little treats are always a crowd-pleaser. They can be made a day ahead of time and stored in a covered container in your refrigerator until ready to serve.

2 cups raw walnuts
1 cup Medjool dates, pitted
4 to 6 tablespoons raw cacao powder

pinch sea salt
shredded organic coconut

Put the walnuts into a food processor fitted with the "s" blade and process until very finely ground and pasty.

Add the dates, cacao powder, and sea salt and continue to process until well combined.

Roll the mixture into small balls and place into a bowl of shredded coconut. Make sure each ball gets coated in coconut, then transfer to a plate. Store in the refrigerator until ready to serve.

Yield: 1½ dozen truffles

RAW SUPERFOOD FUDGE

A decadent dessert that is also nutritious? Yes! This raw fudge recipe serves as a sweet treat and a powerhouse of nutrients, including medium-chain triglycerides from the coconut oil, antioxidants in the raw cacao, vitamin C and amino acids in the goji berries, and essential fatty acids in the chia seeds. Sometimes I will have a little piece of this raw fudge with a green smoothie for breakfast!

¾ cup raw cashew butter

½ cup melted virgin coconut oil

6 tablespoons raw cacao powder

¼ teaspoon organic vanilla powder

pinch sea salt

1 cup pitted Medjool dates

½ cup goji berries

2 to 3 tablespoons white chia seeds

Line an 8.5 x 4.5-inch glass bread pan with unbleached parchment paper.

Place the cashew butter, melted coconut oil, raw cacao powder, vanilla powder, and sea salt into a food processor fitted with the "s" blade and process until a paste forms. Add the dates and process again until smooth. Add the goji berries and chia seeds and pulse to combine. For a smoother fudge, add all ingredients to a high-powered blender except for the goji berries and chia seeds, and blend until smooth. Stir in the berries and seeds.

Using oiled hands, press the fudge mixture evenly into the pan. Transfer the pan to the refrigerator to chill until hardened. Once solid, you can slice the fudge into small squares. Store the fudge squares in your freezer or in your refrigerator.

> **Tip:** Make sure you are using soft, dried dates. Older dates tend to lose moisture and become harder to blend, especially in a recipe like this.

Yield: about 12 to 16 servings

RAW BERRY TART WITH A COCONUT PASTRY CREAM

Be sure to keep this tart refrigerated until ready to serve. You'll need a food processor to make the crust and a high-powered blender for the filling. For the crust, we use truly raw organic almonds that have been soaked for 12 to 24 hours and then dehydrated at a low temperature (this step is optional). This makes the nuts far more digestible; the dehydration process makes them shelf stable. For the fruit, try adding sliced peaches, pitted cherries, or sliced kiwi in addition to the berries if desired.

CRUST

1½ cups raw almonds

½ cup raw pecans

1 cup Medjool dates, pitted

1 tablespoon virgin coconut oil, plus more for greasing the pan

pinch sea salt

FILLING

1 cup raw cashews

¼ cup water

¼ cup freshly squeezed orange juice

3 to 4 tablespoons coconut nectar or honey

¾ cup softened coconut butter

1 to 2 teaspoons nonalcoholic vanilla extract

½ to 1 teaspoon organic almond flavoring

FRUIT

strawberries, halved

raspberries

blackberries

blueberries

To make the crust, first grease a 10-inch tart pan with a removable bottom. Place the nuts into a food processor fitted with the "s" blade and process until finely ground. Add the dates, coconut oil, and sea salt and process again until the dates are ground and evenly incorporated into the nuts. It should stick together; if not, add another tablespoon of coconut oil. Pour the crust mixture into the tart pan and press evenly into the bottom and up the sides of the pan.

To make the filling, place the cashews, water, orange juice, and coconut nectar into a high-powered blender and blend until smooth and ultracreamy, stopping and starting the blender if necessary.

The coconut butter should be soft enough to add if you are living in a hot climate; if not, place it into a small pan and warm on the lowest heat. Add the softened coconut butter to the blender along with the vanilla and almond extracts and blend until smooth.

To assemble the tart, pour the filling into the crust and spread it out evenly. Arrange the berries over the filling in your own unique design. Chill the tart, uncovered, until ready to serve. When ready to serve, push the bottom of the tart pan up through the rim and place onto a platter to serve.

Yield: about 10 servings

CHOCOLATE-RASPBERRY-HAZELNUT TART

This decadent vegan tart can be made with any berry, but I especially like the combination of tart raspberries and sweet chocolate. The tart is best served the day it's made. You can also use a smaller tart pan (an 8-inch works well) and halve the ingredients. Be sure to use the full-fat coconut milk that comes in a can.

CRUST

3 cups hazelnut meal

¾ cup arrowroot powder

¼ cup coconut sugar

¾ teaspoon sea salt

6 tablespoons cold virgin coconut oil, plus more for greasing the pan

2 to 3 tablespoons cold water

FILLING

2 cups raw cashews (soaked for 3 hours)

½ cup raw cacao powder

½ cup pure maple syrup

½ cup full-fat coconut milk

1 to 2 teaspoons nonalcoholic vanilla extract

1 pint fresh raspberries

Preheat the oven to 350°F. Grease an 11-inch round tart pan with coconut oil.

To make the crust, place the hazelnut meal, arrowroot powder, coconut sugar, and sea salt into a bowl and mix together. Add the coconut oil and mix it in, using your fingers or a pastry cutter, until fine crumbs form. Add the water and stir together with a wooden spoon until the mixture forms a ball. Press the dough into the bottom and up the sides of the tart pan. Bake the tart for about 25 minutes, then remove from the oven and cool completely. I like to put it into the refrigerator to speed up the cooling process.

To make the filling, place the cashews into a bowl of water and let soak for about 3 hours; then drain and rinse.

Place soaked cashews into a high-powered blender, add the cacao powder, maple syrup, coconut milk, and vanilla and blend until supersmooth, adding more coconut milk by the tablespoonful if needed.

To assemble the tart, pour the chocolate filling into the cooled crust and chill for 2 hours. Pop the tart out of the pan by pushing it up from the bottom. Transfer to a serving platter. Decorate the top with the raspberries and serve.

Yield: about 10 servings

ZESTY LEMON TART

Serve this simple, nutritious, grain-free, vegan dessert for brunch or after a special occasion meal. The ground turmeric gives the filling a beautiful yellow hue; add more or less depending on how bright you would like the tart to be!

CRUST

1½ cups blanched almond flour

¼ cup arrowroot powder

1 tablespoon coconut flour

½ teaspoon sea salt

¼ cup virgin coconut oil, plus more for greasing the dish

1 tablespoon honey or coconut nectar

2 tablespoons water

FILLING

1½ cups almond or cashew milk

½ cup freshly squeezed lemon juice

⅓ cup honey or coconut nectar

2 tablespoons arrowroot powder

2 teaspoons agar powder

pinch ground turmeric

pinch sea salt

Preheat the oven to 350°F. Lightly grease an 8 x 8-inch baking dish with coconut oil.

To make the crust, whisk together the almond flour, arrowroot, coconut flour, and sea salt in a small bowl. Cut in the coconut oil using your hands or a pastry cutter. Add the honey and water and stir together using a fork.

Form the dough into a ball with your hands and place into the baking dish, pressing it evenly into the baking dish. Bake in the oven for about 25 minutes. Then remove from oven and cool.

To make the filling, place all the ingredients into a blender and blend on high for about 30 seconds. Pour into a 2-quart saucepan and bring to a rapid simmer, whisking constantly. Reduce the heat to medium-low and cook for 5 to 7 minutes. Pour the filling over the cooled crust and place into the refrigerator to set; this should take about 2 hours. Slice the tart and serve. Store any leftovers in the refrigerator for up to a week.

Yield: about 12 small squares

RAW CHOCOLATE–HAZELNUT BROWNIES

These brownies are amazingly fast to prepare and require no baking. You will need a food processor for this recipe. A high-quality cocoa powder can make all the difference with this recipe—we use organic raw cacao powder for the best flavor and highest nutritional value.

---

1 cup raw hazelnuts

½ cup raw almonds

1½ cups Medjool dates, pitted

½ cup raw almond butter

4 to 6 tablespoons raw cacao powder

3 tablespoons shredded organic coconut

Place the hazelnuts and almonds into a food processor fitted with the "s" blade and process until finely ground.

Add the pitted dates, raw almond butter, and cacao powder and process until completely mixed. You can add more or less cacao powder depending on how rich you like your brownies.

Firmly press the mixture evenly into an 8 x 8-inch square pan and sprinkle with shredded coconut. Cut into squares when ready to serve. Refrigerate in a covered container for up to 2 weeks.

Yield: 16 small brownies

> **Tip:** For greater digestibility of the nuts, place them into a bowl of water and soak overnight; drain and rinse. Place nuts into your dehydrator and dehydrate until crispy before using in a raw food recipe like this one.

BLUEBERRY FRUIT PIE WITH RAW NUT CRUST

Don't be fooled by the long list of ingredients. This lively fruit pie is relatively easy and fast to prepare and perfect for a summer picnic when fresh fruit is in season.

CRUST

1 cup raw pecans

1 cup raw almonds

½ teaspoon ground cinnamon

¼ teaspoon ground cardamom

¼ teaspoon ground ginger

1 cup Medjool dates, pitted

BLUEBERRY FILLING

6 tablespoons kudzu, dissolved in 2 to 3 tablespoons water

1½ cups organic berry juice or water

2 cups fresh or frozen blueberries

2 tablespoons pure maple syrup

CASHEW CREAM

1 cup raw cashews

¼ cup pure maple syrup

2 to 3 tablespoons water

2 teaspoons nonalcoholic extract

pinch sea salt

FRUIT TOPPING

1 large ripe mango, peeled and thinly sliced

1 large ripe peach, thinly sliced

2 kiwi fruit, peeled and thinly sliced

1 cup fresh berries

shredded coconut (optional)

To make the crust, place the raw pecans, raw almonds, cinnamon, cardamom, and ginger in a food processor fitted with the "s" blade and process until finely ground. Add the pitted dates and process until well combined. Transfer the mixture to a deep-dish 9-inch pie plate and press evenly onto the bottom and sides of the dish. Chill the crust while you are preparing the filling.

To make the blueberry filling, place the kudzu and water in a small saucepan and let stand for 2 to 4 minutes until the kudzu has completely dissolved. Pour the juice, blueberries, and maple syrup into a blender and blend on high until very smooth.

Pour the berry juice mixture and the kudzu mixture into a saucepan over medium heat and cook, stirring continuously, until thick and clear, 5 to 10 minutes. Remove from the heat and pour into the chilled pie crust. Return the pie to the refrigerator to set; it will take about 2 hours.

To make the cashew cream, rinse out the blender. Put the cashews, maple syrup, water, vanilla, and sea salt in the blender and blend on high until smooth and creamy. Set aside while you prepare the fruit topping.

Once the filling is set, remove the pie from the refrigerator, and spread the cashew cream over the filling. Place the sliced mango, peach, kiwi, and fresh berries in your own unique design over the cashew cream layer. Sprinkle with shredded coconut if desired. Return the pie to the refrigerator until ready to serve. The pie will keep for up to 3 days in the refrigerator. Leftovers make a wonderful breakfast!

Yield: 8 servings

Variation: Use raspberries, strawberries, or cherries instead of blueberries for the filling.

LEMON TEASCAKE

This recipe makes for a delicious vegan and gluten-free dessert. The recipe is adapted from a dessert served at the former Café Ambrosia restaurant in Seattle, Washington. Serve slices of pie with fresh raspberries and sliced kiwi fruit.

FILLING

½ cup uncooked millet

2 cups water

½ cup raw cashews

⅓ cup freshly squeezed lemon juice

½ cup pure maple syrup

2 teaspoons vanilla extract

1 teaspoon organic lemon flavoring

CRUST

1 cup organic gluten-free rolled oats, lightly ground

¼ cup brown rice flour

¼ cup arrowroot powder

½ cup raw walnuts, ground

½ teaspoon sea salt

1 teaspoon vanilla extract

3 tablespoons pure maple syrup

¼ cup melted virgin coconut oil

To cook the millet, rinse the millet in a fine-strainer under cold running water. Transfer the millet and water to a small pot with a tight-fitting lid and bring to a boil then turn the heat down to a low simmer and cook for 45 minutes.

While the millet is cooking prepare the crust. Preheat the oven to 350°F. In a small bowl, mix together the oats, brown rice flour, arrowroot powder, walnuts, and sea salt. In another small bowl, whisk together the vanilla, maple syrup, and coconut oil. Add the wet ingredients to the dry and mix together. Press into a 9-inch pie plate or a 9-inch spring form pan. Bake in the oven for 10 to 12 minutes. Let cool for at least 30 minutes.

Place the cashews, lemon juice, maple syrup, vanilla, and lemon flavoring into a high-powered blender and blend on high for 1 to 2 minutes or until the mixture resembles thick cream. Add the cooked millet to the blender and blend again on high until ultrasmooth, scraping down the blender jar as needed. Pour the filling into cooled crust. Let sit at room temperature for about an hour, then refrigerate for a few hours to set.

Yield: 8 servings

> **Tip:** Always use organic rolled oats, as the nonorganic varieties are sprayed with gut-damaging herbicides. I buy certified gluten-free, organic oats online; see the Resources section (page 429) for more information.

SPICED PUMPKIN PIE

This pie is a nutrient-packed dessert that is as delicious as it is healthy. Agar is a seaweed gel that will cause the filling, when cooked and cooled, to become firm. If I don't have any pumpkin purée on hand I bake a fresh sugar pie pumpkin or butternut squash and then measure out 3 cups of the cooked, mashed flesh. See page 260 for instructions on baking sugar pie pumpkins and other winter squash.

CRUST

- ⅓ cup raw pecans or walnuts
- 1 cup brown rice flour
- ½ cup arrowroot powder
- ½ teaspoon sea salt
- 6 tablespoons organic palm shortening or organic butter
- 4 to 5 tablespoons cold water

FILLING

- ¾ cup raw cashews
- ½ cup water
- 3 cups sugar pie pumpkin purée
- ¾ cup pure maple syrup
- ¼ cup arrowroot powder
- 1¼ teaspoons agar powder
- 2 teaspoons ground cinnamon
- 1 teaspoon ground ginger
- ¼ teaspoon ground nutmeg
- ¼ teaspoon ground cloves

Preheat the oven to 350°F. Set out one deep-dish 9-inch pie plate.

To make the crust, place the nuts, brown rice flour, arrowroot powder, and sea salt into a food processor fitted with the "s" blade and process until the nuts are finely ground into the flour. Add the palm shortening and pulse a few times to incorporate the fat into the flour. Add the water and process until the dough forms a ball. Press the dough into the pie plate, flute edges, and prebake for about 12 minutes.

To make the filling, place the cashews and water in a high-powered blender and blend until smooth. Add the remaining ingredients for the filling to the blender and blend until smooth. If you don't own a high-powered blender, then place the cashew mixture into a food processor, add the remaining filling ingredients, and process until smooth.

Pour the filling into the prebaked crust and bake for about 55 minutes. Let pie set at room temperature for 1 hour to cool, then refrigerate to set fully.

Yield: 8 servings

APPLE-WALNUT CRISP

Serve this simple, nutritious grain-free crisp in autumn when apples are in season. I like to make this dessert and serve it after a hearty meal of roasted organic chicken, root vegetables, and steamed kale.

FILLING

4 to 5 apples, cored and thinly sliced

1 tablespoon arrowroot powder

1 tablespoon pure maple syrup or honey

2 teaspoons ground cinnamon

¼ teaspoon ground nutmeg

TOPPING

2 cups raw walnuts

1 cup Medjool dates, pitted

¼ cup arrowroot powder

2 to 3 teaspoons ground cinnamon

2 to 4 tablespoons virgin coconut oil

⅛ teaspoon sea salt

Preheat the oven to 350°F. Set out an 8 x 8-inch glass baking dish.

To make the filling, place all the ingredients into the baking dish and toss together.

To make the topping, add the walnuts to a food processor fitted with the "s" blade and process until coarsely ground. Add the dates, arrowroot, cinnamon, coconut oil, and sea salt and process again until the dates are very finely ground and the mixture is combined.

Sprinkle the topping over the filling and bake the crisp for 35 to 40 minutes, or until the apples are juicy and bubbling. Serve warm.

Yield: 6 to 8 servings

Variation: Add ½ to 1 cup fresh or frozen cranberries to the filling along with an extra tablespoon of maple syrup or honey.

PEACH-BLUEBERRY CRISP

When purchasing rolled oats, be sure to always buy organic. You can order gluten-free, organic oats online if you can't find them locally. Nonorganic oats (including gluten-free) are sprayed with herbicides that damage the digestive system. You can use this topping with any fruit filling. Try apple-cranberry, blackberry-nectarine, or strawberry-rhubarb.

FILLING

- 4 to 5 medium peaches, sliced
- 2 heaping cups fresh blueberries
- 2 tablespoons coconut sugar or pure maple syrup
- 1 tablespoon arrowroot powder
- ¼ teaspoon cardamom
- ¼ teaspoon ground nutmeg

TOPPING

- 2 cups organic gluten-free rolled oats
- ¼ cup brown rice flour
- ¼ cup arrowroot powder
- 1 teaspoon ground cinnamon
- ⅛ teaspoon sea salt
- ½ cup melted virgin coconut oil or organic butter
- ¼ cup pure maple syrup

Preheat the oven to 375°F. Set out an 8 x 8-inch glass baking dish.

To make the filling, add all the ingredients to the baking dish and gently toss together.

To make the topping, place the rolled oats, brown rice flour, arrowroot powder, cinnamon, and sea salt into a bowl and mix well to combine. Add the melted coconut oil and maple syrup and stir together. Crumble the topping over the fruit.

Bake the crisp for about 40 minutes. Serve warm.

Yield: about 6 to 8 servings

RASPBERRY-RHUBARB COBBLER

I love making this summertime dessert when the raspberries are just coming into season. If raspberries are not available try fresh strawberries, blueberries, or pears!

FILLING

2 heaping cups fresh raspberries

2 cups diced rhubarb

¼ to ½ cup coconut sugar

2 tablespoons arrowroot powder

1 teaspoon finely grated orange zest (optional)

¼ teaspoon ground cardamom

TOPPING

1½ cups blanched almond flour

¼ cup coconut flour

¼ cup arrowroot powder

2 teaspoons baking powder

½ teaspoon sea salt

4 tablespoons organic palm shortening

3 large organic eggs

3 tablespoons pure maple syrup

Preheat the oven to 375°F. Set out an 8 x 8-inch glass baking dish.

To make the filling, add all the ingredients to the baking dish and toss together.

To make the topping, whisk together the almond flour, coconut flour, arrowroot powder, baking powder, and sea salt in a medium mixing bowl. Cut in the shortening using your fingers until pea-size crumbs form. Add the eggs and maple syrup and stir with a fork to combine.

Drop large spoonfuls of the topping onto the filling. I like to drop nine spoonfuls (three rows of three).

Bake the cobbler for approximately 35 minutes. Serve warm.

Yield: 6 to 9 servings

CHEWY CHOCOLATE CHIP COOKIES

These gluten-free cookies use Medjool dates as the main sweetener. Dates are rich in minerals and B vitamins. I always use sprouted brown rice flour when making these, but regular brown rice flour works as well. Serve the cookies with raw almond milk for a healthy treat!

1 cup Medjool dates, pitted

2 tablespoons ground golden flaxseeds

1 cup hot water

¾ cup melted virgin coconut oil, plus more for greasing the cookie sheet

¼ cup coconut sugar (optional)

2 teaspoons vanilla extract

1½ cups brown rice flour

½ cup tapioca flour or arrowroot powder

½ teaspoon baking powder

½ teaspoon baking soda

¼ teaspoon sea salt

½ to 1 cup organic dark chocolate chips

Preheat the oven to 350°F. Grease the cookie sheet with coconut oil.

Place the pitted dates and flaxseeds into a small bowl, cover with the hot water, and soak for about 15 minutes. Then place the soaked dates, flaxseeds, and water into a blender and purée. Add the coconut oil, coconut sugar if using, and the vanilla and blend again.

In a separate bowl, mix together the brown rice flour, tapioca flour, baking powder, baking soda, and sea salt. Add the wet ingredients to the dry and mix together with a wooden spoon or beat with an electric mixer. Fold in the chocolate chips.

Drop the mixture by large spoonfuls onto the prepared cookie sheet. Gently flatten each cookie with oiled or wet hands.

Bake for 14 to 16 minutes; the baking time will depend on what size the cookies are. Larger cookies need a little extra time and smaller cookies a little less. Transfer to a wire rack to cool. Store in an airtight container for up to 4 days.

Yield: 1½ dozen cookies

CHOCOLATE-HAZELNUT–GOJI BERRY COOKIES

This cookie recipe isn't too sweet. It would make a good snack for school or work. Pair a few cookies with some kale chips and raw carrot sticks for a healthy afternoon snack or light lunch!

DRY INGREDIENTS

2 cups raw hazelnuts

⅓ cup raw cacao powder

2 tablespoons coconut flour

¼ teaspoon baking soda

¼ teaspoon sea salt

WET INGREDIENTS

4 tablespoons cold organic butter or virgin coconut oil

¼ cup pure maple syrup

2 large organic eggs

1 teaspoon vanilla extract

½ cup dried goji berries

Preheat the oven to 350°F. Line a cookie sheet with unbleached parchment paper.

Place the hazelnuts into a food processor fitted with the "s" blade and process to a fine meal. Add the remaining dry ingredients and pulse until combined.

Add the butter or coconut oil and pulse. Add the maple syrup, eggs, and vanilla and process to combine. Add the goji berries and pulse briefly just enough to mix them in. Let the dough sit for a few minutes.

Drop the dough by spoonfuls onto the lined cookie sheet. With wet hands, gently flatten each one. Bake for 12 to 15 minutes. Remove from oven and transfer to a wire rack to cool.

Yield: 18 cookies

COCONUT-CASHEW COOKIES

Not only are these cookies gluten-free, but they are also vegan, meaning they contain no dairy or eggs. The combination of the orange zest and shredded coconut gives these cookies a sweet flavor without needing to use a lot of sugar in the recipe.

WET INGREDIENTS

⅓ cup softened virgin coconut oil, plus more for greasing the cookie sheet

¼ cup pure maple syrup

1 tablespoon ground golden flaxseeds

1 to 2 teaspoons vanilla extract

½ teaspoon finely grated orange zest

DRY INGREDIENTS

½ cup raw cashews, ground

1 cup brown rice flour

¼ cup tapioca flour

½ cup shredded organic coconut

½ teaspoon baking powder

¼ teaspoon sea salt

Preheat the oven to 350°F. Grease a cookie sheet with coconut oil or line with unbleached parchment paper.

Place the coconut oil, maple syrup, flaxseeds, vanilla, and orange zest into a medium bowl and blend on high with an electric mixer for about 2 minutes.

Add the cashews to a coffee grinder or mini food processor and process until finely ground.

In a separate bowl, mix together the brown rice flour, tapioca flour, coconut, ground cashews, baking powder, and sea salt. Pour the wet ingredients into the dry and mix together with an electric mixer until well combined.

Form the dough into balls then place on the prepared cookie sheet. Gently flatten each ball with wet or oiled hands. Bake for 12 to 15 minutes. Transfer to a wire rack to cool; the cookies will be somewhat crumbly when hot, but will harden as they cool.

Yield: 1 dozen cookies

GINGERBREAD CUTOUT COOKIES

These amazing little gluten-free cookies are fun to make with children. They can help roll out the dough and cut it into shapes using different cookie cutters. Try pumpkins for Halloween, gingerbread people and stars for Christmas, and hearts for Valentine's Day. Frost with the Cashew-Honey Icing (page 411).

WET INGREDIENTS

½ cup softened virgin coconut oil or unsalted organic butter

2 tablespoons ground flaxseeds

½ cup coconut sugar

¼ cup blackstrap molasses

¼ cup pumpkin purée

2 to 3 teaspoons vanilla extract

DRY INGREDIENTS

1½ cups brown rice flour

½ cup tapioca flour

½ teaspoon baking soda

½ teaspoon sea salt

2 teaspoons ground cinnamon

1½ teaspoons ground ginger

¼ teaspoon ground cloves

¼ teaspoon ground allspice

In a medium mixing bowl, beat together the coconut oil, flaxseeds, coconut sugar, molasses, pumpkin purée, and vanilla with an electric mixer.

In a separate bowl, combine the brown rice flour, tapioca flour, baking soda, sea salt, and spices. Add the dry ingredients to the wet and beat together.

Form the dough into a ball, wrap in waxed paper, and place in the refrigerator to chill for 2 to 3 hours.

Preheat the oven to 350°F. Place a large sheet of unbleached parchment paper onto a flat work surface, such as a countertop or table. Place part of the dough onto the parchment and cover with another sheet. Roll out the dough with a rolling pin to a thickness of about ⅛ inch. Cut out with your favorite cookie cutters. Peel away excess dough around the cut shapes. Carefully move the parchment paper and cookies onto a large cookie sheet.

Bake for about 15 to 16 minutes. Gently remove the cookies from the cookie sheet with a thin spatula and transfer to a wire rack to cool; the cookies will crisp as they cool.

Yield: 1½ to 2 dozen cookies

GINGER MOLASSES COOKIES

I love that these egg-free and grain-free cookies are sweetened completely with nutrient-dense Medjool dates. I always feel good seeing my children pack one of these protein-rich cookies in their school lunches! Serve these cookies with chai tea for a nourishing afternoon snack.

1 cup pitted Medjool dates

2 tablespoons blackstrap molasses

1 teaspoon nonalcoholic vanilla extract

1 cup creamy roasted almond butter

1 tablespoon warm water

2 teaspoons psyllium husk powder

½ teaspoon baking soda

¼ teaspoon sea salt

2 teaspoons ground cinnamon

1 teaspoon ground ginger

¼ teaspoon ground nutmeg

Preheat the oven to 350°F. Line a cookie sheet with unbleached parchment paper.

Place all the ingredients into a food processor fitted with the "s" blade and process until the dates are finely ground and the mixture is combined.

Roll the dough into 1-inch balls and place onto the prepared cookie sheet. Flatten the balls with the palm of your hand. Bake for about 10 to 15 minutes, depending on the size of the cookies. Transfer to a wire rack to cool.

Yield: 1 to 1½ dozen cookies

GRAIN-FREE CHOCOLATE MINI CUPCAKES

Serve these healthy mini cupcakes for a Halloween party, birthday party, or any other celebration. Decorate with the Yam Frosting (page 413) and unsweetened shredded coconut, raw cacao nibs, or finely chopped walnuts.

DRY INGREDIENTS

½ cup coconut flour

6 tablespoons raw cacao powder

¾ teaspoon baking soda

¼ teaspoon sea salt

WET INGREDIENTS

6 large organic eggs

½ cup pure maple syrup

⅓ cup melted virgin coconut oil

2 teaspoons vanilla extract

Preheat the oven to 350°F. Line a 24-cup mini muffin pan with unbleached paper liners.

In a medium mixing bowl, whisk together the dry ingredients. In a separate bowl or blender whisk or blend together the wet ingredients. Pour the wet into the dry and quickly whisk together.

Spoon the batter into the muffin cups, filling them all the way to the top. Bake the cupcakes for 15 to 20 minutes. Transfer to a wire rack to cool completely. Frost and decorate if desired.

Yield: 24 mini cupcakes

VANILLA BEAN CUPCAKES

I like to frost these cupcakes with the Honey–Cream Cheese Frosting (page 412) and decorate them with fresh edible flowers. If you don't have vanilla powder then add 1 tablespoon of vanilla extract to the wet ingredients instead.

DRY INGREDIENTS

2 cups blanched almond flour, packed

¼ cup coconut flour

2 teaspoons baking powder

½ teaspoon baking soda

½ teaspoon sea salt

1 teaspoon organic vanilla powder

WET INGREDIENTS

4 large organic eggs

¾ cup pure maple syrup

½ cup melted virgin coconut oil

Preheat the oven to 350°F. Line a 12-cup muffin pan with unbleached paper liners.

In a medium bowl, whisk together the dry ingredients. In a separate bowl, whisk together the wet ingredients. Add the wet ingredients to the dry and vigorously whisk together until combined.

Spoon the batter into the lined muffin cups. Bake the cupcakes for approximately 25 minutes. Transfer to a wire rack to cool completely before frosting.

Yield: 1 dozen cupcakes

BANANA CAKE

Nobody can tell that this cake is grain and gluten-free! Top it with the Fudgy Coconut Frosting (page 412) just after it comes out of the oven. If you prefer a layered cake, bake the cake in two 10-inch round cake pans instead.

DRY INGREDIENTS

1 cup coconut flour

¾ cup arrowroot powder

2 teaspoons baking powder

¾ teaspoon baking soda

¾ teaspoon sea salt

WET INGREDIENTS

2 cups mashed ripe banana (about 4 to 6 bananas)

1 cup melted virgin coconut oil, plus more for greasing the dish

1 cup coconut sugar

10 large organic eggs

2 teaspoons vanilla extract

Preheat the oven to 350°F. Grease a 9 x 13-inch glass baking dish with coconut oil.

In a medium mixing bowl, whisk together the dry ingredients and set aside.

Add all the wet ingredients to a blender and purée on high until ingredients are thoroughly combined. If you are using a high-powered blender then add the dry ingredients and blend again until combined. If you don't have a high-powered blender, then pour the wet into the dry and vigorously beat together with a wire whisk until completely combined.

Pour the batter into the baking dish and bake for 35 to 40 minutes, or until a knife inserted in the cake comes out clean.

Yield: about 15 servings

CRANBERRY-ORANGE UPSIDE-DOWN CAKE

This recipe is very versatile. Don't like cranberries? Substitute blueberries, apricots, pitted cherries, or sliced apples with cinnamon. The texture and flavor of this cake tastes best the day it is made. Serve it with a mug of warm spice tea at the end of a good meal.

FRUIT

1 tablespoon softened organic butter or virgin coconut oil

1 tablespoon pure maple syrup

1 tablespoon arrowroot powder

2 cups fresh cranberries

DRY INGREDIENTS

6 tablespoons coconut flour

6 tablespoons arrowroot powder

2 teaspoons baking powder

¼ teaspoon sea salt

WET INGREDIENTS

4 large organic eggs

4 tablespoons melted organic butter or virgin coconut oil

¼ cup pure maple syrup

finely grated zest of 1 organic orange

2 tablespoons freshly squeezed orange juice

1 teaspoon vanilla extract

Preheat the oven to 350°F. Place a 9-inch cake pan onto a sheet of unbleached parchment paper and draw a line around the bottom with a pencil. Cut out the circle and place it onto the bottom of the cake pan. Grease the sides of the pan with butter or coconut oil.

To prepare the fruit, mix together the butter or coconut oil, maple syrup, and arrowroot powder in a small bowl. Spread the mixture onto the parchment paper in the cake pan using an offset spatula. Arrange the cranberries on top of the butter-syrup mixture.

Whisk together the dry ingredients. In a separate bowl, whisk together the wet ingredients. Pour the wet into the dry and quickly whisk together until combined. Pour the batter over the fruit and spread evenly with the back of a spoon or spatula.

Bake for 30 to 35 minutes. Transfer to a wire rack to cool for 15 to 20 minutes then carefully invert the cake onto a plate and peel off the parchment paper. Let cool completely and serve.

Yield: 6 to 8 servings

CHOCOLATE–ALMOND BUTTER CAKE

Serve this cake with a dollop of Whipped Vanilla Coconut Cream (page 414) and fresh berries. Double the recipe and bake it in two 9-inch cake pans for a layered cake.

---

1 cup creamy roasted almond butter

2 large organic eggs

⅓ cup melted virgin coconut oil, plus more for greasing the pan

⅓ cup pure maple syrup

¼ cup raw cacao powder

2 teaspoons vanilla extract

½ teaspoon organic almond extract

½ teaspoon baking soda

¼ teaspoon sea salt

Preheat the oven to 350°F. Lightly grease an 8 x 8-inch pan with coconut oil.

Place all the ingredients into a food processor fitted with the "s" blade and process until combined. Pour the batter into the pan and spread out evenly. Bake for about 30 minutes. Cool, slice, and serve.

Yield: about 9 servings

Variation: Add ¼ cup coconut sugar for a sweeter cake.

DECADENT CHOCOLATE BUNDT CAKE

The extra richness in this cake comes from the beets, which provide moisture, sweetness, and added minerals. Serve the cake with fresh organic berries or Warm Berry Sauce (page 359).

DRY INGREDIENTS

2 cups brown rice flour

½ cup tapioca flour

¾ cup raw cacao powder

1½ teaspoons baking soda

½ teaspoon sea salt

WET INGREDIENTS

1 cup warm water

¼ cup ground chia seeds

½ cup melted virgin coconut oil, plus more for greasing the pan

2 large organic eggs

1 cup pure maple syrup

2 tablespoons apple cider vinegar

1 tablespoon vanilla extract

1 cup grated cooked beets (about 1 large beet)

Preheat the oven to 350°F. Oil a Bundt pan with coconut oil.

In a medium bowl, place the brown rice flour, tapioca flour, cacao powder, baking soda, and sea salt and whisk together.

Place the water and chia into a small bowl and whisk together. Set aside for about 5 minutes. Add the chia-water mixture to a blender along with the melted oil, eggs, maple syrup, vinegar, and vanilla and blend on high until smooth. Pour the wet ingredients into the dry and vigorously whisk together. Fold in the cooked grated beets.

Immediately pour the batter into the prepared pan and bake in the preheated oven for 40 to 45 minutes.

Remove the cake from the oven and let cool in the pan for about 10 minutes. Then invert it onto a cake platter or plate. Let cool and serve.

Yield: 8 to 10 servings

Tip: To prepare the 1 cup of grated cooked beets, first trim the ends off a large beet then cut it into quarters. Place the quarters into a steamer basket in a pot filled with about 2 cups of water over medium heat. Place a lid on the pot and steam for about 30 minutes or until beets are very tender. Let cool and then remove the peel and grate. Measure out 1 heaping cup. Alternatively, you could grate a leftover roasted, peeled beet.

GINGERBREAD CAKE WITH
MAPLE-CASHEW SAUCE

This scrumptious dessert will delight gingerbread lovers of all kind. We like to make this cake for either Thanksgiving or Christmas as a special treat. This cake is delicious served on its own or with the cashew sauce.

DRY INGREDIENTS

2 cups brown rice flour

½ cup tapioca flour

2 teaspoons baking powder

½ teaspoon baking soda

½ teaspoon sea salt

2 teaspoons ground ginger

2 teaspoons ground cinnamon

½ teaspoon ground cloves

WET INGREDIENTS

¼ cup ground chia seeds

½ cup warm water

½ cup melted virgin coconut oil, plus more for greasing the dish

½ cup pure maple syrup

½ cup blackstrap molasses

1 tablespoon vanilla extract

SAUCE

½ cup raw cashews

2 to 3 tablespoons pure maple syrup

2 teaspoons vanilla extract

2 to 3 tablespoons water

Preheat the oven to 350°F. Oil an 8 x 8-inch glass baking dish.

Combine the dry ingredients in a medium mixing bowl. In a separate small bowl, whisk together the ground chia and the warm water; set aside for about 5 minutes. Add the chia-water mixture to a blender along with the other wet ingredients and blend until smooth.

Pour the wet ingredients into the dry and mix well with a wire whisk. Pour the batter into the prepared baking dish and bake for about 30 minutes.

To make the sauce, place all the ingredients in a blender and blend until smooth and creamy. Let cake cool for about 10 minutes. When ready to serve, slice the cake and drizzle each piece with maple-cashew sauce.

Yield: 8 to 12 servings

ZUCCHINI SPICE CAKE

Serve a piece of this nourishing cake along with a cup of green tea and a hard-boiled egg for a quick lunch. It also makes a healthy treat for your child's lunch box. Dollop with Whipped Vanilla Coconut Cream (page 414) for a healthy, sweet treat. If you don't have cashew butter on hand, use almond butter instead.

virgin coconut oil, for greasing the pan

1½ cups cashew butter

2 large organic eggs

⅓ to ½ cup coconut sugar

½ teaspoon baking soda

¼ teaspoon sea salt

1 teaspoon ground cinnamon

¾ teaspoon ground ginger

½ teaspoon ground allspice

¼ teaspoon ground nutmeg

1 cup grated zucchini

OPTIONAL ADDITIONS

½ cup raisins or dried currants

½ cup dark chocolate chips

Preheat the oven to 350°F. Grease an 8 x 8-inch pan with coconut oil.

In a medium mixing bowl, beat together the cashew butter, eggs, coconut sugar, baking soda, sea salt, and spices. Beat in the grated zucchini and any optional additions. Let the batter rest for a few minutes, then beat again.

Pour the batter into the prepared pan and bake for about 30 minutes. Remove from the oven and cool for at least 25 minutes before cutting and serving.

> **Tip:** I use a whole 16-ounce jar of Artisana Raw Cashew Butter for this cake.

Yield: about 9 servings

BERRY-PEACH ICED NUT CREAM

This delightful alternative to ice cream uses plant-based ingredients to create a nutrient-dense creamy frozen dessert rich in antioxidants.

½ cup raw cashews

freshly squeezed juice of 1 large Valencia orange

1 teaspoon nonalcoholic vanilla extract

1 small ripe avocado

1 cup frozen raspberries

½ to 1 cup frozen strawberries

½ cup frozen peach slices

If you own a high-powered blender you can blend all of the ingredients in it. Otherwise, use a regular blender to blend the cashews, orange juice, and vanilla until smooth and creamy.

Transfer the cashew mixture to a food processor fitted with the "s" blade and add the avocado, frozen raspberries, frozen strawberries, and frozen peach slices then process until smooth, thick, and creamy.

Serve immediately, or freeze for later use. To serve the frozen nut cream, let it stand at room temperature for about 10 minutes, then place into the food processor and process until soft and creamy.

Yield: 4 servings

CHOCOLATE-BANANA ICED NUT CREAM

Frozen bananas can create the creamiest dairy-free ice cream! Whenever our bananas are getting too ripe I peel them and freeze them whole in large containers; this way we always have a supply for smoothies and sweet treats like this recipe! Serve with fresh berries and raw cacao nibs.

½ cup raw cashews

2 tablespoons water

¼ cup pure maple syrup

3 large frozen bananas, broken into chunks

2 to 4 tablespoons raw cacao powder

If you own a high-powered blender, you can blend all of the ingredients in it. Otherwise, use a blender to blend the cashews, water, and maple syrup until creamy and smooth. Then transfer the cashew mixture to a food processor, add the frozen banana chunks and the cacao powder, and process until smooth, thick, and creamy.

Serve the nut cream immediately, or freeze for later use. To serve the frozen nut cream, let it stand at room temperature for about 10 minutes, then place it into a food processor and process until soft and creamy.

Yield: 4 servings

CHERRY–CHOCOLATE CHIP ICE CREAM

Chilling the coconut milk beforehand helps to solidify it into ice cream during churning. This nutritious dairy-free ice cream is full of beneficial fats found in the coconut milk and hemp seeds. It's quite simple to make your own ice cream, and once you do, you'll likely never go back to the store-bought stuff!

---

two 14-ounce cans full-fat coconut milk, chilled

6 to 8 tablespoons raw honey or coconut nectar

¼ cup hemp seeds, plus more for garnish

1 teaspoon organic vanilla powder

½ teaspoon organic almond extract

1½ cups chopped frozen cherries, plus more for garnish

¼ to ½ cup raw cacao nibs or organic dark chocolate chips, plus more for garnish

---

Place the coconut milk, honey, hemp seeds, vanilla, and almond extract into a high-powered blender and blend until smooth.

Pour the mixture into your ice cream maker, add the chopped frozen cherries and cacao nibs, and process according to the manufacturer's directions. I usually let mine churn for 20 to 25 minutes and then transfer to a container for storing in the freezer.

Freeze for 2 to 3 hours, or until ready to serve. Sprinkle each serving with cacao nibs and hemp seeds, and a fresh cherry or two.

Yield: about 8 servings

AVOCADO-FIG FUDGESICLES

These amazing little treats are perfect for an afternoon summer snack or evening dessert. You will need a set of Popsicle molds for these. You can add more or less cacao powder depending on how rich you would like your fudgesicles.

1 small ripe avocado	4 Medjool dates, pitted
4 fresh black mission figs	2 to 4 tablespoons raw cacao powder

Place all the ingredients in a food processor or high-powered blender and blend on high for 1 to 2 minutes, or until very smooth and creamy, adding just enough water sufficient for blending.

Pour the mixture into Popsicle molds, insert sticks, and freeze for 6 to 8 hours or overnight.

Yield: 4 to 6 fudgesicles

CASHEW-HONEY ICING

Use this simple, nutritious icing recipe to decorate cakes or cookies. Once chilled you can spread it onto cookies and then decorate them, or place it into a cake decorating bag and pipe pretty designs onto your dessert. Add natural food dyes for colored variations. The icing will become soft at temperatures above 75°F, so keep that in mind if you are planning on bringing a decorated cake to a summer picnic in the park.

¼ cup raw cashew butter	¼ teaspoon nonalcoholic vanilla extract
2 tablespoons melted virgin coconut oil	⅛ teaspoon organic almond extract
2 tablespoons raw honey	

Place all the ingredients into a small bowl and mix together using a fork. Chill in the refrigerator for 1 to 2 hours. Stir again before using.

Yield: ½ cup

HONEY–CREAM CHEESE FROSTING

This recipe makes enough frosting to frost a dozen cupcakes. Sometimes I will use lavender honey and omit the orange zest; other times I will add vanilla and almond extracts in place of the orange zest.

---

8 ounces organic cream cheese
3 to 4 tablespoons raw honey

½ teaspoon finely grated orange zest

Place all the ingredients into a mixing bowl and beat together with an electric mixer. Store in the refrigerator until ready to use.

Yield: about 1½ cups

FUDGY COCONUT FROSTING

Use this decadent dairy-free frosting to frost the grain-free Banana Cake (page 402) or drizzle over the Decadent Chocolate Bundt Cake (page 405). You can get coconut cream by refrigerating a can of full-fat coconut milk for a few hours, then opening the can and scooping the hard cream off the top.

---

6 tablespoons virgin coconut oil
3 ounces organic bittersweet chocolate
½ to ¾ cup coconut sugar

3 tablespoons arrowroot powder
⅓ cup coconut cream
2 to 3 teaspoons raw coconut vinegar

In a small saucepan, combine the coconut oil, chocolate, and coconut sugar and whisk over very low heat until melted. Whisk in the arrowroot powder, coconut cream, and vinegar. Pour the mixture into a blender and blend on high for about 60 seconds.

Pour the warm frosting over a sheet cake, or refrigerate the frosting until thickened, then spread onto cupcakes.

Yield: about 1½ cups

YAM FROSTING

This healthy, bright orange frosting gets its color and sweetness from the use of mashed, cooked yams. Use this recipe to frost a cake or cupcakes for Halloween, Thanksgiving, or a birthday party. This recipe makes enough frosting for one dozen cupcakes; double it for a layered cake.

¾ cup cooked, mashed yams (still warm)

6 tablespoons virgin coconut oil

¼ cup pure maple syrup

2 tablespoons unsweetened applesauce

2 tablespoons arrowroot powder

2 teaspoons vanilla extract

pinch sea salt

Place all the ingredients into a high-powered blender and blend until very smooth and creamy. Scrape the frosting from the blender into a container and refrigerate until firm. If you would like it to chill and firm up quickly you can place the container in your freezer for 30 to 40 minutes, stirring every so often, until firm. Spread the frosting onto your favorite cupcakes.

Yield: about 2 cups

Tip: To cook the yams for the frosting, leave the skins on and slice the yams into thick rounds. Place into a small pot and fill about one-third of the way with fresh water. Cover and cook over medium heat until tender. Remove the skins; they will peel off easily once cooked. You can also place large pieces of yam into a steamer basket and steam over medium heat until tender.

WHIPPED VANILLA COCONUT CREAM

Use this simple recipe as a replacement for whipped heavy cream. Dollop it on top of fresh strawberries and blueberries, or use to frost cupcakes. The coconut cream will begin to soften as it sits at room temperature, and will soften quickly on a hot summer afternoon so be sure to keep it chilled. You can easily rewhip it after you remove the container from the refrigerator.

two 14-ounce cans full-fat coconut milk, chilled for 12 hours

1 to 2 tablespoons coconut nectar, honey, or maple syrup

½ teaspoon organic vanilla bean powder

pinch sea salt

After the cans of coconut milk have chilled, open them up and scoop the thick white coconut cream from the top. Pour the watery milk into a jar and reserve to use in your favorite fruit smoothie.

Place the coconut cream, coconut nectar, vanilla, and sea salt into a mixing bowl. Using an electric mixer, whip the chilled cream to soft peaks. Serve immediately, or store in a covered glass container in the refrigerator for up to a week.

Yield: about 1 cup

23

BEVERAGES

Age is an issue of mind over matter. If you don't mind, it doesn't matter.
—Mark Twain

Having a few beverage recipes on hand can be a delicious way to add extra nutrients and phytochemicals to your diet. For example, beverages with lemons and limes contain numerous anticancer compounds, flavonoids, and a healthy dose of vitamin C. The herbal tea recipes in this chapter are cleansing and stimulating to the digestive system, and they provide a rich source of minerals.

Making your own nut milk is actually very easy and the milk recipes provided in this chapter can be used in other recipes as well. Nut milks are so versatile and tasty you'll find that preparing them becomes part of your weekly routine.

RAW ALMOND MILK

Our children love to drink raw almond milk as a snack! I like to pour it over fresh fruit and chopped nuts in lieu of breakfast cereal. You can also make smoothies with almond milk—try blending frozen peaches, raspberries, kale, and almond milk for a refreshing and nutritious smoothie.

½ cup raw almonds (soaked overnight)
3 cups water

1 tablespoon pure maple syrup
pinch sea salt

Place the almonds into a small bowl and cover with filtered water. Soak at room temperature for 8 to 12 hours, or overnight.

After the almonds have soaked, rinse them well under warm running water. Place them in a blender with the water, maple syrup, and sea salt and blend on high for 2 to 3 minutes, or until you have a very smooth milk.

Pour the milk through a fine-mesh strainer lined with a cheesecloth, or through a nut milk bag, into a container and squeeze out as much milk from the pulp as possible.

Store in a covered glass jar in the refrigerator for up to 3 days.

*Yield: **about 3 cups***

> **Tip:** If you live in a warm climate, change the soaking water a few times to keep the nuts from spoiling.

BRAZIL NUT MILK

Did you know that by eating two to three Brazil nuts a day you can get your daily requirement for selenium? Many of our soils are now deplete in this vital mineral so we need to take extra care in getting enough. Selenium helps with immune system function and detoxification. Use Brazil nut milk to make creamy fruit and green smoothies, or pour over your favorite warm, whole-grain cereal for breakfast.

½ cup raw Brazil nuts (soaked overnight)

3 cups water

1 tablespoon pure maple syrup

pinch sea salt

Place the Brazil nuts into a small bowl, cover with filtered water, and let them soak on your kitchen countertop for 8 to 12 hours. Drain off the water and rinse the nuts.

Place the soaked nuts into a blender along with remaining ingredients. Blend on high for 1 to 2 minutes until smooth. Pour the milk through a fine-mesh strainer lined with a cheesecloth, or through a nut milk bag, into a container and squeeze out as much milk from the pulp as possible.

Store in a covered glass jar in the refrigerator for up to 3 days.

*Yield: **about 3 cups***

CASHEW MILK

Cashews are a softer nut, and therefore do not need to be soaked overnight to blend well as almonds or hazelnuts do. Use fresh cashew milk to pour over a cooked whole-grain cereal for breakfast such as the Warming Three-Grain Morning Cereal (page 135) or use it to make fruit smoothies.

½ cup raw cashews

2 cups water

1 tablespoon pure maple syrup

pinch sea salt

Place all the ingredients in a high-powered blender and blend until very smooth. Taste and adjust the sweetness if necessary.

Store in a covered glass jar in the refrigerator for up to 2 days.

Yield: about 2½ cups

HAZELNUT MILK

I love the distinctive nutty flavor of hazelnut milk. Try making smoothies with hazelnut milk. I like to blend frozen wild blueberries or huckleberries with about 1 cup of hazelnut milk for a healthy, refreshing treat.

½ cup raw hazelnuts (soaked overnight)

3 cups water

1 tablespoon pure maple syrup

pinch sea salt

Place the raw hazelnuts into a small bowl and cover with filtered water. Soak at room temperature for about 6 hours or overnight.

After the hazelnuts have soaked, rinse them well under warm running water. Place them in a blender with the water, maple syrup, and sea salt and blend on high for 2 to 3 minutes, or until you have a very smooth milk.

Pour the milk through a fine-mesh strainer lined with a cheesecloth, or through a nut milk bag, into a container and squeeze out as much milk from the pulp as possible.

Store in a covered glass jar in the refrigerator for up to 3 days.

Yield: about 3 cups

HONEY LIMEADE WITH RASPBERRY ICE CUBES

This delicious and colorful drink is wonderful for a summer picnic. Children will love to drink the limeade and eat the raspberries from the melted ice cubes. Limes contain flavonoids called flavonol glycosides, which have been shown to stop cancer cells from dividing. Limes are also an excellent source of vitamin C.

LIMEADE
½ cup freshly squeezed lime juice
¼ cup honey
4 cups water

ICE CUBES
1 ice cube tray
fresh raspberries
water

To make the limeade, place lime juice, honey, and water into a large glass pitcher and stir well. Taste and adjust the sweetness if desired.

To make the ice cubes, place 1 raspberry into each ice cube mold, pour water into the molds to cover, and place in the freezer. Freeze for 6 hours or overnight.

To serve, place the raspberry ice cubes into the pitcher with the limeade. Serve immediately.

Yield: 4¾ cups

STEVIA LEMONADE

I like to have a pitcher of this on hand to drink throughout the day. Our children love this drink also. Both lemons and limes contain potent anticancer compounds called limonoids, which stop cancer cells from proliferating. Lemons are also an excellent source of vitamin C.

½ cup freshly squeezed lemon juice
4 cups water

½ teaspoon liquid stevia

Place all the ingredients into a large glass pitcher and mix well.

Taste and adjust the sweetness if necessary. Stevia is very concentrated so just add a few drops at a time, taste, then add more as needed.

Yield: 4½ cups

HOT MULLED CIDER

We make this in the fall and winter when the chilly weather has set in. Our children love to drink it. Try to find a local organic apple orchard that sells cider and stock up in the fall when the cider has just been pressed. You can freeze it and use it throughout the season.

6 cups organic apple cider
2 large organic orange slices
4 to 5 slices fresh ginger

5 cinnamon sticks
2 teaspoons whole cloves

Place all ingredients into a large pot. Simmer, covered, over low to medium-low heat for about 1 hour.

Strain out the spices by pouring contents through a fine-mesh strainer into another pot.

Keep the pot on warm if you would like to serve it over an extended period of time.

Yield: about 6 cups

CLEANSING ROOT TEA

This tea is actually called a "decoction" because the roots are simmered in water rather than steeped. Licorice root is an adrenal balancer, which is very helpful in times of stress; burdock root helps to purify the blood and stimulate the liver; dandelion root also works to stimulate the liver and purify the blood; and ginger acts as a powerful anti-inflammatory. I like to drink this tea before bed because your body's mechanisms of detoxification are most active during sleep. Sometimes we like to add a little dried nettles and oat straw after the roots have been simmered.

1 tablespoon dried licorice root

2 tablespoons dried burdock root

2 tablespoons dried dandelion root

1 tablespoon chopped fresh ginger

3 to 4 cups water

leafy herbs, such as nettles, oat straw, or red clover (optional)

raw honey (optional)

Place the licorice root, burdock root, dandelion root, ginger, and water into a medium, stainless steel or glass pot, cover, and bring to a gentle boil. Reduce the heat to low and simmer for 20 to 30 minutes.

Remove from heat and add leafy herbs such as nettles, oat straw, or red clover, if desired, and steep for 10 to 20 minutes more with the lid on. Strain tea through a fine-mesh strainer into a widemouthed mason jar. To sweeten, add raw honey. Store any unused tea in the refrigerator in a covered jar.

Yield: about 3 cups

SWEET NETTLE GINGER TEA

Nettles are an amazing source of many different minerals. You can harvest nettles in the springtime when the shoots are small and the leaves are tender. Dry nettle leaves in a food dehydrator and store in a glass jar with a tight-fitting lid. We like to make this delicious and nourishing tea often—our whole family loves it!

1 tablespoon dried licorice root

5 slices fresh ginger

4 cups water

¼ cup dried nettles

Place licorice root, ginger, and water in a medium stainless steel or glass pot, cover, and bring to a gentle boil. Reduce the heat to low and simmer for 20 to 30 minutes. Remove from heat and add the dried nettles and steep for 10 to 20 minutes, or longer, with the lid on.

Strain tea through a fine-mesh strainer into a widemouthed mason jar. Store any unused tea in the refrigerator in a covered jar.

Yield: about 6 cups

DANDELION ROOT CHAI TEA

Dandelion root tea is earthy and slightly bitter. It's excellent for assisting the liver with detoxification as well as stimulating the digestive system. Chai spices are warming and also stimulate digestion. You can find dried dandelion root and the chai spices in the bulk herb section of your local health food store or herb store. Once the herbs have simmered you can add any thick, rich milk of your choice such as homemade raw almond milk, hemp milk, cashew milk, or fresh raw cream (from pastured cows). I usually fill three-quarters of my mug with tea and one-quarter with milk. I then stir in a small spoonful of raw honey to sweeten it.

1 tablespoon dried dandelion root

2 cinnamon sticks, broken into pieces

5 to 6 cardamom pods, crushed

1 teaspoon whole cloves

1 teaspoon whole black peppercorns

one 1-inch piece fresh ginger, thinly sliced

4 cups water

milk of your choice

raw honey

Place the dandelion root and spices into a 2-quart pot and cover with the water; place a lid on the pot. Bring to a boil, then reduce the heat and simmer for 10 to 15 minutes. Strain the tea through a fine-mesh strainer into a quart jar. Pour into mugs, top off with the milk of your choice, and sweeten to taste with raw honey.

Yield: 1 quart

WARMING RASPBERRY LEAF ALMOND DRINK

This drink is intended to nourish breastfeeding mothers, especially immediately following birth and in the early postpartum stage. The fennel seeds and raspberry leaves help to contract the uterus after childbirth and also promote the flow of breast milk. The almonds are very rich and nourishing, providing healthy protein and fats to the new mother. The ginger, cinnamon, and cloves are warming spices that help the digestive systems of both mother and baby.

6 cups water

1 cup raw almonds, ground to a fine powder

one 2-inch piece fresh ginger, sliced

3 cinnamon sticks

4 whole cloves

2 teaspoons fennel seeds

3 tablespoons dried raspberry leaves

⅓ cup raw honey or to taste

Place 4 cups of the water in a pot with the ground almonds and simmer on low for 30 minutes, partially covered. Be very careful not to let the heat get too high, or the ground almonds and water will boil over, which can make quite a mess!

Place the remaining 2 cups of water in a smaller pot with the ginger, cinnamon sticks, cloves, and fennel seeds and simmer for 30 minutes, covered. Remove the pot from the heat and add the raspberry leaves; let steep for 10 to 20 minutes with the lid on.

Strain the herb mixture into a blender and discard the herbs, then add the almond milk mixture and blend on high for a couple of minutes. Add the honey and blend for 1 more minute. Taste and adjust the sweetness if necessary.

Strain the drink through a fine-mesh strainer lined with a cheesecloth.

Yield: about 6 cups

MEASUREMENT EQUIVALENTS

1 tablespoon	=	3 teaspoons		
2 tablespoons	=	⅛ cup	=	1 ounce
4 tablespoons	=	¼ cup	=	2 ounces
⅓ cup	=	5 tablespoons + 1 teaspoon		
½ cup	=	8 tablespoons	=	4 ounces
1 cup	=	16 tablespoons	=	8 ounces
1 pint	=	2 cups	=	16 ounces
1 quart	=	2 pints or 4 cups	=	32 ounces
1 gallon	=	4 quarts	=	128 ounces

RESOURCES

Organic Blanched Almond Flour: www.Nuts.com

Raw Organic GF Buckwheat Groats: www.BobsRedMill.com

Organic Gluten-Free Rolled Oats: www.EdisonGrainery.com

Gluten-Free Whole-Grain Flours: www.BobsRedMill.com

Arrowroot Powder: www.BobsRedMill.com

Sprouted Brown Rice Flour: www.PlanetRiceFoods.com

Sprouted Garbanzo Bean Flour: www.OrganicSproutedFlour.net

Raw Organic Cacao Powder: www.EssentialLivingFoods.com

Maca Powder: www.EssentialLivingFoods.com

Organic Virgin Coconut Oil: www.TropicalTraditions.com; www.Nutiva.com

Chia and Hemp Seeds: www.Nutiva.com

Unpasteurized Organic Raw Almonds: www.OrganicAlmondsRaw.com

Grass-Fed Meats: www.USWellnessMeats.com

Brown Rice Noodles: www.JovialFoods.com

Raw Cashew Butter: www.ArtisanaFoods.com

Roasted Almond Butter: www.ZinkeOrchards.com

Gluten-Free, Soy-Free Miso: www.SouthRiverMiso.com

Kosher Unflavored Gelatin: www.GreatLakesGelatin.com

Agar Powder: www.NowFoods.com

Organic Raw Vanilla Bean Powder: www.DivineOrganics.com

REFERENCES

Introduction

Demmig-Adams B, Adams WW 3rd. Antioxidants in photosynthesis and human nutrition. *Science.* 2002 Dec 13; 298(5601): 2149–53. PMID: 12481128.

Jacka FN, Pasco JA, Mykletun A, et al. Association of Western and traditional diets with depression and anxiety in women. *Am J Psychiatry.* 2010 Mar; 167(3): 305–11.

Pan A, Malik VS, Hu FB. Exporting diabetes mellitus to Asia: The impact of Western-style fast food. *Circulation.* 2012 Jul 10; 126(2): 163–65.

Minich DM, Bland JS. Personalized lifestyle medicine: Relevance for nutrition and lifestyle recommendations. *Scientific World Journal.* 2013 Jun 26; 2013: 129841. PMID: 23878520.

Lucan SC, Barg FK, Long JA. Promoters and barriers to fruit, vegetable, and fast-food consumption among urban, low-income African Americans—a qualitative approach. *Am J Public Health.* 2010 Apr; 100(4): 631–35. PMID: 20167885.

McCann JC, Ames BN. Vitamin K, an example of triage theory: Is micronutrient inadequacy linked to diseases of aging? *Am J Clin Nutr.* 2009 Oct; 90(4): 889–907. PMID: 19692494.

Ames BN. Optimal micronutrients delay mitochondrial decay and age-associated diseases. *Mech Ageing Dev.* 2010 Jul–Aug; 131(7–8): 473–79.

Ames BN. Prevention of mutation, cancer, and other age-associated diseases by optimizing micronutrient intake. *J Nucleic Acids.* 2010 Sep 22; 2010. doi: pii: 725071. PMID: 20936173.

gmoevidence.com/wp-content/uploads/2013/08/BeesYet _Another_Suspect_in_CCD_2_.pdf

de Vendômois JS, Cellier D, Vélot C, et al. Debate on GMOs health risks after statistical findings in regulatory tests. *Int J Biol Sci.* 2010 Oct 5; 6(6): 590–98. PMID: 20941377.

Genuis SJ. What's out there making us sick? *J Environ Public Health.* 2012; 2012: 605137. Epub 2011 Oct 24. PMID: 22262979.

Genuis SJ. Sensitivity-related illness: The escalating pandemic of allergy, food intolerance and chemical sensitivity. *Sci Total Environ.* 2010 Nov 15; 408(24): 6047–61. PMID: 20920818.

The Whole Diet Story

Jin F, Nieman DC, Sha W, et al. Supplementation of milled chia seeds increases plasma ALA and EPA in postmenopausal women. *Plant Foods Hum Nutr.* 2012 Jun; 67(2): 105–10. PMID: 2253852.

college.unc.edu/2012/03/07/dha/#sthash.0Xmh5pMq.dpuf

McElroy KG. Environmental health effects of concentrated animal feeding operations: Implications for nurses. *Nurs Adm Q.* 2010 Oct–Dec; 34(4): 311–19. PMID: 20838176.

Greger M, Koneswaran G. The public health impacts of concentrated animal feeding operations on local communities. *Fam Community Health.* 2010 Jan–Mar; 33(1): 11–20. PMID: 20010001.

Koneswaran G, Nierenberg D. Global farm animal production and global warming: Impacting and mitigating climate change. *Environ Health Perspect.* 2008 May; 116(5): 578–82. PMID: 18470284.

Herrmann W, Schorr H, Obeid R, et al. Vitamin B-12 status, particularly holotranscobalamin II and methylmalonic acid concentrations, and hyperhomocysteinemia in vegetarians. *Am J Clin Nutr.* 2003 Jul; 78(1): 131–36. PMID: 12816782.

Ornish D. Holy Cow! What's good for you is good for our planet: Comment on "Red Meat Consumption and Mortality." *Arch Intern Med.* 2012 Apr 9; 172(7): 563–64. PMID: 22412078.

Ornish D....And the only side-effects are good ones. *Lancet Oncol.* 2011 Sep; 12(10): 924–25. PMID: 21958497.

Hyman MA, Ornish D, Roizen M. Lifestyle medicine: Treating the causes of disease. *Altern Ther Health Med.* 2009 Nov–Dec; 15(6): 12–14. PMID: 19943572.

Ornish D. Mostly plants. *Am J Cardiol.* 2009 Oct 1; 104(7): 957–58. PMID: 19766763.

Boddupalli S, Mein JR, Lakkanna S, et al. Induction of phase 2 antioxidant enzymes by broccoli sulforaphane: Perspectives in maintaining the antioxidant activity of vitamins A, C, and E. *Front Genet.* 2012 Jan 24; 3: 7. PMID: 22303412.

Freed DL. Do dietary lectins cause disease? *BMJ.* 1999 Apr 17; 318(7190): 1023–24. PMID: 10205084.

Yubero-Serrano EM, Gonzalez-Guardia L, Rangel-Zuñiga, et al. Mediterranean diet supplemented with coenzyme Q10 modifies the expression of proinflammatory and endoplasmic reticulum stress-related genes in elderly men and women. *J Gerontol A Biol Sci Med Sci.* 2012 Jan; 67(1): 3–10. PMID: 22016358.

de Lorgeril M. Mediterranean diet and cardiovascular disease: Historical perspective and latest evidence. *Curr Atheroscler Rep.* 2013 Dec; 15(12): 370. PMID: 24105622.

Knoops KT, de Groot LC, Kromhout D, et al. Mediterranean diet, lifestyle factors, and 10-year mortality in elderly European men and women: The HALE project. *JAMA.* 2004 Sep 22; 292(12): 1433–39. PMID: 15383513.

Bray GA, Nielsen SJ, Popkin BM. Consumption of high-fructose corn syrup in beverages may play a role in the epidemic of obesity. *Am J Clin Nutr.* 2004 Apr; 79(4): 537–43. Review. Erratum in: *Am J Clin Nutr.* 2004 Oct; 80(4): 1090. PMID: 15051594.

Masella R, Varì R, D'Archivio M, et al. Extra virgin olive oil biophenols inhibit cell-mediated oxidation of LDL by increasing the mRNA transcription of glutathione-related enzymes. *J Nutr.* 2004 Apr; 134(4): 785–91. PMID: 15051826.

Covas MI, Nyyssönen K, Poulsen HE, et al. The effect of polyphenols in olive oil on heart disease risk factors: A randomized trial. *Ann Intern Med.* 2006 Sep 5; 145(5): 333–41. PMID: 16954359.

Lamont K, Blackhurst D, Albertyn Z, et al. Lowering the alcohol content of red wine does not alter its cardioprotective properties. *S Afr Med J.* 2012 May 23; 102(6): 565–67. PMID: 22668965.

Spaak J, Tomlinson G, McGowan CL, et al. Dose-related effects of red wine and alcohol on heart rate variability. *Am J Physiol Heart Circ Physiol.* 2010 Jun; 298(6): H2226–31. PMID: 20418480.

www.WestonAPrice.org

Michalski MC, Januel C. Does homogenization affect the human health properties of cow's milk? *Trends Food Sci Tech.* 2006 Aug; 17(8): 423–37.

Lee SJ, Sherbon JW. Chemical changes in bovine milk fat globule membrane caused by heat treatment and homogenization of whole milk. *J Dairy Res.* 2002 Nov; 69(4): 555–67. PMID: 12463693.

Schecter A, Haffner D, Colacino J, et al. Polybrominated diphenyl ethers (PBDEs) and hexabromocyclododecane (HBCD) in composite U.S. food samples. *Environ Health Perspect.* 2010 Mar; 118(3): 357–62. PMID: 20064778.

Lam T, Williams PL, Burns JS, et al. Predictors of serum chlorinated pesticide concentrations among pre-pubertal Russian boys. *Environ Health Perspect.* 2013 Aug 16. [Epub ahead of print] PMID: 23955839.

www.ejnet.org/dioxin

Genuis SJ, Beesoon S, Lobo RA, et al. Human elimination of phthalate compounds: Blood, urine, and sweat (BUS) study. *Scientific World Journal.* 2012; 2012: 615068. PMID: 23213291.

Schecter A, Lorber M, Guo Y, et al. Phthalate concentrations and dietary exposure from food purchased in New York State. *Environ Health Perspect.* 2013 Apr; 121(4): 473–94, 494e1-4. PMID: 23461894.

Holtcamp W. Obesogens: An environmental link to obesity. *Environ Health Perspect.* 2012 February; 120(2): a62–a68. PMID: 22296745.

Séralini GE, Claira E, Mesnagea R, et al. Long term toxicity of a Roundup herbicide and a Roundup-tolerant genetically modified maize. *Food Chem Toxicol.* 2012 Nov; 50(11): 4221–31. PMID: 22999595.

Colborn T, vom Saal FS, Soto AM. Developmental effects of endocrine-disrupting chemicals in wildlife and humans. *Environ Health Perspect.* 1993 Oct; 101(5): 378–84. PMID: 8080506.

Lindeberg S. Paleolithic diets as a model for prevention and treatment of Western disease. *Am J Hum Biol.* 2012 Mar–Apr; 24(2): 110–15. PMID: 22262579.

Wigfield YY, Deneault F, Fillion J. Residues of glyphosate and its principle metabolite in certain cereals, oilseeds, and pulses grown in Canada, 1990–1992. *Bulletin of Environmental Contamination and Toxicology.* 1994 Oct; 53(4): 543-547.

Samsel A, Seneff S. Glyphosate's suppression of cytochrome P450 enzymes and amino acid biosynthesis by the gut microbiome: Pathways to modern diseases. *Entropy.* 2013, 15, 1416–63; doi: 10.3390/e15041416.

www.breakingtheviciouscycle.info/p/science-behind-the-diet

Liu Y, Zhang L, Song H, et al. Update on berberine in nonalcoholic fatty liver disease. *Evid based complement. Alternat Med.* 2013; 2013: 308134. doi: 10.1155/2013/308134. Epub 2013 Jun 17. PMID: 23843872.

Han J, Lin H, Huang W. Modulating gut microbiota as an antidiabetic mechanism of berberine. *Med Sci Monit.* 2011 Jul; 17(7): RA164-7. PMID: 21709646.

van Alphen LB, Burt SA, Veenendaal AK, et al. The natural antimicrobial carvacrol inhibits Campylobacter jejuni motility and infection of epithelial cells. *PLoS One.* 2012; 7(9): e45343. PMID: 23049787.

Jönsson T, Olsson S, Ahrén B, et al. Agrarian diet and diseases of affluence—do evolutionary novel dietary lectins cause leptin resistance? *BMC Endocr Disord.* 2005 Dec 10; 5: 10. PMID: 16336696.

chriskresser.com/rhr-what-science-really-says-about-the-paleo-diet-with-mat-lalonde

Choi YJ, Seelbach MJ, Pu H, et al. Polychlorinated biphenyls disrupt intestinal integrity via NADPH oxidase-induced alterations of tight junction protein expression. *Environ Health Perspect.* 2010 Jul; 118(7): 976–81. PMID: 20299304.

The Whole Food Sensitivity Story

Genuis SJ. Sensitivity-related illness: The escalating pandemic of allergy, food intolerance and chemical sensitivity. *Sci Total Environ.* 2010 Nov 15; 408(24): 6047–61. PMID: 20920818.

Genuis SJ, Sears M, Schwalfenberg G, et al. Incorporating environmental health in clinical medicine. *J Environ Public Health.* 2012; 2012: 103041. PMID: 22675371.

Genuis SJ. What's out there making us sick? *J Environ Public Health.* 2012; 2012: 605137. PMID: 22262979.

Volta U, De Giorgio R. New understanding of gluten sensitivity. *Nat Rev Gastroenterol Hepatol.* 2012 Feb 28; 9(5): 295–99. PMID: 22371218.

Di Sabatino A, Corazza GR. Nonceliac gluten sensitivity: Sense or sensibility? *Ann Intern Med.* 2012 Feb 21; 156(4): 309–11. PMID: 22351716.

Sapone A, Bai JC, Ciacci C, et al. Spectrum of gluten-related disorders: Consensus on new nomenclature and classification. *BMC Med.* 2012 Feb 7; 10: 13. PMID: 22313950.

Carroccio A, Mansueto P, Iacono G, et al. Non-celiac wheat sensitivity diagnosed by double-blind placebo-controlled challenge: Exploring a new clinical entity. *Am J Gastroenterol.* 2012 Dec; 107(12): 1898–906; quiz 1907. PMID: 22825366.

Thompson T, Lee AR, Grace T. Gluten contamination of grains, seeds, and flours in the United States: A pilot study. *J Am Diet Assoc.* 2010 Jun; 110(6): 937–40. PMID: 20497786.

Lidén M, Kristjánsson G, Valtysdottir S, et al. Self-reported food intolerance and mucosal reactivity after rectal food protein challenge in patients with rheumatoid arthritis. *Scand J Rheumatol.* 2010 Aug; 39(4): 292–98. PMID: 20141485.

Harlan DM, Lee MM. Infant formula, autoimmune triggers, and type 1 diabetes. *N Engl J Med.* 2010 Nov 11; 363(20): 1961–63. PMID: 21067389.

Olivier CE, Lorena SL, Pavan CR, et al. Is it just lactose intolerance? *Allergy Asthma Proc.* 2012 Sep–Oct; 33(5): 432–36. PMID: 23026186.

Oranje AP, Wolkerstorfer A, de Waard-van der Spek FB. Natural course of cow's milk allergy in childhood atopic eczema/dermatitis syndrome. *Ann Allergy Asthma Immunol.* 2002 Dec; 89(6 Suppl 1): 52–55. PMID: 12487205.

Lill C, Loader B, Seemann R, et al. Milk allergy is frequent in patients with chronic sinusitis and nasal polyposis. *Am J Rhinol Allergy.* 2011 Nov–Dec; 25(6): e221-4. PMID: 22185729.

El-Hodhod MA, Younis NT, Zaitoun YA, et al. Cow's milk allergy related pediatric constipation: Appropriate time of milk tolerance. *Pediatr Allergy Immunol.* 2010 Mar; 21(2 Pt 2): e407-12. PMID: 19555354.

Høst A. Cow's milk protein allergy and intolerance in infancy. Some clinical, epidemiological and immunological aspects. *Pediatr Allergy Immunol.* 1994; 5(5 Suppl): 1–36. PMID: 7704117.

Ho MH, Wong WH, Chang C. Clinical spectrum of food allergies: A comprehensive review. *Clin Rev Allergy Immunol.* 2012 Nov 16. [Epub ahead of print] PMID: 23229594.

Digestive Health

Malterre T. Digestive and nutritional considerations in celiac disease: Could supplementation help? *Altern Med Rev.* 2009 Sep; 14(3): 247–57. PMID: 19803549.

Leeds JS, Hopper AD, Hurlstone DP, et al. Is exocrine pancreatic insufficiency in adult coeliac disease a cause of persisting symptoms? *Aliment Pharmacol Ther.* 2007; 25: 265–71.

Domínguez-Muñoz JE. Pancreatic enzyme therapy for pancreatic exocrine insufficiency. *Gastroenterol Hepatol* (NY). 2011 Jun; 7(6): 401–3. PMID: 21869872.

Konkel L. The environment within: Exploring the role of the gut microbiome in health and disease. *Environ Health Perspect.* 2013 Sep; 121(9): A276–81. PMID: 24004817.

Guinane CM, Cotter PD. Role of the gut microbiota in health and chronic gastrointestinal disease: Understanding a hidden metabolic organ. *Therap Adv Gastroenterol.* 2013 Jul; 6(4): 295–308. PMID: 23814609.

Ridaura VK, Faith JJ, Rey FE, et al. Gut microbiota from twins discordant for obesity modulate metabolism in mice. *Science.* 2013 Sep 6; 341(6150): 1241214. PMID: 24009397.

Spreadbury I. Comparison with ancestral diets suggests dense acellular carbohydrates promote an inflammatory microbiota, and may be the primary dietary cause of leptin resistance and obesity. *Diabetes Metab Syndr Obes.* 2012; 5: 175–89. PMID: 22826636.

Heidelbaugh JJ, Goldberg KL, Inadomi JM. Overutilization of proton pump inhibitors: A review of cost-effectiveness and risk [corrected]. *Am J Gastroenterol.* 2009 Mar; 104 Suppl 2: S27–32. PMID: 19262544.

Frech EJ, Go MF. Treatment and chemoprevention of NSAID-associated gastrointestinal complications. *Ther Clin Risk Manag.* 2009 Feb; 5(1): 65–73. PMID: 19436617.

Metsälä J, Lundqvist A, Virta LJ, et al. Mother's and offspring's use of antibiotics and infant allergy to cow's milk. *Epidemiology.* 2013 Mar; 24(2): 303–9. PMID: 23348066.

Weed HG. Review: Probiotics prevent C. difficile–associated diarrhea in patients using antibiotics. *Ann Intern Med.* 2013 Oct 15; 159(8) PMID: 24126668.

Erb Downward JR, Falkowski NR, Mason KL, et al. Modulation of post-antibiotic bacterial community reassembly and host response by Candida albicans. *Sci Rep.* 2013 Jul 12; 3: 2191.

Dutton DJ, Fyie K, Faris P, et al. The association between amalgam dental surfaces and urinary mercury levels in a sample of Albertans, a prevalence study. *J Occup Med Toxicol.* 2013 Aug 29; 8(1): 22. [Epub ahead of print] PMID: 23984857.

Mutter J. Is dental amalgam safe for humans? The opinion of the scientific committee of the European Commission. *J Occup Med Toxicol.* 2011 Jan 13; 6(1): 2. PMID: 21232090.

Clayton EM, Todd M, Dowd JB, et al. The impact of bisphenol A and triclosan on immune parameters in the U.S. population, NHANES 2003–2006. *Environ Health Perspect.* 2011 Mar; 119(3): 390–96. PMID: 21062687.

Jeffery IB, O'Toole PW. Diet-microbiota interactions and their implications for healthy living. *Nutrients.* 2013, 5(1), 234–52.

De Filippo C, Cavalieri D, Di Paola M, et al. Impact of diet in shaping gut microbiota revealed by a comparative study in children from Europe and rural Africa. *PNAS.* 2010 Aug 17; 107(33): 14691–96.

Policy Statement—Chemical-management policy: Prioritizing children's health. Council on Environmental Health. *Pediatrics*; originally published online April 25, 2011; DOI: 10.1542/peds.2011-0523.

The Whole Toxicity Story

www.environmentaldefence.ca/prepolluted

www.ewg.org/news/videos/10-americans

Grandjean P, Landrigan PJ. Developmental neurotoxicity of industrial chemicals. *Lancet.* 2006 Dec 16; 368(9553): 2167–78. PMID: 17174709.

Environmental Working Group. 2005. *Body burden: The pollution in newborns.* Washington, DC.

Environmental Working Group. 2009. *Pollution in people: Cord blood contaminants in minority newborns.* Washington, DC.

Eskenazi B, Chevrier J, Rauch SA, et al. In utero and childhood polybrominated diphenyl ether (PBDE) exposures and neurodevelopment in the CHAMACOS study. *Environ Health Perspect.* 2013 Feb; 121(2): 257–62.

Qiu J. Tough talk over mercury treaty. *Nature.* 2013 Jan 10; 493(7431): 144–45. PMID: 23302836.

www.oecd.org/newsroom/environmentactnoworfacecostlycon sequenceswarnsoecd.htm

www.nbcnews.com/id/27704012/ns/world_news-world _environment/t/brown-clouds-dim-asia-threaten-worlds -food/#.UfXVLqVk-oM

www.scientificamerican.com/article.cfm?id=price-of-coal -in-china-climate-change

www.akaction.org/Publications/Coal_Development/Toxic _Trade_Map_poster_mercury_final_8x10.pdf

news.sciencemag.org/2013/01/nations-agree-global-mercury -limits?ref=hp

Clarkson TW, Magos L, Myers GJ. The toxicology of mercury— current exposures and clinical manifestations. *N Engl J Med.* 2003 Oct 30; 349(18): 1731–37. PMID: 14585942.

www.briloon.org/uploads/documents/hgcenter/gmh/ gmhSummary.pdf

Meyer J, Michalke K, Kouril T, et al. Votalisations of metals and metalloids: An inherent feature of methanoarchea? *Syst Applied Microbiol.* 2008 June; 31(2): 81–87.

www.whfoods.com/genpage.php?tname=george&dbid=103

www.iaomt.org/find-a-doctor/search-for-dentist-physician

Adams JB, Baral M, Geis E, et al. Safety and efficacy of oral DMSA therapy for children with autism spectrum disorders: Part A—Medical results. *BMC Clinical Pharmacology.* 2009 Oct 23; 9: 16. www.biomedcentral.com/1472-6904/9/16.

www.nmenv.state.nm.us/fod/LiquidWaste/pharm%20paper.pdf

water.usgs.gov/wrri/10grants/progress/2010NE207B.pdf

Ji K, Kho Y, Park C, et al. Influence of water and food consump- tion on inadvertent antibiotics intake among general popula- tion. *Environ Res.* 2010 Oct; 110(7): 641–49. PMID: 20624619.

Cooney CM. Study detects trace levels of pharmaceuticals in U.S. drinking water. *Environmental Science & Technology.* 2009 43 (3), 551–551. pubs.acs.org/action/showCitFormats? doi=10.1021%2Fes803457y.

www.nrdc.org/health/atrazine/files/atrazine.pdf

Schecter A, Cramer P, Boggess K. et al. Intake of dioxins and related compounds from food in the U.S. population. *J Toxicol Environ Health A.* 2001 May 11; 63(1): 1–18. PMID: 11346131.

www.chej.org/wp-content/uploads/Documents/American% 20Peoples%20Dioxin%20Report.pdf

Duty SM, Ackerman RM, Calafat AM, et al. Personal care product use predicts urinary concentrations of some phthal- ate monoesters. *Environ Health Perspect.* 2005 Nov; 113(11): 1530–35. PMID: 16263507.

Dodson RE, Nishioka M, Standley LJ, et al. Endocrine disrup- tors and asthma-associated chemicals in consumer prod- ucts. *Environ Health Perspect.* 2012 July; 120(7): 935–43.

Gomez E, Pillon A, Fenet H, et al. Estrogenic activity of cosmetic components in reporter cell lines: Parabens, UV screens, and musks. *J Toxicol Environ Health A.* 2005 Feb 27; 68(4): 239–51.

James-Todd T, Stahlhut R, Meeker JD, et al. Urinary phthalate metabolite concentrations and diabetes among women in the National Health and Nutrition Examination Survey (NHANES) 2001–2008. *Environ Health Perspect.* 2012 Sep; 120(9): 1307–13.

Teitelbaum SL, Mervish N, Moshier EL, et al. Associations between phthalate metabolite urinary concentrations and body size measures in New York City children. *Environ Res.* 2012 Jan; 112: 186–93. PMID: 22222007.

Carwile JL, Luu HT, Bassett LS, et al. Polycarbonate bottle use and urinary bisphenol A concentrations. *Environ Health Per- spect.* 2009 Sep; 117(9): 1368–72.

Angle BM, Do RP, Ponzi D, et al. Metabolic disruption in male mice due to fetal exposure to low but not high doses of bisphenol A (BPA): Evidence for effects on body weight, food intake, adipocytes, leptin, adiponectin, insulin and glucose regulation. *Reprod Toxicol.* 2013 Jul 25. pii: S0890- 6238(13)00231-1. PMID: 23892310.

Gayrard V, Lacroix MZ, Collet SH, et al. High bioavailability of bisphenol A from sublingual exposure. *Environ Health Per- spect.* 2013 Aug; 121(8): 951–56.

Alonso-Magdalena P, Ropero AB, Soriano S, et al. Bisphenol-A: A new diabetogenic factor? *Hormones* (Athens). 2010 Apr–Jun; 9(2): 118–26. PMID: 20687395.

www.ejnet.org/dioxin

Lee DH, Lee IK, Song K, et al. A strong dose-response rela- tion between serum concentrations of persistent organic pollutants and diabetes: Results from the National Health and Examination Survey 1999–2002. *Diabetes Care.* 2006 Jul; 29(7): 1638–44. PMID: 16801591.

Crinnion WJ. The role of persistent organic pollutants in the worldwide epidemic of type 2 diabetes mellitus and the pos- sible connection to Farmed Atlantic Salmon (*Salmo salar*). *Altern Med Rev.* 2011 Dec; 16(4): 301–13. PMID: 22214250.

www.ewg.org/news/news-releases/2003/07/30/first-ever-us -tests-farmed-salmon-show-high-levels-cancer-causing-pcbs

www.earth-policy.org/plan_b_updates/2013/update114

www.sites.google.com/site/envirodiabetes/home/contam/pops

www.vancouversun.com/Quest+life+without+plastic/ 9000202/story.html

Crinnion WJ. Organic foods contain higher levels of certain nutri- ents, lower levels of pesticides, and may provide health ben- efits for the consumer. *Altern Med Rev.* 2010 Apr; 15(1): 4–12.

Benbrook C. Are organic foods safer or healthier? *Ann Intern Med.* 2013 Feb 19; 158(4): 296–97. PMID: 23420244.

Bloom MS, Jansing RL, Kannan K, et al. Thyroid hormones are associated with exposure to persistent organic pollutants in aging residents of upper Hudson River communities. *Int J Hyg Environ Health.* 2013 Sep 25. [Epub ahead of print].

Park JD, Zheng W. Human exposure and health effects of inor- ganic and elemental mercury. *J Prev Med Public Health.* 2012 Nov; 45(6): 344–52.

Wang B, Du Y. Cadmium and its neurotoxic effects. *Oxid Med Cell Longev.* 2013; 2013: 898034. doi: 10.1155/2013/898034. Epub 2013 Aug 12. PMID: 23997854.

Bassig BA, Zhang L, Tang X, et al. Occupational exposure to trichloroethylene and serum concentrations of IL-6, IL-10, and TNF-alpha. *Environ Mol Mutagen.* 2013 Jul; 54(6): 450–54. doi: 10.1002/em.21789. Epub 2013 Jun 25.

Policy Statement—Chemical-management policy: Prioritiz- ing children's health. Council on Environmental Health.

Pediatrics; originally published online April 25, 2011; DOI: 10.1542/peds.2011-052.

Lu C, Toepel K, Irish R, et al. Organic diets significantly lower children's dietary exposure to organophosphorus pesticides. *Environ Health Perspect.* 2006 Feb; 114(2): 260–63.

Environmental Working Group. 2005. *Body burden: The pollution in newborns.* Washington, DC.

Grandjean P, Landrigan PJ. Developmental neurotoxicity of industrial chemicals. *Lancet.* 2006 Dec 16; 368(9553): 2167–78. PMID: 17174709.

Crinnion WJ. Organic foods contain higher levels of certain nutrients, lower levels of pesticides, and may provide health benefits for the consumer. *Altern Med Rev.* 2010 Apr; 15(1): 4–12.

Brandt K, Leifert C, Sanderson R, et al. Agroecosystem management and nutritional quality of plant foods: The case of organic fruits and vegetables. *Crit. Rev. in Plant Sci.* 2011; 30: 177–97.

Smith-Spangler C, Brandeau ML, Hunter GE, et al. Are organic foods safer or healthier than conventional alternatives?: A systematic review. *Ann Intern Med.* 2012 Sep 4; 157(5): 348–66.

www.huffingtonpost.com/2012/09/13/stanford-organics-study -public-health_n_1880441.html

Benbrook C, McCullum-Gómez C. Organic vs conventional farming. *J Am Diet Assoc.* 2009 May; 109(5): 809,811. PMID: 19394464.

Landrigan PJ, Lambertini L, Birnbaum LS. A research strategy to discover the environmental causes of autism and neurodevelopmental disabilities. *Environ Health Perspect.* 2012 Jul; 120(7): a258–60. PMID: 22543002.

Lu C, Toepel K, Irish R, et al. Organic diets significantly lower children's dietary exposure to organophosphorus pesticides. *Environ Health Perspect.* 2006 Feb; 114(2): 260–63.

Roberts EM, English PB, Grether JK, et al. Maternal residence near agricultural pesticide applications and autism spectrum disorders among children in the California Central Valley. *Environ Health Perspect.* 2007 Oct; 115(10): 1482–89.

healthland.time.com/2011/04/21/exposure-to-pesticides-in -pregnancy-can-lower-childrens-iq

www.foodandwaterwatch.org/reports/superweeds

www.organicconsumers.org/articles/article_17602.cfm

Gassmann AJ, Petzold-Maxwell JL, Keweshan RS, et al. Field-evolved resistance to Bt maize by western corn rootworm. *PLoS One.* 2011; 6(7): e22629. Epub 2011 Jul 29.PMID: 21829470.

Larson RL, Hill AL, Fenwick A, et al. Influence of glyphosate on Rhizoctonia and Fusarium root rot in sugar beet. *Pest Manag Sci.* 2006 Dec; 62(12): 1182–92.

Normile D. Vietnam turns back a "tsunami of pesticides." *Science.* 2013 Aug 16; 341(6147): 737–38. PMID: 23950527.

Organics, Your Health, and the Planet

www.biointegrity.org/report-on-lawsuit.htm

www.nongmoproject.org/learn-more

www.aaemonline.org/gmopost.html

Malatesta M, Caporaloni C, Gavaudan S, et al. Ultrastructural morphometrical and immunocytochemical analyses of hepatocyte nuclei from mice fed on genetically modified soybean. *Cell Struct Funct.* 2002 Aug; 27(4): 173–80.

Ewen SW, Pusztai A. Effect of diets containing genetically modified potatoes expressing *Galanthus nivalis* lectin on rat small intestine. *Lancet.* 1999 Oct 16; 354(9187): 1353–54. PMID: 10533866.

Vecchio L, Cisterna B, Malatesta M, et al. Ultrastructural analysis of testes from mice fed on genetically modified soybean. *Eur J Histochem.* 2004 Oct–Dec; 48(4): 448–54. PMID: 15718213.

Jasper R, Locatelli GO, Pilati C, et al. Evaluation of biochemical, hematological and oxidative parameters in mice exposed to the herbicide glyphosate-Roundup(®). *Interdiscip Toxicol.* 2012 Sep; 5(3): 133–40. PMID: 23554553.

Séralini GE, Clair E, Mesnage R, et al. Long term toxicity of a Roundup herbicide and a Roundup-tolerant genetically modified maize. *Food Chem Toxicol.* 2012 Nov; 50(11): 4221–31. PMID: 22999595.

www.organic-systems.org/journal/81/8106.pdf

Aris A, Leblanc S. Maternal and fetal exposure to pesticides associated to genetically modified foods in Eastern Townships of Quebec, Canada. *Reprod Toxicol.* 2011 May; 31(4): 528–33.

www.ucsusa.org/food_and_agriculture/our-failing-food-system/genetic-engineering/failure-to-yield.html

Charles M Benbrook. Impacts of genetically engineered crops on pesticide use in the U.S.—the first sixteen years. *Environmental Sciences Europe* 2012, 24: 24. www.enveurope.com/content/24/1/24

www.nongmoproject.org/learn-more

www.ewg.org/release/americans-eat-their-weight-genetically -engineered-food

www.nongmoshoppingguide.com

The Basics of a Whole Foods Diet

Demmig-Adams B, Adams WW 3rd. Antioxidants in photosynthesis and human nutrition. *Science.* 2002 Dec 13; 298(5601): 2149–53. PMID: 12481128.

Egger J, Carter CM, Soothill JF, et al. Oligoantigenic diet treatment of children with epilepsy and migraine. *J Pediatr.* 1989 Jan; 114(1): 51–58. PMID: 2909707.

Egger J, Carter CM, Wilson J, et al. Is migraine food allergy? A double-blind-controlled trial of oligoantigenic diet treatment. *Lancet.* 1983 Oct 15; 2(8355): 865–69. PMID: 6137694.

Xiao S, Fei N, Pang X, et al. A gut microbiota-targeted dietary intervention for amelioration of chronic inflammation underlying metabolic syndrome. *FEMS Microbiol Ecol.* 2013 Sep 30. [Epub ahead of print].

Costabile A, Kolida S, Klinder A, et al. A double-blind, placebo-controlled, cross-over study to establish the bifidogenic effect of a very-long-chain inulin extracted from globe artichoke (*Cynara scolymus*) in healthy human subjects. *Br J Nutr.* 2010 Oct; 104(7): 1007–17. PMID: 20591206.

Wallace IR, McEvoy CT, Hunter SJ, et al. Dose-response effect of fruit and vegetables on insulin resistance in people at high risk of cardiovascular disease: A randomized controlled trial. *Diabetes Care.* 2013 Oct 15. [Epub ahead of print] PMID: 24130354.

Sherry CL, Kim SS, Dilger RN, et al. Sickness behavior induced by endotoxin can be mitigated by the dietary soluble fiber, pectin, through up-regulation of IL-4 and Th2 polarization. *Brain Behav Immun.* 2010 May; 24(4): 631–40. PMID: 20138982.

Deopurkar R, Ghanim H, Friedman J, et al. Differential effects of cream, glucose, and orange juice on inflammation, endotoxin, and the expression of Toll-like receptor-4 and suppressor of cytokine signaling-3. *Diabetes Care.* 2010 May; 33(5): 991–97. PMID: 20067961.

Morris MC, Evans DA, Tangney CC, et al. Associations of vegetable and fruit consumption with age-related cognitive change. *Neurology.* 2006 Oct 24; 67(8): 1370–76. PMID: 17060562.

Jenkins DJ, Kendall CW, Marchie A, et al. Direct comparison of dietary portfolio vs statin on C-reactive protein. *Eur J Clin Nutr.* 2005 Jul; 59(7): 851–60. PMID: 15900306.

Panico S, Mattiello A, Panico C, et al. Mediterranean dietary pattern and chronic diseases. *Cancer Treat Res.* 2014; 159: 69–81. PMID: 24114475.

Brooks JD, Ward WE, Lewis JE, et al. Supplementation with flaxseed alters estrogen metabolism in postmenopausal women to a greater extent than does supplementation with an equal amount of soy. *Am J Clin Nutr.* 2004 Feb; 79(2): 318–25. PMID: 14749240.

Fowke JH, Longcope C, Hebert JR. Brassica vegetable consumption shifts estrogen metabolism in healthy postmenopausal women. *Cancer Epidemiol Biomarkers Prev.* 2000 Aug; 9(8): 773–79. PMID: 10952093.

Rakoff-Nahoum S, Paglino J, Eslami-Varzaneh F, et al. Recognition of commensal microflora by toll-like receptors is required for intestinal homeostasis. *Cell.* 2004 Jul 23; 118(2): 229–41. PMID: 15260992.

Wintergerst ES, Maggini S, Hornig DH. Contribution of selected vitamins and trace elements to immune function. *Ann Nutr Metab.* 2007; 51(4): 301–23. PMID: 17726308.

Metso S, Hyytiä-Ilmonen H, Kaukinen K, et al. Gluten-free diet and autoimmune thyroiditis in patients with celiac disease. A prospective controlled study. *Scand J Gastroenterol.* 2012 Jan; 47(1): 43–48. PMID: 22126672.

Rasmusson AM, Schnurr PP, Zukowska Z, et al. Adaptation to extreme stress: Post-traumatic stress disorder, neuropeptide Y and metabolic syndrome. *Exp Biol Med* (Maywood). 2010 Oct; 235(10): 1150–62. PMID: 20881319.

Tomiyama AJ, Mann T, Vinas D, et al. Low calorie dieting increases cortisol. *Psychosom Med.* 2010 May; 72(4): 357–64. PMID: 20368473.

Carter P, Gray LJ, Troughton J, et al. Fruit and vegetable intake and incidence of type 2 diabetes mellitus: Systematic review and meta-analysis. *BMJ.* 2010 Aug 18; 341: c4229. PMID: 20724400.

Liu RH. Dietary bioactive compounds and their health implications. *J Food Sci.* 2013 Jun; 78 Suppl 1: A18–25. PMID: 23789932.

Vinson JA, Su X, Zubik L, et al. Phenol antioxidant quantity and quality in foods: Fruits. *J Agric Food Chem.* 2001 Nov; 49(11): 5315–21. PMID: 11714322.

Brent GA. Environmental exposures and autoimmune thyroid disease. *Thyroid.* 2010 July; 20(7): 755–61. doi: 10.1089/thy.2010.1636 PMID: 20578899.

Dal Maso L, Bosetti C, La Vecchia C et al. Risk factors for thyroid cancer: An epidemiological review focused on nutritional factors. *Cancer Causes Control.* 2009 Feb; 20(1): 75–86. PMID: 18766448.

www.whfoods.com/genpage.php?tname=foodspice&dbid=11

Lee YP, Puddey IB, Hodgson JM. Protein, fibre and blood pressure: Potential benefit of legumes. *Clin Exp Pharmacol Physiol.* 2008 Apr; 35(4): 473–76. PMID: 18307744.

He K, Song Y, Belin RJ, et al. Magnesium intake and the metabolic syndrome: Epidemiologic evidence to date. *J Cardiometab Syndr.* 2006 Fall; 1(5): 351–55. PMID: 17679786.

Menotti A, Kromhout D, Blackburn H, et al. Food intake patterns and 25-year mortality from coronary heart disease: Cross-cultural correlations in the Seven Countries Study. The Seven Countries Study Research Group. *Eur J Epidemiol.* 1999 Jul; 15(6): 507–15. PMID: 10485342.

Ros E. Health benefits of nut consumption. *Nutrients.* 2010 Jul; 2(7): 652–82. PMID: 22254047.

Macdonald LE, Brett J, Kelton D, et al. A systematic review and meta-analysis of the effects of pasteurization on milk vitamins, and evidence for raw milk consumption and other health-related outcomes. *J Food Prot.* 2011 Nov; 74(11): 1814–32. PMID: 22054181.

www.pcrm.org/search/?cid=1202

Daley CA, Abbott A, Doyle PS, et al. A review of fatty acid profiles and antioxidant content in grass-fed and grain-fed beef. *Nutr J.* 2010 Mar 10; 9: 10. PMID: 20219103.

Crinnion WJ. The role of persistent organic pollutants in the worldwide epidemic of type 2 diabetes mellitus and the possible connection to Farmed Atlantic Salmon (*Salmo salar*). *Altern Med Rev.* 2011 Dec; 16(4): 301–13. PMID: 22214250.

www.authoritynutrition.com/pastured-vs-omega-3-vs-conventional-eggs

Holick MF. Vitamin D deficiency. *N Engl J Med.* 2007 Jul 19; 357(3): 266–81. PMID: 17634462.

Thorne-Lyman A, Fawzi WW. Vitamin D during pregnancy and maternal, neonatal and infant health outcomes: A systematic review and meta-analysis. *Paediatr Perinat Epidemiol.* 2012 Jul; 26 Suppl 1: 75–90. PMID: 22742603.

Chandrasekaran VR, Hsu DZ, Liu MY. Beneficial effect of sesame oil on heavy metal toxicity. *JPEN J Parenter Enteral Nutr.* 2013 Jun 6. [Epub ahead of print].

Kanimozhi P, Prasad NR. Antioxidant potential of sesamol and its role on radiation-induced DNA damage in whole-body irradiated Swiss albino mice. *Environ Toxicol Pharmacol.* 2009 Sep; 28(2): 192–97.

Blomhoff R, Carlsen MH, Andersen LF, et al. Health benefits of nuts: Potential role of antioxidants. *Br J Nutr.* 2006 Nov; 96 Suppl 2: S52–60. 2006. PMID: 17125534.

Kelly JH Jr, Sabate J. Nuts and coronary heart disease: An epidemiological perspective. *Br J Nutr.* 2006 Nov; 96 Suppl 2: S61–67. PMID: 17125535.

INDEX

ABOUT THE AUTHORS

Alissa Segersten received her bachelor of science in nutrition from Bastyr University in Kenmore, Washington. She is the previous owner of a personal chef business in Seattle, Washington, that successfully addressed the health and lifestyle needs of many families with her delicious, healthy cooking. She is currently a cooking instructor, empowering people with cooking skills and knowledge of whole foods so that they may reconnect with the pleasure in eating delicious, nourishing food. Her popular recipe blog, www .NourishingMeals.com is filled with healthy, wholesome gluten-free recipes.

Tom Malterre MS, CN holds both a bachelor's and master's degree in nutrition from Bastyr University. Tom is a faculty member of the Autism Research Institute and a clinical nutritionist for Whole Life Nutrition. He has been invited to speak at the Washington Association for Naturopathic Physicians, the Ontario Association for Naturopathic Physicians, the British Columbia Association for Naturopathic Physicians, the International College of Integrative Medicine, the National College for Naturopathic Medicine, Boucher Institute for Naturopathic Medicine, the Southwest College of Naturopathic Medicine, and Bastyr University. Tom has trained with the Institute for Functional Medicine for over 7 years. Tom specializes in whole body wellness—looking at all factors of a person's life to bring about healing. Stress, environmental toxicants, nutritional deficiencies, and epigenetics all contribute to a decline in health. Whole Life Nutrition encompasses all aspects of life to get to the root of the health issues.